Praise for *Chronic Condition*

WINNER OF THE DONNER PRIZE
SHORTLISTED FOR THE SHAUGHNESSY COHEN PRIZE
SHORTLISTED FOR THE DAFOE PRIZE

"This book deals with the most pressing public-policy issue facing Canadians. *Chronic Condition* should inspire a national debate on the future of Canadians' most cherished social program."
—Donner Prize jury citation

"A refreshing new look at health care in Canada."
—*The Vancouver Sun*

"*Chronic Condition* is a great guide to models from around the world to be considered for reforms in Canada. Readers will find the lessons of history, global comparisons, abundant domestic data sets and the wisdom of one of Canada's foremost commentators to guide them."   —*The Globe and Mail*

"What [Simpson] has written is arguably the most comprehensive tour d'horizon of the Canadian healthcare system available."
—*Queen's University Alumni Review*

"It's hard to argue with a writer like Simpson, who has such impeccable credentials…"   —*The Gazette* (Montreal)

PENGUIN

CHRONIC CONDITION

JEFFREY SIMPSON has been *The Globe and Mail*'s national affairs
columnist for more than twenty-five years. He is an award-
winning author of eight previous books—including *Discipline of
Power*, which won a Governor General's Award—and is an officer
of the Order of Canada. He has also won the Hyman Solomon
Award for excellence in public-policy journalism and is a senior
fellow at the University of Ottawa's Graduate School of Public and
International Affairs. He lives in Ottawa.

JEFFREY SIMPSON

CHRONIC CONDITION

WHY CANADA'S HEALTH-CARE SYSTEM
NEEDS TO BE DRAGGED INTO
THE 21ST CENTURY

PENGUIN

an imprint of Penguin Canada Books Inc.

Published by the Penguin Group
Penguin Canada Books Inc.
90 Eglinton Avenue East, Suite 700, Toronto, Ontario, Canada M4P 2Y3

Penguin Group (USA) Inc., 375 Hudson Street, New York, New York 10014, U.S.A.
Penguin Books Ltd, 80 Strand, London WC2R 0RL, England
Penguin Ireland, 25 St Stephen's Green, Dublin 2, Ireland
(a division of Penguin Books Ltd)
Penguin Group (Australia), 707 Collins Street, Melbourne, Victoria 3008, Australia
(a division of Pearson Australia Group Pty Ltd)
Penguin Books India Pvt Ltd, 11 Community Centre, Panchsheel Park,
New Delhi – 110 017, India
Penguin Group (NZ), 67 Apollo Drive, Rosedale, Auckland 0632, New Zealand
(a division of Pearson New Zealand Ltd)
Penguin Books (South Africa) (Pty) Ltd, 24 Sturdee Avenue, Rosebank,
Johannesburg 2196, South Africa

Penguin Books Ltd, Registered Offices: 80 Strand, London WC2R 0RL, England

First published in Allen Lane hardcover by Penguin Canada, 2012
Published in this edition, 2013

3 4 5 6 7 8 9 10 (WEB)

Copyright © Jeffrey Simpson, 2012
Epilogue copyright © Jeffrey Simpson, 2013

Manufactured in Canada.

Library and Archives Canada Cataloguing in Publication data
available upon request to the publisher.

ISBN: 978-0-14-318100-2

Visit the Penguin Canada website at www.penguin.ca

Special and corporate bulk purchase rates available; please see
www.penguin.ca/corporatesales or call 1-800-810-3104, ext. 2477.

For Wendy, Tait, Danielle and Brook

CONTENTS

Introduction   1

PART ONE

1   Hospital Days   21

PART TWO

2   Health Care's Early History   57

3   Medicare in Saskatchewan   74

4   The Father of Medicare   96

5   The Liberals and Medicare   112

6   The Canada Health Act   129

PART THREE

7   How Good Is Medicare?   155

8   How Much Does Medicare Cost?   172

9   Can Efficiencies Save Medicare?   195

10   Is Private Health Care the Answer?   221

11   Dr. Duval's Option   238

12   Can We Make Ourselves Healthier?   254

13   What Does the Public Think?   270

14   What about Other Countries?   286

PART FOUR

REMEDIES

15   Doctors and Nurses   313

16   Hospitals   328

17   Drugs   345

18   Conclusion   365

Epilogue   373

Appreciation/

Acknowledgments   383

Index   387

INTRODUCTION

Medicare is the third rail of Canadian politics. Touch it and you die. Every politician knows this truth. Yes, politicians talk about health care, usually to promise more of it. Such talk is not part of a reasoned debate but essentially a bidding war. Many of them understand that a health-care system that costs about $200 billion a year in public and private money cannot continue as it is, that the system is inadequately structured for an aging population and has costs that grow faster than government revenues. Discussing these realities, however, risks shortening political careers.

Canadians embrace their public health-care system, medicare, more passionately than any other public program. Poll after poll has underscored their passion. Medicare has become a national icon that politicians dare not question. In public, they can only claim undying fidelity to medicare; in private, many of them acknowledge that it cannot continue as delivered, administered and financed, at least at current levels of taxation.

In 2009, Canadians spent 11.7 percent of their national income on health care. It is estimated that each year the health-care system is used about 400 million times by a population of 34 million. You might think that such an expensive and all-pervasive system would provoke people to think and politicians to talk about what needs to be done to preserve it. No such luck. The entrenched interests within the health-care system are so strong, the ideological prisms through which defenders observe the system so fixed, the public's embrace so passionate, its fears of change so pervasive and its aspirations for the system so contradictory that having an adult conversation seems next to impossible.

The French language and culture define the distinctiveness of Quebec. Elsewhere, health care reflects what Canadians believe to be one of their unique values: not to be American. Public-opinion polls asking Canadians how they differ from Americans place gun control and health care atop the list. Nowhere else in the world does public health care play such a defining role in shaping a national self-identity. In other countries, health care is a system, a program, a policy, unquestionably of considerable importance. In Canada, especially outside Quebec, health care is all these things and a great deal more.

Public policies in a democracy can be attacked and changed without citizens getting too upset about somehow losing their collective identity. Icons, however, have existential qualities that make them immune from serious debate. To question an icon is to probe something sacramental, definitional and deeply funda-mental. When any Canadian wants to start a debate about the fundamentals of medicare, or even ask more modest but essen-tial questions about whether the system can be sustained and by which means, the speaker risks being slapped down as somehow "un-Canadian" or wanting U.S.-style private health care.

Across the country, many elected officials and senior civil servants have looked at the costs of the system versus govern-ments' ability to keep paying for it at current levels of taxation. They understand that health care is devouring budgets, taking an increasing share of spending each year. They know that other government programs are suffering as more money gets shov-elled into health care. In the past thirty-three years, health-care costs grew faster than the national economy nineteen times, at the same rate five times, and at a slower rate nine times. When medicare began, health care claimed 7 percent of the country's economy; today it eats up 11.7 percent. According to a study for the C.D. Howe Institute by David Dodge, former governor of the Bank of Canada, deputy minister of finance and deputy minister of health, health care will consume 15.4 percent of the national economy in two decades—assuming huge efficiency gains—and 18.7 percent without them.

Dodge's projections were roughly in line with those offered by the Organisation for Economic Co-operation and Development (OECD), which in 2010 looked ahead to 2050. An aging population will not cripple medicare, as some scaremongers have suggested. No "grey tsunami" threatens, but an aging population will unavoidably increase costs: for pharmaceuticals, long-term care facilities, home care and hospitals. Aging will mean fewer people not working compared with the number of those in the workforce, so the tax burden of the future will be more narrowly shared. Today's health-care deficits will become more burdensome for tomorrow's generation unless we do something today.

In a system admirably built on equity of access, it is worth asking also about intergenerational equity, or obligations to our children. If we are not willing to tax ourselves, or find some other means to make medicare sustainable, we will place additional burdens on future generations, hardly an equitable arrangement.

Health-care budgets have been rising, and will continue to rise, faster than the rate of inflation adjusted for population growth, faster than provincial government revenues or spending on any other program, faster than nominal economic growth (growth plus inflation). Since government revenues generally grow in tandem with nominal economic growth, if health care grows faster than nominal economic growth, government budgets will be pinched. Health care today consumes 42 to 45 percent of provincial program spending. If no change is made to the spending trajectory of health care, in two decades the share will be 55 to 65 percent. The wealthier a country becomes, the more its citizens want to spend money, either directly or through the state, on health care. Fine, except that in Canada we restrict severely what people can spend on themselves for essential medical care, and we are reluctant to pay more tax. We have boxed ourselves in.

The OECD's 2010 conclusion, in its survey of the Canadian economy, put the issue squarely: "The key policy question is whether the growing imbalance between health care and revenue sources is sustainable at current policy settings. The very real possibility that provincial health-care spending will outstrip revenue growth raises the prospect of enormous future fiscal deficits, requiring i) cuts in other spending, ii) tax increases, iii) delisting of public health-care services (privatization), or iv) finding savings within health care itself. Higher federal transfers, the historically preferred solution, do not seem likely, given the federal government's own fiscal problems." In plain English, Canada has to make choices, none of them easy.

Around any provincial cabinet table, elected officials have responsibilities for health care, but they must also fund education, justice, training, roads, public transit, social housing, welfare and environmental protection, among other services. Around the federal cabinet table, politicians have to consider regional transfers, defence and foreign affairs, agriculture, pensions, aboriginals, university research, national transportation, immigration and a host of other matters. Legitimate, competing priorities crash against the political imperatives and incessant financial demands of health care. It doesn't matter whether a province has raised taxes, as in Ontario and Quebec, or reduced them, as in Alberta and British Columbia. The health-care conflict is inescapable between revenues and expenditures. This is the family secret plaguing every provincial government. The details vary according to province; the challenge does not. The challenge, however, only reluctantly and furtively speaks its name.

A few politicians have offered timid warnings. British Columbia's finance minister Colin Hansen said in his 2010 budget, "If health care continues to grow at the current pace, it will increasingly crowd out spending in other areas." Ontario's finance minister Dwight Duncan said in his 2010 budget, "So the question now facing us is: How do we fund the best health care without compromising our investments in schools, helping the vulnerable or protecting the environment?" Quebec's finance minister Raymond Bachand said in his 2010 budget, "Accounting for 31 percent of program spending in 1980, health-care spending now represents 45 percent. If nothing is done to change this dynamic, spending could represent two-thirds of program expenses in twenty years." These ministers raised the health-care sustainability question, implicitly and/or explicitly. Doing something is another matter.

It is one thing for a finance minister to offer occasional warnings; it is quite another for governments to launch a serious and sustained debate with citizens, inviting them to choose among hard, even unpalatable, options to make health care sustainable, which means operating the system at current tax rates and without gutting other programs. Without this debate, Canadians will sleepwalk toward even harder decisions—or irresponsibly pass on the hard questions (and higher costs) to future generations.

The provincial spending pattern is similar across the country. Health care grows faster than any part of a provincial budget. Other programs get systematically squeezed; revenue pots are scoured to find resources. Ontario, for example, originally launched lotteries and gaming establishments to provide money for culture and recreation programs. The province now puts almost all these revenues, $1.5 billion of $1.7 billion in 2011–12, into health care. (Actually, the government puts the money into the general pot of revenues, and they claim to be spending $1.5 billion on health care.) Other provinces have done the same to find money for health care without having to raise taxes. Health care is now hooked on gambling.

Having lobbied for the assignment, former Saskatchewan premier Roy Romanow was asked by Prime Minister Jean Chrétien to study ways of improving medicare. It was hardly surprising, with that mandate, that his 2002 report trashed private health care. It was disappointing, however, that a former provincial premier who had admirably balanced his province's books gave such short shrift to the long-term problem of making medicare sustainable. He offered some useful suggestions about improving the existing system, and he certainly made the case for spending a lot more money on medicare. But he called the impact of health-care spending on other government spending "overheated rhetoric," and he larded his report with phrases worthy of a politician and invocations worthy of a churchman. Medicare was not just a vital public service, he wrote, but a "right of citizenship," a "defining aspect of our citizenship," a "moral enterprise," a "public trust," "the Canadian way." Moving into rhetorical overdrive, Romanow called for a health-care covenant between Canadians and their governments, thereby elevating health care, like religion, to something akin to a compact between God and his Chosen People. It's no wonder, then, that a calm conversation about health care is difficult, if not impossible, since to begin asking hard questions would apparently be apostasy.

Canadians therefore carry on their love affair with medicare oblivious to what medicare is doing to public finances, resistant to paying higher taxes but opposed to any limitations to medicare's reach. They even demand more from medicare, while worrying that somehow it won't be there for them when needed. They are especially alarmed that any major change might lead down the slippery slope toward two-tier U.S.-style health care.

Canada is unique in the Western world in the way it organizes health care, although that uniqueness is not generally known to the public. Many other countries have more extensive public-health systems that offer such services as eye care, dentistry, home care and pharmaceuticals. The Canadian system, by contrast, offers deep but narrow coverage for the costs of hospitals and physicians only, with a mixed bag of public and private coverage for pharmaceuticals, some home care and acute long-term care, depending on age and province, and very little, if any, public coverage for eye care and dentistry.

Cost sustainability is one worry about medicare. Another ought to be that Canada's health-care system isn't very good when stacked up against what is spent. Canadian health care produces only average value for money. Politicians and some health-care experts insist that Canadian health care is the best in the world. In fact, Canadian health care is regularly rated at average or slightly below average in international comparisons. Perhaps Canadians believe the mythology about their system because politicians like to repeat it so often, or because they compare medicare only with the U.S. system.

Beyond North America are other systems that deliver at least comparable levels of health services and, in many cases, superior services, at lower costs. Given the self-congratulation in Canada, it is sobering to realize that the country stands nowhere near the top in any international comparative study. We have a Chevrolet health-care system by international comparative standards, but the Canadian public thinks we have a Cadillac. Put another way, our results are those of a Chevrolet compared with outcomes in countries with largely public systems, but we pay at Cadillac costs, since Canada stands near the top of the spending list of countries with largely public systems.

Comparisons with the United States distort Canadians' thinking about their society. Swinging between moral superiority and inherent inferiority, Canadians measure themselves exclusively against the United States, the multiply-by-ten behemoth next door. When U.S. filmmaker Michael Moore, chastising his own country's health-care system in his 2007 film *Sicko*, heaped excessive praise on Canada's, he did Canada no favours. Seldom, if ever, do Canadians get beyond the shadow of the United States to see themselves through another prism. Canadians know dribs and drabs about other societies' health-care systems, but they almost never draw inspiration from them. That myopia is a pity for many reasons, since we might learn from others and, in so doing, be less fearful of change to the chronic condition of medicare. No country's experience can be bolted to another's without taking into consideration the differences of culture, history, economy, demographics and politics. No other country's public health-care system could be imported holus-bolus into Canada, replacing medicare, even if the outcomes of another's system are better on balance. But Canadians should at least consider other systems, which is why this book will explore those of Australia, Sweden and the United Kingdom.

Why not examine U.S. health care? It's the one Canadians know best, or rather, think they know best, even if in fact they don't know it very well. U.S. health care is, of course, the hidden secret of Canadian medicare. Episodically, if embarrassingly, provinces have sent patients to the United States when their own systems cannot cope—for urgent cancer treatments, for example. Canadians go to the United States for faster treatment and diagnostic tests if they can afford it. Much as the U.S. system is reviled by defenders of Canadian medicare as costly and socially unjust, these criticisms do not stop some Canadians from entering the American private health-care universe. The number is small, though: a survey of more than two thousand Canadians carried out by the Deloitte consulting firm in 2009 found only 2 percent of respondents had gone to the United States for treatment. Only 7 percent of respondents in that survey said they would "definitely" be willing to travel outside their country for elective procedures, suggesting that the lure of the United States, while powerful for a very small minority, does not figure much in the health-care decisions of many Canadians.

U.S. health care is so different that comparisons are of limited value. Canadians will definitely not adopt a variant of U.S. health care. Why should they? The United States spends about half again as much of its gross domestic product on health care as Canada does—17.6 percent for the United States compared with 11.7 percent for Canada—but does not receive better aggregate health-care outcomes. Both countries ration health care, although *ration* is a word seldom heard on either side of the border. Canada rations care by triage, which means figuring out who needs help most urgently and causing others to wait. The United States has historically rationed health care by not providing health-care insurance to about 15 percent of its population, requiring unlucky people to depend on public hospitals. The lack of insurance often means care that arrives too late in an illness for the most effective treatment. President Barack Obama's complicated health-care reforms are supposed to push down the number of those uninsured. Lawsuits and political struggles surround his reforms.

That no other country in the world uses the U.S. health-care model, and that U.S. health care regularly scores well below Canadian medicare in aggregate outcomes, means we waste our time contemplating the U.S. system. To certain Canadians, such as former Newfoundland and Labrador premier Danny Williams, who went to Florida for heart surgery, and to Canadian companies that routinely send their senior manage-ment team to U.S. clinics for checkups and to other people with money, the U.S. system apparently works better than medicare. For the most part, the U.S. model offers an unfortunate distrac-tion and a false comparison. Defenders of medicare use the U.S. model to scare Canadians into believing that debate here would lead inexorably to U.S.-style medicine, even though no political figure in Canada has recommended that system in our lifetime. Still, the comparison serves political purposes, as when former prime minister Jean Chrétien quipped, "Down there, they check your wallet before your pulse." Canada is lucky to live beside the United States for many reasons. When it comes to health care, Canada lives next to the wrong neighbour with the wrong model. It would shock Canadians, however, to be told that they actually have U.S.-style medicine for part of their health-care needs. The OECD made this very point: that outside of hospitals and doctor services, the Canadian system, in the fields of drugs, nursing care, long-term care, home care, rehabilitation and physiotherapy, is uncoordinated, costly and not at all respon-sive to the needs of the public—that is, a U.S.-style system. The OECD suggested provocatively, but not inaccurately, that Canada blends a rigid system for some health-care needs and a costly U.S.-style system for other needs, the worst of both health-care worlds.

The U.S. model is a wonderful bogeyman for unreconstructed defenders of Canadian medicare. How many politicians such as Chrétien and health-policy experts who defend medicare to the nth degree have incessantly compared the Canadian and U.S. systems, always to Canada's benefit? These comparisons make Canadians feel better about their country, but they also mean we close our eyes to the hard choices confronting medicare. After all, Canadians can complacently say to themselves, "Since our system is so superior, why worry about things here?" The first intellectual requirement for any meaningful conversation about Canadian health care is to stop Canada–United States comparisons. To suggest that a debate about medicare will inexorably lead to U.S.-style medicine is fear-mongering. We are not going to adopt U.S.-style health care, nor should we. Full stop. We can learn, of course, from particular aspects of the U.S. system. We can and do benefit hugely from U.S. medical research. We can study particular U.S. examples of delivering care. We can be inspired by U.S. clinical evaluations. But when it comes to the overall organization of health care, Canada–United States comparisons serve only political objectives.

There is no right amount of money a society should spend on health care. We could spend more than we do today on health care as a share of our national economy, and almost certainly will in future. Canada is rich, and rich countries spend more of their gross domestic product on health care than do poor ones. Spending a lot on health comes with having the money to spend on it, for individuals and societies.

Canada is not alone in wrestling with rising health-care costs. They are going up as a share of the national economy in every advanced industrial economy. Canada is luckier than some of those countries because our economy is in better shape, our deficits are lower and our future economic prospects brighter. So we could spend more, even much more, on health care—if we were willing to pay for it. We could raise taxes and put all the additional money into health care. We could stop spending as much on other public goods (transit, education, social welfare, the environment and so on) so tax levels would remain the same while health-care budgets rose. We could let people spend more of their own money to buy essential health services. We could require people to pay directly for some portion of the health care that the state now finances. We could implement a combination of some of these changes. We just have to choose.

What we cannot do is continue to demand more from medicare without being willing to tax ourselves more to pay for it or reduce spending on other public goods. We could, of course, insist that health care become more efficient, and there is wisdom in that insistence. Indeed, most of the public debate around health care, and most citizens' fondest hopes for avoiding serious change, centres on solving the sustainability challenge and improving health-care outcomes through efficiency gains. These are available, urgent, necessary and insufficient. Efficiency gains from a massive public system of any kind defy the way those systems are organized and the nature of incentives within them. The lure of efficiency is enticing, and the need for greater efficiency is urgent, but efficiency alone will not allow us to improve the chronic condition of medicare.

Canada suffers from health-care myopia. All the health-care experts, the commissions and the legislative studies when studying health care examine only health care. They do not look at health care as one public service among many. They just assume it should have first claim on public resources—because that is what polls suggest citizens insist is their most important public priority—without giving much concern for what that spending does to other programs.

Roy Romanow said bluntly in his 2002 report, "The system needs more money," including a minimum threshold for federal transfers to provinces. The extra money, Romanow explained, would ease the transition to needed health-care changes. These included "better management practices," more focus on prevention of illness and "more agile and collaborative institutions," whatever that meant. A few recommendations were specific; most were vague.

Prime Minister Paul Martin and the provincial premiers disregarded some of Romanow's recommendations but heeded his call for more money. They signed what Martin called a "fix it for a generation" deal, starting in the fiscal year 2003–2004, worth $41 billion for health care from Ottawa over a decade—with federal transfers indexed at 6 percent a year. The federal money produced some modest improvements to the system, especially in reduced wait times for a limited number of procedures. But the new money also stalled reforms that would likely have occurred had money been tighter. Romanow argued that more money was needed to "buy change." The new money mostly bought time.

Indexing yearly health-care transfers at 6 percent sounds generous. Who among us would not like our incomes indexed at 6 percent? Which company would not like that sort of profit growth year after year? No other government program enjoys that kind of indexing. And yet the 6 percent increase just kept the system afloat, since provincial health-care spending rose in the 7 percent range from 2000 to 2010, according to the Canadian Institute for Health Information. The 6 percent index prevented the health-care system from getting worse, because anything less than a 6 percent transfer would have meant less money in real terms, since that was the rate of health-care inflation. The public apparently did not think all the additional money had done much to improve the system. According to an Ipsos Reid survey for the Canadian Medical Association published in the summer of 2011, 15 percent of respondents thought the extra money had improved the system, 47 percent thought the system had remained the same and 36 percent believed it had gotten worse.

In the final days of 2011, the government of Prime Minister Stephen Harper announced how it would address health care. It promised to extend the 2003–2004 accord beyond its ten-year time frame for three more years, that is, until 2016–17, with a 6 percent annual index. After that, the government said federal transfers would fall to something approximating the real growth in the economy plus inflation, or perhaps 4 percent. Most of the provinces squealed, as provinces often do, with the only contented ones being British Columbia, Alberta and Saskatchewan. The others had become accustomed to the 6 percent indexation; anything less would mean harder choices, and what politician would not like to avoid those?

Why has health-care spending grown so rapidly? Aging is a small factor, although it will become a bigger one. The population grows, and there is always some inflation. Both obviously add to health-care costs. But the two biggest reasons are Canadians' increased use of medical services, especially pharmaceuticals, plus pay increases above inflation for those who work in the system. Seventy percent of a hospital's costs, for example, are for wages, salaries and benefits. If these rise faster than the growth in government revenues, which in turn influence transfers to hospitals, the budgetary pressure is intense. If physicians get increases above the increase in governments' revenues, as they have been receiving recently, these increases augment budgetary pressures.

Here is the health-care spending dilemma for every government: a system that is labour intensive but with lower productivity rates than the economy as a whole.

A further cost pressure arises from a system where no one has to pay to see a doctor or visit a hospital, because there is no constraint on demand (other than the rationing of waiting), and that can lead to overuse in some instances. Patients who do not pay, and doctors who do not charge, invite at least the possibility of what economists call "moral hazard," the overuse by provider and consumer of a good or service priced at zero.

So we are left with choices, hard ones today, harder ones tomorrow—the ones citizens would prefer not to hear about. Polling data repeatedly show that people do not want to pay higher taxes, and certainly do not want to pay from their own pockets to access the system, as with user fees. The Quebec government proposed user fees tied to income, with no fees at all for low-income citizens. The government withdrew the idea after the finance minister said that the "Quebec political culture" was not ready for this initiative. He could have been speaking about all of Canada.

Citizens do not favour the public system dropping any services, although a few provinces have done this to save money. Nor, of course, does the public want less money spent on other programs. No new taxes. No fees or private payments. No fewer services—indeed, more if possible. No cuts elsewhere. All the painful options—the ones politicians are reluctant to outline— have been pushed off the table. Politicians are left to resolve health-care dilemmas by pursuing the easiest one to articulate and the hardest one to achieve—the dream of efficiency gains.

This book tries to look at choices and options. It is not

designed to trash medicare. Medicare has been, and remains, an important Canadian national accomplishment. Just as the railway was a ribbon of steel that linked Canada in the nineteenth century, medicare might be thought of as a bond that has linked modern Canada. It has improved the health of Canadians and therefore the life chances of many citizens. Although this book is not about medicine per se, the medical achievements inside the system are often wonderful. When Canadians do gain access to the system, they report high levels of satisfaction.

Medicare's foundation is equity, the notion that we are all better off when the risks of illness are shared, because no one knows where those risks will fall. That there should be a publicly financed system, available to all regardless of income or illness or chance, is a cornerstone of most liberal democracies, including Canada.

This book is about the choices surrounding health care in Canada. To understand those choices better, it asks three questions. How did Canada get this system? How is the system working when measured against actual health outcomes and costs, and the insistence that medicare is the best system in the world compared with other systems? What should we do?

Medicare is the only system that most Canadians have known. They do not remember health care before medicare. Medicare's evolution is a gripping story full of controversy and critical turning points. Nothing was preordained. The history of how we got this unique system, therefore, is worth remembering for its own sake. History also reminds us that today's controversies have antecedents that contribute to making reforms difficult.

How the system works is what concerns most Canadians. History might be interesting or instructive. Policy planners and health-policy experts can build their models and do their studies, but patients want high-quality service now, they want it free and they want it effective. They pay their taxes for a health-care system that is among the most expensive in the world. They are not getting enough value for that money. Why not?

Necessary changes will be hard, but we cannot even consider them without a serious conversation, which is difficult in a world of blogs and Twitter and the generalized decline in quality media coverage of important public matters, the partisan rhetoric, federal–provincial finger pointing, interest-group assertions and political fears around a subject that Canadians say they care passionately about but are not eager to debate. There are no easy answers, and simple solutions to complex problems are invariably wrong. But we must ask hard questions, because the status quo should not endure.

PART ONE

ONE

Hospital Days

D r. Jeffrey Turnbull glances at the top line of the patient's chart. He blocks with his hand the subsequent lines that describe the patient's condition and treatment since being admitted the night before. "I know the rest," Turnbull predicts.

The patient, R, is a ninety-four-year-old male. Turnbull's quick assessment: "This will cost about $50,000 for the twenty to thirty days he is here." Turnbull reads the rest of the chart. R came from a retirement home. He was given a battery of tests after being admitted to the Ottawa Hospital. The chart, all handwritten by nurses and residents, shows R's vital signs are acceptable, but he has a urinary-tract infection, lesions (likely malignant) on his back and a form of dementia.

"That man should never have come into an acute-care hospital," Turnbull observes. "Someone should have made arrangements a month ago for him to go somewhere, but now it's happened." Turnbull continues: "There are maybe 160 people in the hospital at $1100 a day waiting for long-term care. So we're spending maybe $180,000 a day for care that is crappy, not in their best interests. In a nursing home, it would be about $200 a day. The care itself here isn't crappy, but this man won't have rehab. He's not going to have his family around.

"They've done ten tests so far. What will happen now is that we will treat his urinary-tract infection. We'll stabilize his condition. We'll call the family and we'll agree that he should be sent to a long-term care facility, and then he'll wait for a bed. We'll transfer him to our waiting unit, and then he'll wait."

Turnbull's Monday-morning prediction introduced me, in the fall of 2011, to a week learning what goes on in the Ottawa Hospital, one of the largest teaching hospitals in Canada, with an annual budget of about $1 billion, and a template for similar institutions across Canada. The week allowed me to watch one part of Canadian health care across wards, operating rooms, the emergency department, administrative offices, inner-city outpatient care. It became evident throughout the week that at the Ottawa Hospital, as at other large acute-care hospitals across Canada, brilliant medicine is practised, caring staff offer succor and support, technologies and drugs unheard of several decades ago help patients with their ailments. Some of the very best features of the Canadian health-care system were on display; so were some of the worst.

A hospital is a complicated institution, and a teaching hospital the most complicated health-care institution of all. It is the apex of Canadian health care, a source of immense community pride, a magnet for medical talent, an institution to which Canadians head for all sorts of health problems. The Canadian health-care system was originally designed around hospitals and, to a fault, it remains so today—a system whose hospitals struggle to cope with changing patient demand, an aging population (R, for example), higher costs, global budgets imposed by provincial capitals, fast-developing technologies, rigid rules, new drugs and the social inequities that lead to poor health.

Turnbull, an internal-medicine specialist, is the Ottawa

Hospital's chief of staff. When I spent time with him, he had just completed a year (2010–2011) as president of the Canadian Medical Association, during which the CMA mobilized a public campaign to draw attention to the health-care system's challenges. Turnbull believes fiercely in the public health-care system and brought immense passion to his one-year post.

Turnbull did not spend his presidency pleading for more money for physicians or echoing publicly their various complaints, let alone preaching for private health care. He understood that the profession had recently done so well financially that it would have been indecent of physicians to complain. Instead, he asked his profession, and the Canadian public, to debate a CMA document that he helped to craft, "Health Care Transformation in Canada." "The founding principles of Medicare are not being met today either in letter or in spirit," it charged. "Canadians are not receiving the value they deserve from the health care system ... Canada cannot continue on this path ... Nothing less than one of Canada's most cherished national institutions is at stake. Unwillingness to confront the challenges is not an option." Of all recent reports on Canadian health care, his diagnosis—from a passionate believer in medicare—was among the starkest.

Turnbull is back full-time in the hospital now, although he remains in demand as a speaker, a doctor *engagé*. He breaks away each year to work in Bangladesh and Africa at clinics he helps to finance. He is what every patient would wish his or her doctor to be: smart, caring and personable. Having analyzed the health-care system's weaknesses, he broke the taboos too many other defenders of Canadian medicare try to impose on debate. His bottom line: medicare, as now structured, financed and administered, is not good enough.

Turnbull continues his Monday-morning rounds, a preliminary review of about two dozen patients. His survey completed, he joins residents, other doctors, medical students, a pharmacist and an assignment nurse around a table in a nondescript conference room. This daily meeting allows everyone to review the roster of patients: their treatment and needs and conditions, how long they should remain on the ward, where they might go thereafter.

New patients arrive every night, if there is room for them. Other patients leave during the day, sometimes to be discharged from the hospital, often transferred to a ward in the hospital called the APU, the Awaiting Placement Unit, where they will wait, and wait, and wait some more for a more appropriate and cheaper place outside the hospital. Patient A arrived overnight, and so shows up as a new patient on the chart along with ninety-four-year-old R. Patient A had become involved in an altercation in a parking lot. He claimed that a driver had run over his foot with a car and his finger got jammed in the door in the ensuing dispute. Crying, fearful of losing his foot, afflicted by a history of drinking, he was demanding that fluid be drained from his foot. He was giving the nurses a hard time, a medical student reported.

Another patient, S, "presented" (the verb used in hospital circles) with multiple problems: Crohn's disease, a form of dementia, blindness, shaking all over, an alcoholic. Later that day, Turnbull gently approaches S on the ward and asks how much alcohol she consumes a day. "About thirteen ounces," she replies. Her pallor is grey, and she is still shaking. Who buys the alcohol? Turnbull asks the blind woman. Her husband. If she returns home, Turnbull continues, will she stop drinking? Yes, she would like that, S answers.

Turnbull turns away. If Patient S did go home, he observes, her husband would still be there, so she would resume her habit.

She should go into some form of long-term care facility, except that she would have to agree, and no places are available anyway. We will stabilize her condition. She will return home. She will be back, he predicts.

At the morning meeting, most of the patients under discussion are elderly. Excessive alcohol consumption played a role in perhaps a quarter of the cases. Two had fallen in their homes, several had forms of dementia, most had multiple problems, often chronic. These patients would likely remain for a while in internal medicine wards. They form an indicative but not necessarily representative profile of hospital patients. A patient list in orthopaedics, cardiology, endocrinology or oncology would be different, although they too would all be tilted toward an older clientele. Some medical disciplines get people in and out of hospitals fast, especially after routine surgeries and after childbirth without complications. Internal medicine must deal with the impact of aging as forcefully as any specialty. Whether seniors should be treated in a hospital, and whether they should remain on wards such as internal medicine as long as they do, is another matter.

It also became clear at the morning meetings throughout the week that medical personnel spend as much time discussing patients' social and economic conditions as their physical health needs. What often brought patients to the internal medicine ward were the results of their unsatisfactory social and economic conditions. Most of them were old and often frail. They frequently did not have much money, lived in precarious family arrangements (if there was a family at all) and had presented to hospitals before. Sending them home, even if they were technically well enough, did not seem like the best option because of familial or housing conditions. Discussions among medical staff around the table often sounded much like a session among social workers.

Every patient on the list required pharmaceuticals, and often lots of them. Patient need comes first, obviously, so a sometimes breathtakingly long list of pharmaceuticals was prescribed for patients with multiple conditions. In the Canadian system, pharmaceuticals outside hospitals are not free. Patients pay for them, either a small sum if they are seniors or very poor, out of their own pocket, or the drugs are covered by private insurance. It's a hodgepodge of coverage, in other words. Inside hospitals, however, pharmaceuticals are free, because everything is free inside hospitals under the Canadian system, from entry to exit.

Around the table, therefore, no one discusses cost. Such a discussion could lead to exploring moral hazard—exploitation of a service paid for by another party. The potential for moral hazard permeates the Canadian system, from patients over-using the system to doctors prescribing excessive treatment. But the incidence of moral hazard is low. Patients as a general rule do not go to the hospital for fun; doctors do not overprescribe medications or order too many tests for the joy of it. Nonetheless, there has been an explosion of testing, partly because new diagnostic tools are available (magnetic resonance imaging [MRI] machines, for example), and an increase in the use of new drugs (cholesterol-lowering drugs, for example) that have driven up health-care costs, although some new drugs improve health and treat ailments outside institutional settings, thereby saving the health-care system money. Asked about all the drugs being prescribed, Turnbull says he tries to take costs into account and to restrict prescriptions to those that are absolutely necessary. Sometimes, he blocks diagnostic tests that he feels are of limited or no value. It's a rearguard struggle, however. Tests can be ordered to cover potential legal challenges. Patients demand them, having heard these tests were available. Their tax dollars have purchased the machines, and they want them to be used.

Orders were given for a few patients who needed to go elsewhere that day or soon. Where to go? Inside the conference room, the case of a seventy-one-year-old man with type 2 diabetes, hypertension and other ailments had been discussed. Outside the room, Turnbull commented, "He should have gone straight to a long-term care facility or, better still, a long-term care facility attached to a nursing home with family doctors involved. Chronic disease management, which is now 57 per cent of the action, should be built around things outside the hospital, but the acute-care system is being used for that purpose. This man should never have come into an acute-care hospital."

R's case comes up. "What will happen now is that we will treat his urinary infection," Turnbull says after the discussion. "He's horribly demented. We'll call in the family. We'll say that he is best cared for in another environment. Then we'll agree that he should go to a long-term care environment. Then he'll wait for a bed. We'll transfer him from here to our waiting place and he'll wait. They want to do some tests on the cancerous lesions on his back. I'll try to put an end to that." The lesions will not kill him before other frailties.

The Ottawa Hospital produces a patient flow monitor (PFM) document throughout the day. It identifies how many patients are in the hospital, overnight admittances, patients waiting for assignment, critical-care occupancy and the number of ALCs, or alternative level of care patients. In a properly organized health-care system, these ALC patients should not remain in hospital for more than a few days. They should go as quickly as possible to nursing homes, long-term care facilities or a supervised home-care program.

Turnbull asks for the PFM at noon. It shows 1022 patients in the hospital's two main campuses, the Civic and the General, and 135 ALCs. Thirteen percent of the beds, therefore, are occupied by people who, under ideal circumstances, should not be in the hospital. These are the "bed blockers" that are every large hospital's nightmare across Canada. They prevent other patients' access to beds on admission, eat up huge daily costs and put pressure on hospitals' global budgets. They are the front-line evidence of a health-care system that history bequeathed, top-heavy with hospitals, short on other, cheaper facilities. Turnbull gets updates throughout the day. At 2:30 P.M., overall occupancy is 1005, ALCs 136; at 4:30 P.M., overall occupancy stands at 985 (some patients have been discharged throughout the afternoon), ALCs 139.

The PFMs reveal a hospital wrestling hourly with more patients than its budget permits. Every hour of the day, the number of patients exceeds available beds. The number of patients in existing beds exceeds the number for whom the hospital has been given money by the provincial health ministry. The hospital copes as best it can. Beds are temporarily placed in halls for patients awaiting places in wards. A conference room is converted into a temporary space for several beds. Turnbull starts a conversation with a non-medical colleague whose job involves finding space for patients. "Last week, it was terrible," she says with a sigh. "We haven't been under 100 percent in I don't know how long. I started in mid-May. I came back from retirement. I'm an interim manager." (The overcrowding did improve somewhat in 2012. The hospital reduced the number of cancelled surgeries, assigned case workers to the frail and elderly as soon as they arrived to plan post-hospital care, and sent some patients home after pre-surgery preparations rather than occupying beds.)

Later, in his office, Turnbull ruminates about the system. "Let's make the system as efficient as it can possibly be and then look for more money if we need it," he says. "If somebody came to me for more dollars for the existing system, I'd say not a penny more—and I'm in the system. I'd say, 'Are you kidding? You're asking me to pay more for a bad car.'"

Hospitals are being used in too many instances for the wrong purposes, because the overall system is poorly structured and organized.

"I'll give you an example of why we have a good system and a bad system," he recounts. "About three weeks ago, there was a fifty-year-old man who got sick at work. We got patched in at the hospital and were warned that this wasn't going to be pretty. He had collapsed at work. By the time he arrived, he was ashen, not completely gone but almost. He arrests at the same moment he gets here: no blood pressure, no pulse. CPR. Chaos. A nurse was assigned to run his blood. There are orderlies on standby to take him wherever he needs to go. X-rays and radiology are notified. The guy goes up from emergency because he has ruptured his ventricle because he had a heart attack. The guy is here, diagnosed, over to the Heart Institute [for surgery] and in two hours he's fixed. That's what we do very well.

"That same day," he continues, "a ninety-year-old patient comes in with pneumonia. The pneumonia is something that could easily have been cared for in another setting. She waits twelve or twenty-four hours before a decision is made. Then she waits another day or two for a bed. She gets into a bed and is treated. She spends so much time in the hospital environment without physiotherapy. Off she goes to long-term care.

"The first is what we do well; the second, because the chronic disease management system had failed, is what we don't do very well. We've got the mindset of more tests, more drugs. She's ninety. She's frail and elderly. She should just have been given the antibiotics at the nursing home or at home."

Before he departs, Turnbull receives a report on R, the ninety-four-year-old patient with the urinary infection and dementia. A PSA test has come back showing prostate cancer. The chief resident and Turnbull decide that nothing should be done, given R's advanced age and other ailments. But R's family has assembled. Some of them want action—a CT scan to check for a stroke, for example. R's daughter wants aggressive treatment of the cancer. R's wife and granddaughter are present. R's wife is not sure about further treatment. The chief resident gently and persuasively explains that aggressive treatment will do no good. He says that a place will eventually be found for R outside the hospital, but he will never go home again. Finding that location will take some time.

Dr. Guy Hebert heard about the car crash on his way to work. He and the patient from the crash arrived at the hospital at about the same time. She had suffered broken bones, one of which pierced her skin. She was groaning in agony in a trauma unit of the emergency department. Four hours after arrival, the woman underwent surgery to repair those breaks. Two days later, she was discharged, a small triumph among many for the emergency department. As Hebert, a transplanted Acadian and a senior member of the hospital emergency medical team, said later, "She was fortunate in her mishap."

She had not been Hebert's patient. Instead, as she was being treated in trauma, Hebert studied the monitor screens on the wall. They provided an overview of patients stretching from the waiting room outside the emergency department to the post-operative recovery rooms.

"We've got fourteen people in the waiting room," he says. "The majority are waiting to get into the stretcher bay area. Look at the breakdown of patients in the observation area, their ages. There's one person at twenty-one years of age, then sixty-one, seventy-eight, eighty-eight, sixty-six. There's one person with multiple psychiatric problems at seventy-three, then seventy-six, seventy-nine, a younger person, then seventy-eight, seventy-nine, eighty-four, ninety-four, eighty-three."

These emergency patients will wait to see a physician, according to a priority established by the triage nurse. They could wait for hours. The provincial target for time spent in a hospital emergency department is four hours for minor or uncomplicated conditions, eight hours for complex ones. According to a June 2011 report, the province had not met those targets. Instead, average time spent had been 4.3 and 10.8 hours. At the Ottawa Hospital, depending on which of the two emergency departments were analyzed, the times for the month of June 2011 were 5.8 to 6.1 hours for minor problems and 16 to 19.5 for complicated ones.

Compared with those numbers, this was a good day. "If we start at eight in the morning, the volumes will start to creep up significantly," Hebert says. "We'll get a little bit of a slowdown in the early afternoon, and then later afternoon to early evening, we get another peak. Roughly around midnight, it starts to quiet down until the next morning."

This day unfolds as Hebert predicted. By late afternoon, he could report, "Right now, six patients are waiting for emergency admittance, two for cardiac monitoring. We have seven people waiting to get into the observation ward. Observation is full. We have no beds. So this is where the backlog starts to accumulate. They are going to work at moving some of these patients out if they can.

"This morning, the entire department had forty-five patients. Right now, we are at eighty-five. A lot of patients are waiting to be seen here in urgent care. And we can see that there are patients who are on stretchers waiting to go into the stretcher bay area.

"We've got sixteen patients out front. This number sometimes goes up to thirty or thirty-five. That's when the waiting room gets really bad. But nobody has been waiting more than three hours up to now. So we're still meeting our physician-initial-assessment time of getting them seen. Right now, we're still on track."

One hundred and forty thousand persons show up at the hospital's two emergency departments each year. Hebert's emergency unit sees about 70,000 annually. That volume perplexes him, because the department was renovated and expanded in 2003. "We went from an emergency department that was supposed to see about 30,000 patients a year, but we are now seeing about 70,000 a year," he says. "We used to be backed up ten to fifteen patients. We have all this additional capacity, yet we are as backed up as ever, because the patients are still not going up to the ward. The daily reality is that we are backed up twenty to twenty-five patients."

What's happened? How could the number of emergency patients have risen proportionately much more sharply than the population of Ottawa, when family clinics have opened that are supposed to take some of the pressure off emergency departments? Hebert struggles for an answer. Hospital CEO Jack Kitts confirms that the number of emergency department patients has risen 6 percent a year for the past five years. "I think it's the aging population," he says, although the overall population is by no means aging that fast. Certainly the cases displayed on the television monitors in emergency suggest age is definitely a factor. Another would be the lack of access to family physicians, which sends people to the emergency department.

Hebert suggests another possibility. "There are a number of patients who come into the emergency department because they are getting frustrated with the wait times out there. If your family doctor orders an MRI, the wait time can be three to six weeks to explore a back pain. So if you can't work and are at home in pain, and you're told you have to wait and you're losing money and you can't pay the bills, what are you supposed to do?

"If I see twenty-five patients here a day, you might surmise that three to five patients in that group may have come to the emergency department because they felt they weren't getting active service elsewhere. Maybe they felt they needed to see a specialist. Maybe the wait time to see a specialist was three months. Maybe they felt they needed to have a test.

"It doesn't necessarily mean that emergency will go along with your desires. They could determine that there is no urgent problem. We might get you in sooner, or we might not." (Hebert is right about limited access to family physicians driving some patients to ERs. An Ontario Ministry of Health study in September 2010 found that 15 percent of patients with a family physician went to emergency because the physician was unavailable.)

Television shows about hospitals focus on the high dramas of ERs: stretchers being pushed here and there, nurses and physicians running alongside, everything breathless and life-threatening—cases like the one involving the morning's car-accident patient. Predictably, those shows don't capture what really happens, as Hebert explains.

"We have scoring based on the Canadian Triage and Acuity Scale [CTAS]," he says. "The triage nurse, based on that information, will categorize patients who want to be seen between 1 and 5, with 1 being the most serious and 5 a cut on the finger. The 4s and 5s account for 15 percent of our visits; the 3s for maybe 65 percent; the 2s at 15 percent; the 1s at 5 percent."

The ER is a hospital's front end. If the back end is filled up with bed-blockers, the jam they cause works its way back to the front end. It's an endemic problem with large hospitals across the country: too many patients at the front end; too many in the wards; too few discharges.

"This is one of the realities we live with day in and day out," Hebert says. "We are significantly overcrowded. The hospital gets blocked, and unfortunately we have backlogs into our emergency department." He checks the wall monitor. "In the clinical exam areas, we have forty-two beds. Nineteen are being taken by people waiting for admission. And I can tell you that to have nineteen is a very good day. Many days, it's thirty or thirty-five."

He continues: "We have only forty-two units, so when we get busy, they all start to back up into the waiting room and on the ambulance runway. Through this door over here, the ambulances arrive, and if we have no place to put the patients, the ambulance drivers have to wait out front with their patients either in the ambulance, or they line them up with stretchers in the hallway ... We can't stop the tap. We can't stop patients from walking through our doors. We can't stop ambulances from arriving."

The patients Hebert sees that day in the ward, however, are all suffering from very minor problems, the 4s and 5s. They shouldn't really be in an ER.

Some hospitals across Canada have a family-health clinic on site; others have one nearby. Hospital ERs ought to be able to steer people immediately away from their door to one of those clinics where service might be faster and would certainly cost less. Hebert worries about sending people to a clinic somewhere else in the city.

"We worry about being medically and legally responsible for diverting people, because someone can come in complaining of a minor ache in their thigh, for instance, and at the end of the day they can turn out to have a ruptured artery," he says. "If we send that patient home or to a walk-in clinic down the street, you never know what might happen." If, as a society, we will not accept this kind of risk, and are ready to launch legal actions against medical personnel who take such reasonable risks, then making the system more flexible and efficient just became harder.

Still, time spent in the waiting room explains why patients chafe at what they find. They register, and they are seen by a triage nurse who asks questions about their condition. The worst go first; the rest wait, and wait. Waiting is wearing enough, but no updated information is given about how long and why. Patients get frustrated. "We don't have the personnel to do that because the nurses are so busy," Hebert explains. "In an ideal world, that would be something to strive for. And it's not something that we have not thought of. It's certainly not a novel idea. We've been limited by the amount of resources that we could direct to that type of activity. It would do wonders for patient satisfaction."

Later in the afternoon, Hebert breaks away from seeing patients and explains what he sees on the ubiquitous monitors. He wants to know how long patients have been in the department. He begins reciting, "The person here the longest has spent 69 hours in emergency. So that person has been here for almost three days, waiting for a bed upstairs. The shortest period of time for admitted patients: 14 hours, 4 hours. Some of them might have been admitted an hour or two ago." He scans further: "28 hours, 23, 22. Hold on, here's one who's been here 118 hours. Perhaps this person requires an isolation bed upstairs. Finding an isolation room is a particular challenge."

He picks up Jeffrey Turnbull's theme: "This is a daily occurrence for us," he says. "This is why the hospital is at 105 percent capacity. I can't remember the last time when I saw us in the 90 percent range. Oh, maybe we were 99 percent for a short while—sorry." (The hospital reduced its occupancy rate to about 100 percent in the spring of 2012.)

Joel Werier is on pre-surgery rounds. Today, an operating room is available to him for two surgeries, one scheduled to last for two hours, the other perhaps six. Of course, Werier can do various orthopaedic surgeries. His specialty, however, is sarcomas, cancers of the soft tissues and bones, one of which killed Terry Fox. They are often insidious tumours, hard to extract, draped around bones, embedded in muscles or joints. Only a handful of surgeons in Ontario do sarcoma surgeries. Since the surgeries can take a very long time, the government has adjusted the payment schedule for this handful of physicians, recognizing their surgeries are not assembly-line affairs.

Werier, originally from Winnipeg, is a gentle bundle of energy. A short man, he bounces on his feet a lot. He has a leprechaun's smile, as if he knows something funny that you don't, and a reassuring demeanour, a useful characteristic in someone who deals with what the author of a book about cancer called the "emperor of all maladies."

A woman in her early fifties extends her hand, palm down. Werier places her hand in his to observe a walnut-sized lump on the top. She is alone and outwardly quite calm. The surgery will take a maximum of two hours, he tells her. I am confident it will go well. Any questions? No, she replies. She is ready and composed.

The next patient is not, and for understandable reasons. She is thirteen and a half years old and has been undergoing chemotherapy for several months. She has lost her hair and some weight. Her Arab-Canadian father and mother have their arms around her, consoling their girl as she weeps uncontrollably. She is shaking with fear. The parents tell her that everything will be fine, and in so doing they are trying to reassure themselves. Like all parents confronted with the prospect of unimaginable loss, they want desperately to believe that this tumour deep in their daughter's leg, this obscene invasion of a young girl's body that has already caused so much grief and pain, will be removed by this man, and that through him, his training, his skill and this hospital, she will survive.

This is the easy part, Werier tells her and her parents. What you have gone through so far, that's been tough. You're not going to feel anything, he reassures her, and everything will be all right. She nods through her sobs. How many terrors has she already known? And now this? Her parents soak up Werier's reassurance. He tells them that they can go home and come back later. He must know that they will not leave. As the day stretches on, other family members will join the parents in the family lounge, supporting each other, vicariously rooting for the girl on the operating table to whom fate has dealt such a cruel blow but who has been delivered by the Canadian health-care system into Werier's skilled hands.

Canada's health-care system does many things well, once access is gained to it. The acute-care hospitals are the apex of the system. The care inside them is usually good to very good by international standards, even if the organization of hospitals, and their place within the wider health-care system, leaves much to be desired. The children's hospitals, such as the Children's Hospital of Eastern Ontario where this girl is a patient, are world-class treatment centres, the pride of their communities. The girl has been transferred for surgery to the Ottawa Hospital, because surgeons such as Joel Werier do their work there. She will return to CHEO after the operation for more chemotherapy to try to stop any cancer that remains after the surgery from spreading. If all goes well, Werier says before the operation, he will excise the entire tumour, even though it is lodged in a difficult place, and the chemotherapy will work. The girl will be monitored periodic-ally for some years, the cancer will not return, she might have a slightly weakened limb, but she will survive and live a normal life. She is young, and that helps. The odds are in her favour, even though this cancer is an aggressive variety. We won't know for sure for a decade, he concludes.

An operating room is a place of technical majesty. Seven persons attend the two surgeries: Werier, a visiting physician from Saudi Arabia, a fifth-year surgical resident, a medical student, an anaesthetist and two operating-room nurses. "Are you okay with blood?" Werier asks me. Actually, there is very little blood as the resident opens the top of the hand of the first patient. Their objective is a tumour that had swelled up from beneath the tendons of the hand and wrapped itself around several of the bones. The incision made, clips hold back the skin so that deeper cuts can be made. Other instruments hold aloft tendons so that the scalpels can cut around the tumour below. The surgeons chat partly about the task before them, partly about nothing in particular, as if they were sitting on a bus together heading to the office. It's an intricate surgery because of the tumour's location. In forty-five minutes, they have winkled it from her hand and plopped it in a tray. Werier let the resident do much of the work. He offered occasional instructions and sometimes picked up the surgical instruments himself. The hard part done, he wanders around the operating room while the resident sews up the incision. Unless there are unlikely post-operative complications, he observes, the woman will go home that day. The tumour will be sent to the pathology lab. A few days later, the results come back. Unexpectedly, the pathology revealed that the tumour had been benign.

A break ensues to prepare for the day's most challenging case: the thirteen-and-a-half-year-old girl. The surgeon from Saudi Arabia and the surgical resident begin what will be a long operation. The tumour is very deep in the leg. The screen on the wall shows the magnetic resonance image of the tumour, and Werier periodically consults the image as he directs the operation. He is more intensely involved in this surgery, especially as the cutting goes deeper and deeper. Among the surgery's many challenges is to avoid slicing any major arteries, veins and nerves. Occasionally, Werier looks up and explains what this or that manoeuvre means in the grand scheme of the operation. Then he ducks his head again, either cutting by himself or showing his younger colleagues where and how to cut, and why. Five long hours later, the tumour is removed, the girl is sent to recovery and the anxious parents are told that the operation has been a success. No one, not even Werier, can foretell the long-term prognosis. Two weeks later, the girl would resume chemotherapy treatments for another six months. Werier said a month after the operation that his "gut" told him she would be fine.

These were complicated surgeries, for such is the nature of sarcomas. They were executed by superbly trained staff in expensively outfitted operating rooms. These ORs are the crown jewels inside a hospital. Administrators try to keep patients flowing through them; surgeons angle for operating time in them. Neither group succeeds as it would like, nor as patients would presumably want. In 2011, the Ottawa Hospital did 24,795 surgeries, and cancelled 604 for lack of beds, which is one consequence of the hospital beds being occupied on average at 105 percent capacity Monday to Friday throughout the year.

There is an evident problem across Canada with the way operating rooms are used. On the one hand, there is large unmet demand for surgeries, witness to which are long wait times; on the other, there is large unused capacity, witness to which are the yawning hours when the operating rooms are idle. When unmet demand meets unused supply, something ought to be done to match better available supply to evident demand. First-year economics textbooks instruct undergraduates on available solutions to this matching challenge. Within the Canadian health-care system, however, this matching does not happen enough—to the frustration of patients and surgeons alike—because the system does not allow for the kind of market economics found in the textbooks. It relies instead on making hospitals work within global budgets, regardless of demand. As a consequence, the Canadian health-care system, by international comparative studies, has the longest wait times among Western industrialized countries.

The Ottawa General has one hundred operating rooms. Four of them are kept open twenty-four hours a day, seven days a week, for emergency surgeries. Sometimes these four are not all needed; nonetheless, they are prudently kept available. The other ninety-six operating rooms open, as the one did for Werier's surgeries, at 8 A.M. and close at 4 or 5 P.M., unless a particular surgery runs late. The ninety-six are closed Saturdays and Sundays. By cheeky contrast, Walmart is open from 7 A.M. to 11 P.M., seven days a week. Banks that decades ago opened at 10 A.M. and closed at 3 P.M., Monday to Friday, now offer seven-day-a-week service at some branches from 9 A.M. to 5 P.M.

Do the math. Twenty-four hours in a day for seven days means 168 hours. Since there are one hundred ORs, that means 16,800 available hours, theoretically, for surgeries. But since only four ORs are open 24/7 and the other ninety-six for only nine hours a day, five days a week, that means actual use of the OR rooms amounts to 4992 hours, or slightly less than one-third of the time.

Nobody suggests twenty-four-hour-a-day use. There wouldn't be enough staff, even if there were enough money. Suppose, for the sake of argument, however, that the ORs could be kept open on weekends for nine hours per day. Very few patients would object to an operation on Saturday or Sunday as opposed to Wednesday if it meant a shorter wait. Ninety-six rooms kept open nine hours a day for two days would mean another 1728 hours of operating time. Too much? How about three more hours a day, then, for five days a week for half of the rooms, or 720 total hours?

Play with numbers any way you want. The point is simply that unmet demand is not meeting unused capacity when so many rooms remain idle for so long. There are ways of dealing with this chronic problem, but the Canadian system forbids some of them, such as deploying any unused operating-room time for patients willing to pay privately. Governments are very tentatively finding the courage to try what other health-care systems have implemented, such as letting money follow patients, thereby creating incentives for hospitals to do more procedures. Nor can they break union rules that make surgeries happen to fit the convenience of providers instead of patients, an endemic problem everywhere in the Canadian system. A system that boasts brilliant surgeons such as Joel Werier, accomplished staff, wonderfully furnished facilities but uses them only a fraction of the available time in the face of unmet demand is a system straitjacketed by ideology.

The usual group of medical staff, including Turnbull, has gathered around the boardroom table mid-morning Thursday, working through the list of patients. A particular patient sparks another social-work discussion: what to do with the seventy-seven-year-old man with cirrhosis of the liver who does not speak English? His wife has been away but will be back tomorrow. Should they discharge the patient or wait another day for the wife to return? The patient speaks only Polish. The Polish-language speaker from the translation firm that the hospital uses is unavailable.

Anybody know a friend who speaks Polish? While batting around options, an "urgent" message appears on Turnbull's pager. It reads: "extreme occupancy." Turnbull barely glances at the pager, despite the words *urgent* and *extreme*. A resident in receipt of the same message jokes, "It's the 8:30," by which he means this message usually arrives earlier in the morning to inform staff that the hospital is desperately overcrowded. Staff should therefore discharge patients if at all possible. As for the Polish-speaking patient, Turnbull decides that given the bed shortages in the hospital, he should be sent home.

These decisions about when and where to send patients are sometimes difficult. During afternoon rounds, a doctor's assistant, a man who left the Canadian military for this new career, pulls Turnbull aside in the corridor. Turnbull listens while the assistant painstakingly describes an evolving case.

A patient who has already spent fifty-five days in the hospital is ready to be discharged, the assistant recounts. The patient has been seen by physiotherapy, occupational therapy, neurology. Staff agrees that he should go home, a recommendation with which the patient agrees. He suffers from excessive alcohol consumption and periodic depression, but the hospital can do little about either problem. It's time for him to leave, except that his wife, who is a trained psychologist, is furious at the hospital's decision.

The assistant explains that the wife came to the hospital yesterday, threw a telephone at a secretary and verbally abused the staff, whom she accused of not caring for her husband. Plaintively, the doctor's assistant explains that the staff has done everything they can do. He had summoned all his inner reserve to deal with the wife's tantrums.

Turnbull nods and offers a supporting word. "I'll call her," he promises. A few minutes later, he places a call, listens to an obviously perturbed voice on the other end and explains in measured tones the hospital's decision. The conversation ends, but perhaps not the saga. The wife's parting words, according to Turnbull, were "this is not the last you are going to hear from me."

What could happen next, he is asked? "She has already complained to the patients' complaints committee. She could launch legal action. She could complain to the College of Physicians and Surgeons." She has obviously been a pain, but Turnbull evinces some sympathy for his verbal abuser: "She's at the end of her tether with an alcoholic husband. She dreads him coming home. She wants him kept here or somewhere other than at home. It's 70 percent likely that he will be back on the bottle."

Physician assistants, like the man who briefed Turnbull about this patient, are new in health care. They overlap to some extent with nurse practitioners, who spend additional time beyond standard nursing training to be qualified to perform certain tasks previously the sole domain of physicians. Most health-care reformers favour these moves, reckoning that tasks performed by lesser-trained personnel than doctors will save the system money. Greater specialization is the way of modern medicine. There are specialties and subspecialties within nursing; increasing specialties, subspecialties and sub-subspecialties among physicians. It is not therefore axiomatically apparent that this specialization actually saves money, since for every nurse practitioner who does something at a lower cost than a physician, there is a sub-subspecialist doctor doing something technical, demanding and more expensive. Put another way, what appears at first glance like a cheaper system does not necessarily turn out that way.

Turnbull carries an iPad and uses it frequently. When on rounds, however, he is immersed in paper. In this age of computers and digital communication, the hospital is behind the times. Over the next three years, the hospital is supposed to give all staff what Turnbull has. For the moment, clipboards, pens and handwritten charts prevail. Ontario was supposed to have launched a comprehensive e-health system, something every commission, study and report had recommended, but the implementation got botched and mired in scandal. Patient records and internal hospital communications should be entirely electronic, but Canada stands dead last among leading Western countries in the use of electronic records. When it is remarked that newspapers moved fully into the computer age three decades ago, Turnbull smiles, writes on another clipboard and moves on. Things are getting better, he asserts. Undoubtedly they are, but a system that even partly still runs on paper is a system that is obviously very hard to change.

Turnbull darts away from the hospital for a few hours Thursday, as he did Tuesday, to a part of his practice designed to keep people away from the hospital. Not just any people, but the most disadvantaged people in Ottawa, those who would place a heavy burden on already-stressed institutions. Both times, he is joined by Wendy Muckle, the director of Inner City Health, charged with delivering medical care to the homeless, addicted and those afflicted with mental illness—the silent sufferers whom many Canadians banish from their minds. They are everywhere among us but, at best, at the margin of our collective consciousness, except perhaps for the person squatting on a street corner holding out a cap, or someone who taps on our car window.

At 10:30 A.M., Turnbull arrives at the Oaks, a converted hotel used as a hostel for alcoholics. The Oaks has fifty-five rooms, always full. The men and women here have tried to stop drinking. They've passed through treatment centres, been counselled and helped, but theirs is an insidious addiction. As Turnbull enters, fill-up time has started. Perhaps fifteen men and women are lined up for their drinks. Each has an allocated amount of diluted wine, poured from a beer spigot into a measuring cup held by staff, then ladled into their mugs or cups. Some of those in line have walkers, several are in wheelchairs. The amount of their drinking is controlled, but the drinking addiction controls them. Drinks in hand, many go outside to a sitting area for a smoke and a chat. The ritual will be repeated in several hours.

While Turnbull discusses medical cases with the nurses, Muckle, a trained nurse who sometimes works with Turnbull overseas, explains the psychology of alcoholism. "The people here believe, despite all the evidence to the contrary, that alcohol is a good thing," says Muckle. "They understand objectively that this is not a valid belief, but at the end of the day their brains are hard-wired. We've had people who were dying—*dying*—who could not reliably find a bathroom but who could hide a bottle in the ceiling and find it right away. Their brains have an unbelievable wiring for their addiction."

The city has various treatment centres for alcoholics. The Oaks residents have been through them, often many times. The idea of requiring them to abstain, or punishing them for drinking, is folly. "For addictions like this, the only thing that works, or has a chance of working," Muckle says, "are four- or five-year outpatient programs. Running these people through twenty-eight-day programs won't work. Twenty-eight days is not enough time for the receptors in their brains to change."

Some of the residents are pleased to see Turnbull and Muckle. They put an arm around one or the other, banter, offer tidbits about life at the Oaks, recite their health complaints. A trust has evidently developed. That health needs are treated here and at other institutions served by Inner City Health keeps some residents away from hospitals.

"We had a study done a few years ago," Turnbull says, "that showed we saved $3 million just by not having people like this go to emergency rooms, by moving the chronic disease management out of the hospital into the community."

The Oaks is the Ritz hotel for this community. Earlier in the week, Turnbull and Muckle had made the rounds at the Shepherds of Good Hope, the Salvation Army, the Union Mission. Challenges at these institutions are even more complicated than at the Oaks: physical ill health of all kinds, mental health problems, drugs, alcohol, prostitution, homelessness. Here, within sight of the Peace Tower on Parliament Hill, drinking is not always controlled.

Muckle explains what sometimes happens. "The clients go up to Parliament Hill. They get all tanked up on Purell. They go up there when it opens. There are hand-wash dispensers every-where. They drink Purell. Then they come back absolutely tanked on it. They're usually back by nine."

Muckle and Turnbull are mingling now. "How have you been, Wendy?" they ask. "How are you doing?" she replies. Turnbull turns to a man and asks how much he has been drinking. "Understand it was four or five bottles [of wine], then you got into the hard stuff," he says. The man replies, "Six or seven bottles, and then the hard stuff. A couple of twelve-ouncers." Turnbull asks, "Were you drinking Listerine or Purell?" "I didn't like Listerine," the man replies.

Asked about another man with whom she had been conversing, Muckle explains. "He was having about five ounces of wine every hour from seven in the morning until eleven at night ... We get them down to about two bottles a day, which is about a quarter of what they would drink on the street. If we find he's worse in the evening, we'll give him a little more."

The duo moves through the shelters, with Turnbull checking those who need medical help and instructing the nurses. Many of the people have multiple problems that grow from mental illness.

We leave a room where a middle-aged man, once a junior and American Hockey League player, appears in bad shape, unwilling even to rise from bed. He took a lot of "head shots," Muckle says, "and everything came from that."

An Asian man wanders down the corridor. He presented to the hospital without a health card. "Nobody knew where he came from," Muckle explains. "He has very serious health problems. He doesn't speak English. He had no ID, and he needs quite a lot of medication. He's apparently been in Canada for forty years. He's eighty." He occupies one of about two hundred beds in the Salvation Army Shelter. "It's full all the time," Muckle says. "People are sleeping on the floor every night." There are five general shelters in the system, plus two shelters for youth, and one for aboriginals—about nine hundred beds in total. The average cost per person is about $200 a day, "but that's pretty cheap compared with having them in the hospital."

In addition to mental illness and addictions, there is diabetes. Muckle laughs. "We're drowning in diabetes. We lead the wave in diabetes. We are way ahead of the general population, and we have a large aboriginal population that is more susceptible. We have many of our people taking psychiatric medications that make them more susceptible to metabolic disorders, of which diabetes is one."

And AIDS? "The medical success against AIDS never found its way down to the homeless population," Turnbull adds. "So we created a clinic for them. We make sure they take their meds, and we give them the meds. We don't ask them to go up to the hospital." And there is a hospice where the homeless are given palliative care and a half-decent place to die.

"The age-adjusted mortality rate of somebody in the shelter is four to seven times that of the housed population," Turnbull says. "The incidence of hepatitis C in our drug users is 80 percent. So that's an epidemic. A lot of the indices that we see here are those we would expect to see in sub-Saharan Africa."

Jeffrey Turnbull, Wendy Muckle, the nurses and staff of Inner City Health are providing dedicated, indeed saintly, services to those most in distress in Ottawa. They are doing something medicine seldom provides any more: bringing services to patients, rather than making patients come to the service. They are saving the health-care system, and therefore taxpayers, a lot of money. If health care were not provided in this way to these distressed people, more would turn up in emergency wards. This small program, in one Canadian city, illustrates that the more patients can be steered away from acute-care hospitals, the better for them and the hospital. What we might call the dehospitalization of the health-care system is an imperative to provide better care at lower cost.

Another lesson impresses itself on those who visit the shelters. Although many people are in need of health care, and all are in need of help, the formal health-care system, with all its institutions, technologies and skilled personnel, is less likely over the long haul to reduce the incidence of health-related distress than the evolution of a less-unequal society. Illness of any kind can strike at random, and aging cannot be escaped. But every study known to health-care policy agrees that the poor are more likely to burden the health-care system than the rich; that their health-care needs will likely be more frequent and complex; that the costs therefore of caring for these challenges will be greater than for those of the affluent. And every study confirms, too, that despite all the pressures to spend even more money on the health-care system per se, a dollar spent on reducing inequality would do more for that system's sustainability over the long term than another machine, nurse, doctor or hospital bed. Alleviating poverty is complicated, not politically alluring and takes time, whereas the demands for more health care are straightforward, short term, politically powerful and therefore difficult to resist.

Jeffrey Turnbull is ruminating on the last day of the week about the public health-care system that, as head of the Canadian Medical Association, he tried to spark a debate about changing.

"If I were the minister of health, I'd be absolutely terrified," he says. "You have a budget of something like $49 billion. You have a ministry that is the size of a big city. It's a complex field that takes decades to understand. You're there for maybe two years, and then you'll move on. You never really understand it.

"You try to develop a long-term, strategic plan and it goes out the window. You're trying to respond to the issue of the day, and at the same time your finance minister is saying, 'We've got to get control of this beast.' And then you start to make stupid decisions, like cutting immunizations. You can't trust the doctors, you can't trust the nurses, because they have their own interests. So who do you turn to?"

Getting "control of the beast" means, in part, slowing down the rate of cost increases that Turnbull acknowledges are squeezing other government programs. When he criss-crossed Canada as CMA president, seeking to encourage a national dialogue, the sustainability issue of health care "didn't come up." The public, predictably, wanted more services but offered few ideas about how to pay for them.

"Everybody was in favour of expanding the scope of service: pharmacare, long-term care, home care. They frankly don't understand why we don't have them," he recalls. "The money side, they knew, was expensive business, but it was not the problem. The public, I thought, was incredibly bright in many regards, but they did not say we had to bring the costs down or that we are losing so many public services." No politician has told the public the fiscal facts, he acknowledges.

Turnbull, like so many other ardent believers in Canada's system, is convinced that efficiency gains are everywhere apparent but seldom grasped. He cites a 2010 OECD study that suggested Canada could save 2.5 percent of its gross domestic product through efficiency gains, bringing health care as a share of the national economy below 10 percent from just below 12 percent, where it stands now. Turnbull's efficiency dream is shared by many health-care-policy experts, fierce defenders of the existing medicare system, administrators and senior civil servants. It's a dream, alas, that always seems to crash against the realities of the health-care system—and of public administration more generally.

Ontario, like provincial governments across Canada, created regional health authorities, Local Health Integration Networks (LHINs), as part of the efficiency drive. They were supposed to coordinate health care, ration and triage services better and bring acute-care hospitals and community care closer together. No more institutional silos. No more egos getting in the way. LHINs and regional health authorities across Canada were going to bring more rational planning, more efficiencies, improved service at a lower cost. How have these LHINs worked? "We have a LHIN. I'm the chief of staff at the hospital," Turnbull recounts. "I wouldn't even know that there is a LHIN. Nothing has changed in my life. It's not one little bit different." In early 2012, the Ontario government announced that the LHINs would be given more authority, especially over family practitioners. It remains to be seen what kind of authority the LHINs will exercise, and how successful this change will be.

The Ottawa Hospital operates largely within a global budget assigned by the provincial health ministry. The hospital is not paid according to how many patients it processes. Administrators do the best they can, but they have no incentive to make any additional money for their institutions by seeing more patients or selling services to those willing to pay. They operate within a rigid system that forces hospitals to do too much and at too high a cost.

They also operate with a strange model whereby the most expensive and important employees—doctors—are not paid by the hospital or the LHIN but by a faraway government agency. Administrators cannot control the doctors' remuneration and struggle to define their work within the institution. The hybrid system would be akin to trying to run a university if the administration lacked control over the faculty's pay, promotion, tenure or other elements of employment. Or a pharmacy chain in which the owners did not pay the pharmacists who worked for it. The deal struck at the beginning of medicare in Saskatchewan— doctors would be autonomous entrepreneurs within a public system—remains largely in place half a century later. It leads to dysfunctional and inadequate cost control.

Hospitals also face other cost pressures over which they have no control, such as union wage agreements representing two-thirds of the hospital's budget. The Ontario government asked public sector unions to take a zero percent agreement in 2010, given the province's dire fiscal situation. Predictably, the unions refused and provincial arbitrators concurred with them, rejecting the government's inability-to-pay argument. The result for the Ottawa Hospital: a $14 million additional bill. When employees' pay rises faster than revenues, something has to give. This reality, coupled with Ontario's doleful fiscal situation, finally led the McGuinty government to get tough with the doctors, demanding a pay freeze and cutting fees for certain services such as cataract removal and diagnostic imaging, the costs of which have gone down.

Tentatively, Ontario is moving to a system already adopted all over the world (and in British Columbia), a system Turnbull endorses, whereby money for hospitals follows patients. The more procedures and patients, the more money the hospital receives. "Every patient who now comes through the door represents X number of dollars," he says. "We should start to think differently about every patient. The patient should be a revenue source, not a cost." Incentives, however, are hard to find within the top-down bureaucratic model that Canada adopted from Britain's National Health Service half a century ago. Britain has moved decisively away from the old NHS model in recent decades, with improved results in reducing wait times. Canada remains wedded to it. But beware of simple solutions. A money-following-the-patient model might be more expensive, because more patients would be seen, assuming no other changes were made in hospital procedures. Without the right rules, hospitals might cherry-pick patients who bring in the most money, not necessarily those in most need.

Turnbull despairs. "The health-care system is slipping away in front of us. I really believe that." He has devoted his entire career to public medicine, as practitioner, administrator, inner-city physician and head of the CMA. His passion cannot mask sorrow and alarm: "People have come to expect mediocrity in some aspects of medical care because they don't pay for it. People wouldn't put up with mediocrity if they were paying for it."

He puts a human face on the system. "You're a business guy. You live a busy life. You've got a knee problem. You finally get to see the specialist, and that has taken many months. He says you need an MRI. That can take up to three months in Ottawa. So you wait six months to see the specialist. You wait three more months to get the MRI. Then the specialist says he's putting you on the list for surgery. And now the twenty-six-week wait starts. There's a huge economic cost, and there's a huge personal cost."

Turnbull is not exaggerating. The provincial average wait for an MRI is 98 days, but in eastern Ontario's Champlain Health Authority LHIN the wait can extend to 213 days; for CT scans, the provincial average is 38 days, but in the Champlain LHIN it is 53; cancer surgery's provincial standard is 60 days, but in the Champlain LHIN it is 70 days. In Ottawa, the LHIN meets the provincial target of 14 days for radiation to start only 48 percent of the time, and chemotherapy 49 percent. These delays are unacceptable by any reasonable standard, and illustrate why Canada's wait times are the longest, according to the OECD.

The health-care system's costs keep rising. So do government contributions, but there still never seems to be enough money. "We are budgeted for 92.5 percent occupancy in the hospital," Turnbull says. "Every patient over that is looked on as a cost. To close the gap, we try for efficiencies. We scrimp and we save, close beds, postpone operations, close in the summer … It's a game of chicken. Do you hold the public hostage? Who's going to blink first?"

As for R, the ninety-four-year-old patient who appeared on Turnbull's chart Monday morning, Turnbull predicted what would happen when he first glanced at the first line of the man's chart. R had indeed been moved to the APU, awaiting placement unit, because no place in the health-care system outside the hospital could be found. He remained there for twenty-five days. The total cost to the hospital for his care: $20,318, plus perhaps $3000 or $4000 that doctors billed for their services treating R.

PART TWO

TWO

Health Care's Early History

The Ottawa Hospital, and all others across Canada, can date their origin to March 3, 1665, when seventeen men and their families in what is now Montreal signed a contract with a master surgeon. The contract obliged the master surgeons (another had joined the first) to "well and truly service the hospital of Ville-Marie, to treat, dress, and physic all the sick persons who may be there, and this for periods of three months each in turn and to visit such sick persons assiduously at about seven o'clock each morning and at such other hours as may be necessary." Thus was born the hospital physician's early-morning rounds of the kind Dr. Jeffrey Turnbull does at the Ottawa Hospital, and a contractual commitment, doctor to patient, to treat the sick for an agreed-on prepayment negotiated in advance, an insurance policy, if you like.

Medical personnel tend to be status conscious. In 1710, barber-surgeons and surgeon-apothecaries persuaded the colonial governor to forbid practice by anyone not already established in New France—an early closed shop. The edict was never enforced. Forty years later, however, formal mechanisms were created to evaluate credentials and expertise, to prevent "evil" from "strangers whose ability is unknown."

The British, after assuming control of New France in 1759, had scant regard for these French barber-surgeons and

surgeon-apothecaries. They authorized British-trained practitioners to form a licensing board. Anything remotely like an
organized profession with serious certifying boards lay far in the
future. Until well past the halfway mark of the nineteenth century,
health-care delivery remained rudimentary. Doctors worked
without serious licensing bodies in an atmosphere of generalized
skepticism about formal medicine.

The Canadian Medical Association was created in 1867. It
devised a code of ethics, and groups of doctors won the right in
self-governing colleges to discipline members for "infamous or
disgraceful conduct in a professional respect." Self-policing was
intended to prevent doctors from advertising successful cases
in the newspapers, guaranteeing cures and generally bragging
about themselves—limitations that remain today. By the end of the
nineteenth century, doctors in most provinces had won, or would
soon win, the profession's right to self-government. An early
attempt by populists in Ontario for the province to set doctors'
fees was defeated—a harbinger of fights over fee schedules and
other methods of paying physicians that continue to this day.

Doctors considered nurses to be second-class medical
practitioners. Doctors' spokesmen decried nurses who make "ill-
directed excursions beyond their proper latitude." The jostling
between doctors and nurses about their respective capabilities
and responsibilities began early and has not completely stopped.

That Germany under Chancellor Otto von Bismarck became
the first industrialized country, in 1883, to adopt health insurance meant little to Canadians. The German scheme, politically
designed to lure the working class from socialist politics (the
conservative Bismarck called it a "bribe to the working class"),
was organized as a compulsory contribution from both workers
and employees to an insurance fund. Prepaid social insurance
remains the foundation of today's German health-care system,

one of the best in the world, although it takes a slightly larger share of the national economy than Canada's, while providing a wider range of services. Social insurance exists in various European countries whose health-care systems compare very favourably with Canada's.

Britain, Canada's point of comparison, took until 1911 to act. Various working men's societies, lodges of skilled workers and municipalities had been hiring general practitioners on contract. Doctors worked for a salary with the group that hired them, a practice that specialists disliked because they preferred (and still do in Canada) to be paid for each procedure. The British government, trying to expand and bring coherence to this hodgepodge, proposed a national sickness-insurance plan. Doctors were divided. Some saw higher salaries, others feared government interference in their practice. The British Medical Association adopted a formal position against national sickness insurance, but it came into force in 1912 anyway, covering 15 million wage earners, with a fillip to the doctors when the government increased their stipend.

More doctors then joined the scheme, and most enjoyed higher incomes than before its introduction (which is what happened decades later in Canada after the introduction of medicare). The Canadian Medical Association, however, was unimpressed. Its president declared in 1913, "The future outlook of Canadian medicine demands a strong association to confront legislation that would make us a despised arm of the civil service." For the next seven decades, the fear that doctors would become glorified civil servants defined the public position of the Canadian medical profession.

As in Britain, clumps of Canadian workers banded together to insure themselves. In 1883, Glace Bay miners in Nova Scotia agreed to deductions from their pay in exchange for insurance against doctors' costs and hospitalization charges. The deductions were compulsory and were paid to the hospital and doctor of the employee's choice. Similar arrangements followed in mining and lumbering towns such as Timmins, in Ontario, and Port Alberni and Trail, in British Columbia. None involved government. They were voluntary schemes and highly localized. They left out the majority of the Canadian population, who paid for health care as best they could, relied on charity or used the services of municipal hospitals financed to serve the "sick poor."

The First World War changed thinking. It did not escape the attention of recruiters that so many would-be soldiers were turned down because of ill health or ailments. In British Columbia, for example, more than 8500 "able-bodied" men were considered unfit for military duty. Those who served abroad experienced better medical care than anything available at home. On returning, at least some of them wondered why such care did not exist in Canada. The fear of big government seemed absurd to those who had fought in the war and, in too many cases, had had to rely on government medical services.

Political and social movements channelled the sacrifices of the war and the yearning for a better postwar society into agendas for reform, including health care. Some of these movements took their cause to the streets. The Winnipeg General Strike of 1919 spawned smaller sympathy strikes in other cities. New political parties arose, such as the Independent Labour Party in Ontario, which elected twelve members in 1917. United Farmers parties grew in Ontario and Alberta; Progressives took root in Manitoba.

The federal Liberals in 1919 elected Mackenzie King as their leader, a man who considered himself an expert on social policy and something of a reformer, a self-appraisal that always clashed with his innate political caution. He told delegates that he favoured a national sickness plan, the start of three decades of rhetorical commitments never backed by sustained action. As he was not one for direct commitments when indirect ones would suffice, King's promise contained four qualifications—timing, finance, scope and federal–provincial relations. These qualifications shaped subsequent debates about health care.

Commissions were struck to study reform possibilities, the first in British Columbia in 1919. Since that initial B.C. study, health care has spawned more Royal Commissions, commissions, legislative committee reports and studies than any other public-policy issue in Canada. No decade since has been without at least one public examination—and in some decades, several. Commissions on health care have provided employment for many and controversy for all.

The B.C. commission sprang from the memory of the war. The leader of the Soldier Party in the legislature (there was such a party) introduced a motion favouring the principle of compulsory state health insurance. He was supported by Labour Party members, and a dissident Liberal, Major J.W. McIntosh, a physician, a war veteran, a former president of the Vancouver Medical Association and a forceful advocate for public health insurance. Pressure on the government came from labour unions, church groups and, perhaps most important, veterans' groups.

The commission spent two years pondering the situation and proposed a very modest health-insurance scheme, but the general public seemed apathetic and the medical profession largely hostile. When presented with the report, the B.C. government opted for what would become a familiar strategy: it punted the issue to the federal government. Ottawa, read a resolution of the B.C. legislature in 1922, should "give early consideration to legislation providing for an adequate system of insurance against sickness." It took four and a half decades for Ottawa to do just that.

To B.C. should go the honour of being the first Canadian province where something at least approximating a serious debate about public health care occurred, although today most Canadians would likely think that distinction belongs to Saskatchewan, the province with the first universal health-care system.

A watered-down version of the commission's original scheme made it to the legislature, supported by unions, women's and church groups, left-wing Liberals and the Co-operative Commonwealth Federation (CCF, the western coalition of progressive, labour and socialist interests that was the precursor of the New Democratic Party), but opposed by boards of trade, chambers of commerce and doctors. This division of forces would mark many subsequent debates about health care. A bill passed, by twenty-five votes to fourteen, but the battle resumed outside the legislature. The cash-strapped government had withdrawn coverage for the unemployed and pensioners in the watered-down bill. Doctors, fearing for their incomes, cast themselves as defenders of the excluded, while wanting higher fees for treating the poor. The B.C. Medical Association got so worked up that it described the bill as the "first step to suicide" for the profession. Doctors paid for rallies, dinners and radio broadcasts lambasting the scheme—a foretaste of future strategies by doctors fighting state-run health care—and the government relented. In the 1937 election, voters were asked in a plebiscite if they were "in favour of a comprehensive Health Insurance Plan, progressively applied." Fifty-nine percent answered yes, to which the government responded that health care needed federal leadership and cash, neither of which were forthcoming. Mackenzie King was back in power in Ottawa, and he was in no hurry to do anything. Thus ended B.C.'s effort.

British Columbia was not alone in groping toward some form of extended, if not extensive, public health care. The Depression laid waste to the incomes of many doctors, especially those in rural areas. Municipalities were often desperate, unable to support their hospitals. In rural Saskatchewan, some doctors were themselves in the relief queues. Payments to them were given in kind rather than cash. A survey of doctors in Hamilton, Ontario, in 1932 found half their patients were not paying, and half the doctors complained that they could not provide for their families. A survey of New Brunswick doctors revealed the same results. A merry-go-round of pleas and accusations ensued: doctors pleaded with municipalities for help, municipalities turned to provincial governments, provinces insisted that only Ottawa had enough money, Ottawa declared that health care was a provincial responsibility. When a delegation of doctors went to see Conservative Prime Minister R.B. Bennett, he expressed concern but said, "The matters you have presented are strictly the business of the provinces."

Winnipeg doctors, three decades before the 1962 doctors' strike in Saskatchewan, found their incomes plummeting by 40 to 60 percent. In the face of doctors' complaints, the Manitoba legislature requested a study by a committee, which recommended that most Canadian of solutions—a Royal Commission! The recommendation was never acted on.

Winnipeg doctors became increasingly angry, even desperate. They formed political action committees and their own study group urging the government to pay them half the profession's normal rates for seeing those who could not pay. Having threatened to withdraw services if some payments from government were not forthcoming, the doctors made good on their threat, so about fifty thousand citizens on relief were without the services of Winnipeg's doctors. A somewhat bizarre political marriage ensued. The unemployed and the doctors marched together in the streets, with police intervening in one case with tear gas. Finally, the city council capitulated and agreed to the doctors' demands that a special fund be established to pay them for treating the indigent, at rates well below the doctors' normal ones. Even the lower rates for what became known as the Greater Winnipeg Medical Relief Plan proved too much for the council, because after one year the council was demanding still-lower rates for the doctors. At least the doctors were receiving some payment, which was better than nothing.

The enthusiasm that doctors showed in Winnipeg during the strike, and elsewhere, for limited government payment for health care reflected the stresses of the Depression. When better economic times returned, doctors remained happy that governments paid them for treating the poor. The rest of the population's health care, they argued, should remain in the hands of private insurance companies, doctors' own insurance plans or individual patients.

The farther east one moved across Canada in the 1920s and '30s, the less interest governments and citizens seemed to show for full-scale public health care. There were scattered voluntary insurance schemes, public health programs and some public money for hospital construction, but nothing more. The deeply traditionalist political cultures of the Maritimes kept public health care off the agenda, as it remained in Ontario. In Quebec, where the Catholic Church ran social policy, including hospitals, governments remained completely uninterested. On the prairies, where the Depression struck with particular force and where political cultures were less encumbered by tradition, the movement toward some form of extended public health care developed, albeit haltingly.

In 1932, the Alberta legislature authorized a study of health care. It had taken the United Farmers of Alberta eleven years following its election in 1921 to get to this point, caught as the UFA was between its desire to use government for the public good and its desire to keep expenditures and public debt at the lowest levels possible. The appointed commission declared that "adequate medical services will never be available to all people of Alberta until income earners, through a system of compulsory contributions contribute a monthly sum sufficient to provide adequate medical services to all the people of the province." Compulsory contributions from all the people for health care for all the people. That concept went beyond what had been proposed in British Columbia, where a mixed voluntary/ compulsory scheme had been advanced. In 1935, therefore, the United Farmers of Alberta government proudly passed the Act Respecting Health Insurance. It was a groundbreaking scheme from a government on its political deathbed. Had the UFA government survived the 1935 election, its scheme might have set the example for other provinces, thereby propelling Canada down another path to a form of public health care.

The scheme was ingenious. It would have been an interesting mix of decentralization and centralization and, as such, previewed some of what came much later in other public health plans. A government-appointed commission would have run the scheme (centralization) based on per capita payments by municipalities and provinces, and contributions (a kind of health premium) from employers and employees (decentralization). Citizens would have paid the per capita premium to their municipality—$2.11 of the $11.28 that municipalities had to pay the commission. This payment was toward a service rendered—a dedicated tax of the sort that exists in some provinces today but remains deeply controversial wherever it is applied.

Albertans would have received from this UFA scheme all

necessary hospital, medical, nursing, dental, diagnostic services and drugs. It would have been a comprehensive plan, including a large public-health program for babies and children, vaccinations and physical examinations, something public-health advocates are still striving for today. Social Credit, the party elected in 1935, had other ideas, most of them startlingly crazy, about combating the Depression by printing more money and exhorting everyone to become more Christian as an antidote to public misery. Public health care was not for them.

In Saskatchewan, doctors were battered by the Depression. Their tumbling incomes turned them into enthusiasts for state-sponsored health care for the poor, from whom doctors could not otherwise get payment. Many doctors were receiving government assistance to carry on their practices. Some communities hired doctors on salary; some municipal hospitals paid them. There were a few municipal health-insurance plans, but the Saskatchewan government was broke. As long as Ottawa remained impervious to pleas for help, little could be done by the provincial government acting alone. All that would change in 1943 when the CCF arrived in office in Regina.

The CCF, an avowedly socialist party in its infancy, grew up in the 1930s, the political manifestation of left-wing groups agitating to change the capitalist system that in their opinion had so evidently failed during the Depression. Perhaps the most prominent of these institutions was the League for Social Reconstruction, a group of intellectuals who advocated socialist reforms of the Canadian state. The league's seminal document, *Social Planning for Canada*, remained for many years a basis for subsequent shadings of socialist thought.

Social Planning for Canada demanded, among other reforms,

a "completely socialized health services under the control and direction of the provincial governments." All services would be publicly financed and organized, including pharmaceuticals and dentistry. It did not matter to the league whether funding came from general taxation or employers' contributions, since under a socialist system, employers "would in many cases come to be the State." Surprisingly, the socialist group favoured some measure of private medicine, because "doctors should not be confined to practice under the plan of state medicine, but should be allowed to do private practice outside of it, for those persons who demand more attention than the state scheme authorizes." To use the league's own word, *socialist*, today's Canadian medicare is therefore a more socialist plan than the league's proposal, since no doctor today can work outside the public plan and be paid by the plan, or charge more than the fee schedule negotiated with a provincial government. What the socialists of the 1930s countenanced is today verboten, even by most free-enterprise politicians.

Other groups pushed a similar health-care message, including the Montreal Group for the Security of the People's Health, one of whose key founders was Norman Bethune, perhaps best known to Canadians as the doctor who worked for the Republicans in the Spanish Civil War and for the Communist Chinese during their revolution. He wrote to the CCF leader, J.S. Woodsworth, about the Montreal Group, describing it as comprising "communists, CCFers, and humanitarians of no political hue but of progressive views." His position as chief of the tuberculosis unit at Sacré-Coeur hospital gave him a pulpit from which he preached against private medicine and for public health care. In a 1936 speech, Bethune declared, "The people are ready for socialized medicine. The obstructionists to the people's health security lie within the profession itself. Recognize this fact. It is the all-important fact of the situation. These men with the mocking face of the reactionary ... proclaim their principles under the guise of 'maintenance of the sacred relationship between the doctor and patient'... These are the enemies of the people and make no mistake. They are the enemies of medicine too."

Legendary as Bethune was to become, largely for his work overseas, neither Quebec nor other Canadian doctors heeded his call, nor indeed did many Canadians. Quebeckers in particular seemed immune from socialized medicine, since the mere mention of "socialism" sent the Catholic Church into rhetorical overdrive against secularism, statism and anti-spirituality, much more powerful messages for francophone Quebeckers than anything Bethune and his ilk offered.

With all this intellectual action on the left, and the Liberal government of Mackenzie King making noises about doing something, the details of which were never very clear, the opposition Progressive Conservative Party in Ottawa figured that it should at least be seen as studying the health-care issue. Their new leader, John Bracken, had been Manitoba premier during the Winnipeg doctors' strike. He thought of himself as something of a reformer, even insisting that the word *Progressive* be affixed to *Conservative* as part of his price for becoming leader in 1942. Bracken therefore asked Charlotte Whitton, a woman far ahead of her time in many respects and later a colourful mayor of Ottawa, to look into public health care on behalf of the Progressive Conservatives. Whitton had been a professor at Queen's University during the First World War and a member of the Canadian Council on Social Development, where she campaigned for the care of juvenile immigrants and neglected children. In 1943, she duly produced not a memo but a book, *The Dawn of an Ampler Life*, that went far beyond anything Bracken's party would accept, and beyond the thinking of most social activists in the country.

She had read Britain's 1942 Beveridge Report, a seminal document by Lord Beveridge, a Liberal peer, on social insurance that became the framework for the British Labour Party's social policies after it took office in 1945. She was also familiar with two national reports in Canada that advised public health-insurance systems financed by employee contributions. That kind of system, in those days, would have been considered cutting-edge policy, but Whitton went further. She recommended what would emerge decades later, a health-care model—a "social utility" she called it—administered and financed by general revenues, not employee contributions. She suggested that health care be financed through taxation because she did not think it should be tied to employment. Would this be "state or socialized medicine?" she was asked. Yes, both, she defiantly responded. A publicly funded system, she argued, was "inevitable in health care in Canada." She anticipated the essence of financing to come, with one exception. She wanted a board, chaired by a federal minister with representatives from the provinces, municipalities, medical professionals and not-for-profit groups, to recommend each year how much money should be transferred from Ottawa to the provinces for social services, including health care. That idea, wonderful in theory, could never survive the endemic tensions between Ottawa, the paymaster, and provinces that delivered health care. But the essence of her idea—payments by Ottawa to the provinces—became part of the fabric of Canadian postwar hospital and health-care arrangements. *The Dawn of an Ampler Life* was supposed to provide guidance to the Progressive Conservatives. It did not; for at least another two decades, the party remained closely aligned with the doctors' view of how to provide health care.

Just as the First World War had provided an impetus for some who sought a fairer society, so the Second World War produced fresh thinking about reordering a fairer postwar society. Whereas government had seemed helpless during the Depression, it mobilized a massive national effort to prosecute the war. The state, having expanded enormously to combat perils abroad, could be mobilized to tackle injustices at home. The vision of an activist state was central to the trade union movement, whose political party, the CCF, rose to almost 30 percent in mid-war public-opinion polls. In Ontario in 1943, the CCF jumped from zero to thirty-four of ninety legislative seats; in 1943, the CCF formed the government in Saskatchewan. Union membership doubled during the war.

Even a few doctors caught the direction of the wind. In 1942, a former president of the Canadian Medical Association declared that opponents of state health insurance were as those "who opposed prison reform, asylum reform, emancipation of slaves and other greater movements." The president of the Winnipeg Medical Society, a city where doctors had gone on strike ten years before, asserted that "the socialization of medicine is coming as surely as tomorrow's dawn. It is the natural result of public demand for adequate, complete medical service." These medical voices favouring full-scale public health care remained in a minority. Most doctors wanted state medicine only for the poor.

The CCF favoured what its health planning committee called "a state medical service" financed through general taxation without premiums or other contributory mechanisms. All doctors would eventually be on salary, although at the outset general practitioners could supplement their salaries with fees for services rendered. The CCF also envisaged a Canada-wide network of community health centres. Apart from the idea of putting all doctors on salary, the CCF's vision would eventually prevail over all the others.

Faced with agitation from reform-minded groups and the rise of the CCF, Mackenzie King did what came naturally: he delayed while appearing to move. In what was by then a pattern, he created another Royal Commission, the Rowell-Sirois commission, to study federal–provincial relations, especially fiscal relations. A lengthy tome eventually emerged, but the section on health care was scant. The commission recognized that Ottawa could collect premiums from employers for health care but thought health insurance was really a provincial matter, a position that suited King. He was more preoccupied with prosecuting the war and worrying about the state of the nation's finances than launching a bold new social policy.

King fretted about what a health scheme might cost. He also feared strident opposition to anything like a "state medical service" from large provinces such as Quebec and Ontario. King therefore sought something that could be afforded and made acceptable to as many provinces as possible. He offered proposals far short of what the CCF, social activists, labour and farm groups and a few more reform-minded Liberals had wanted—health grants from Ottawa for particular problems such as mental health, venereal disease and crippling childhood illnesses; financial assistance in hospital construction; and a modest federal subsidy for provincial health insurance. Saskatchewan under the CCF wanted more, of course, but was happy with the offer. So was Manitoba. British Columbia and Alberta were lukewarm; the other provinces were opposed.

Some of the modest momentum for state-sponsored health care had been lost because doctors had stepped partially into the role of insurance providers. During the Depression, and before, doctors had wanted the state to insure the poor, and for private insurance or citizens themselves to pay for the rest of the population. When federal–provincial negotiations went only a small way toward public health care, the doctors began to reckon that perhaps they could forestall any future movement, make friends with the voters and fill a genuine need. Across the country there sprang up doctor-administered and -owned insurance plans that in the beginning covered only a small minority of Canadians. More and more citizens joined these plans (later linked together in seven provinces into the Trans-Canada Medical Plans). When these doctors' plans were coupled with those offered by private insurers like Blue Cross, it suggested to doctors, many citizens and provincial governments such as those in Ontario and Alberta that a combination of private insurance, doctor-administered insurance and a government-subsidized plan for the poor might provide the kind of widespread health coverage that citizens seemed to want—without the cost to the treasury and loss of professional freedom that doctors feared from state health care.

In 1949, a Gallup poll asked Canadians if they would approve of a national health plan with a flat monthly payment (a kind of insurance plan rather than a tax-financed one) in exchange for medical and hospital care. Eighty percent said yes. It was against this yet-unfocused preference for public health care that the medical profession focused its efforts, money and considerable political clout. As one CMA president told his comrades, "Socialized Medicine means a crushing burden on the taxpayer. Socialized Medicine meant an inferior medical service, staffed ... by inferior men. Socialized Medicine is the first step and a long step towards the Gehenna of the Welfare State" (*Gehenna* being an Old Testament term for hell).

Nationally, in the immediate postwar period, it appeared that the Gehenna of public health care had been postponed, if not indefinitely then for a long time. The biggest provinces seemed more or less contented with the private/doctors' insurance model, as were the doctors, while the smallest provinces lacked the financial wherewithal to consider anything remotely ambitious. The federal Liberals were focusing on hospital construction and subsidies that fell far short of comprehensive health care. As long as Mackenzie King prevailed, caution would trump action. Shrinking the state after its enormous wartime expansion seemed sensible policy to many voters.

But for one poor province, flattened as no other by the Depression, willing to take a political chance on a form of agrarian socialism, there might never have been the model for what became Canadian medicare. The project was born in Saskatchewan amid intense controversy, a doctors' strike and fierce ideological struggle. We think today that medicare quickly triumphed in Saskatchewan, whereas, in fact, its realization was protracted and, toward the end of the drama, a near-run thing.

THREE

Medicare in Saskatchewan

O n July 23, 1962, representatives of the CCF government of Saskatchewan and the Saskatchewan College of Physicians and Surgeons signed what became known as the Saskatoon Agreement. The agreement allowed doctors to save face, but little else. The concessions that the doctors won were immaterial and did not long survive in practice; the defeat they suffered would later be repeated across Canada. Ten years later, doctors everywhere in Canada became part of national medicare modelled on the scheme that emerged in Saskatchewan. Public health care became law in Saskatchewan after a fractious non-violent twenty-three-day doctors' strike, something almost unimaginable from a profession dedicated to healing. If the doctors had prevailed in their Saskatchewan struggle — and many of them believed that they would — Canada's health-care history would have been written quite differently.

Saskatchewan provided the first crucible for complete public health care in North America. Until the CCF won election in Saskatchewan in 1944, no government had been fully committed to public health care. Tommy Douglas, the CCF premier, under-scored his party's commitment by also becoming minister of public health, having pledged in the campaign to make medical, dental and hospital services "available to all without counting the ability of the individual to pay."

Eighteen years passed between the CCF's first election and the realization of provincial medicare. The party's heart was always willing; the province's revenues were not. Serious but incremental steps toward the ultimate objective were all that Saskatchewan had been able to afford. In a province where every farmer's nightmares included going deeply into debt, a political culture developed, to which the CCF completely subscribed, that the provincial government should avoid debt too. From 1945–46 to 1961–62, the Douglas governments presented only one deficit budget. This fiscal prudence was assisted, it must be said, by assorted federal transfers that covered 30 to 36 percent of the provincial budget.

Ideas need a personal spark and fertile ground to spring to life. Tommy Douglas provided the spark, Saskatchewan the fertile ground—fertile in a manner of speaking, because the Great Depression had dried out the land, bankrupted many farmers and thrust people together to defend their interests as best they could. Confronted with the political order in Ottawa and Regina, the mercenary railways, grain companies, farm-implement manufacturers and banks, the evil caprices of the weather and modest means if not spirit, residents wondered about fundamental political change. What did Saskatchewan have to lose, after all its torments?

A Liberal Party political machine had governed for a long time (from 1905 to 1944, except for one five-year period), dispensing patronage, presiding over the pre-Depression growth of the province, identifying itself with the glorious future that always seemed just over Saskatchewan's horizon. When the Depression struck, the provincial Liberals were at sea, as were governments everywhere. They knew how to govern, for they had been in power a long time; they just did not know what to do. In 1937, relief spending exceeded combined provincial and municipal spending on other matters by 63 percent.

In the Regina Manifesto of 1933, the birth cry of the CCF, a brief section had put the case for public health care. It was one of the few parts of the manifesto that eventually became, almost intact, the law of Canada: "The maintenance of a healthy population has become a function for which every civilized community should undertake responsibility. Health services should be made at least as available as are educational services today. But under a system which is still mainly one of private enterprise, the costs of proper medical care, such as the wealthier members of society can easily afford, are at present prohibitive for great masses of people. A properly organized system of public health services including medical and dental care, which would stress the prevention rather than the cure of illness, should be extended to all people."

A fledgling network of public health-care institutions had grown up before the CCF took power. Parallel to the co-operative movement in the economy was an initiative by people in rural municipalities who agreed to tax themselves to pay a salaried doctor to provide medical services. These municipal schemes began in 1914 and spread across rural Saskatchewan. Municipal hospital plans came later. Municipalities, fearful that tuberculosis might break out indiscriminately in one or more of them, pooled resources to buy insurance. The provincial government created a Cancer Commission with nominal costs to patients and a roster of surgeons whose services would be paid for by the commission. The CCF built on these pre-existing foundations.

Tommy Douglas had contracted chronic osteomyelitis in his leg as a child in Scotland. He was in and out of hospital for three years. "My father was an iron molder and we had no money for doctors," he later recounted. "After we emigrated to Canada, the pain in my knee came back. Mother took me to the outdoor clinic of a Winnipeg hospital. They put me in the public ward as a charity patient and I still remember the young house doctor saying that my leg must be cut off.

"But I was lucky. A brilliant orthopaedic surgeon, whose name was Smith, came through the ward looking for patients he could use in teaching demonstrations. He examined my swollen knee and then went to see my parents. 'If you'll let me use your boy to help teach medical students,' he said, 'I think I can save his leg. His knee may never be strong again but it can be saved.' I shall always be grateful to the medical profession for the skill that kept me from becoming a cripple, but the experience of being a patient remains with me.

"Had I been a rich man's son, the services of the finest surgeons would have been available. As an iron molder's boy, I almost had my leg amputated before chance intervened and a specialist cured me without thought of a fee."

Douglas reflected later that "I made a pledge with myself long before I ever sat in this House, in the years when I knew something about what it meant to get health services when you didn't have the money to pay for it. I made a pledge with myself that someday, if I ever had anything to do with it, people would be able to get health services just as they are able to get educational services, as an inalienable right of being a citizen of a Christian country."

Tommy Douglas grew up amid the industrial turbulence of Glasgow in the early twentieth century, where he heard the incandescent oratory of the union leaders associated with the nascent

Scottish Labour Party. When his family emigrated, they landed in Winnipeg during the General Strike of 1919. There, he listened to the fiery speeches of labour leaders and Social Gospel adherents such as J.S. Woodsworth. Douglas's working-class parents insisted that he pursue higher education. He went to Brandon College, associated with the Baptist Church, where he won gold medals in oratory and debating and became head of the student body in his final year. He had done some supply preaching at the Baptist church in Weyburn, Saskatchewan. When his studies ended, the congregation invited Douglas to be their minister, which he became in 1930 at the age of twenty-five.

Religion inspired Douglas; political activity attracted him. He got involved in social movements in and around Weyburn soon after his arrival. He organized the unemployed into the Weyburn Labour Association, addressed the United Farmers of Saskatchewan, toured farm districts and kept in touch with Labour MPs, as they then were known nationally and in Saskatchewan. In 1934, Douglas ran for the CCF in Weyburn, finishing third but getting back his deposit. He had learned a few tricks in the campaign, one being that dry explanations of policy sold less well than narratives about himself, friends and neighbours, especially if the stories were peppered with wit.

Douglas told himself after the defeat that politics could wait. He wanted to do a Ph.D., and an offer came from a parish in Milwaukee, the acceptance of which would allow him to do his academic work in Chicago. As the 1935 federal election approached, however, friends and supporters pressed Douglas to run again. He rebuffed them, until a senior Baptist official suggested that if he did ever run again, that would be the end of his ministry in the church. He chose politics over the church, then and there, and never looked back, winning the Weyburn seat. He would be in and around electoral politics provincially and nationally for another forty-seven years, usually elected, occasionally defeated. When the Canadian Broadcasting Corporation in 2004 asked viewers to vote for "The Greatest Canadian," the largest number of respondents supported Tommy Douglas, champion of medicare, the Canadian icon.

Douglas, as premier and health minister after the CCF took power in 1944, began almost immediately the step-by-step policies that led to the final implementation of medicare eighteen years later, over the objections of striking Saskatchewan doctors. The Cancer Commission's mandate and budget were expanded. Complete hospital and medical care was extended to the province's twenty-nine thousand pensioners and spouses. Four mental-health clinics were established. On January 1, 1949, the Douglas government became the first one in North America to introduce complete public coverage for all hospital services, the first seeds of a health-care system centred on hospitals.

Tommy Douglas struggled, as responsible leaders always do, with how to finance his dream. He governed one of Canada's least affluent provinces (in those days), and during his years in power the provincial budget swelled by a factor of five. He was committed to balanced budgets but expansive government. Federal transfers greatly aided squaring this circle, but even these transfers were insufficient. He needed something more than government taxation revenues; he needed contributions from individuals for certain services. Moreover, as he said, individuals receiving a public service should be reminded through a payment for that service that the service was not "free."

From the beginning, therefore, the CCF implemented what we would call "user fees" for hospital admissions and premiums to pay for health services, although premiums were sometimes called a per capita health tax. For the Hospital Services Plan, each person or family head had to pay an annual insurance premium: $5 a person to a maximum family cost of $30. These could later be credited against federal income tax. The money from these premiums, or health taxes, covered about half the cost of the hospital insurance plan, general tax revenues the rest. Much later, when Ottawa committed itself to paying half the costs under a national reimbursement scheme, the share of total Saskatchewan health-care costs derived from premiums fell to 37 percent. Premiums, however, remained so central to financing the public scheme that the Douglas government raised them three times for families, with even larger increases for individuals.

Today, the imposition or increase of health-care premiums is guaranteed to wound politically any provincial government. Premiums are seen by the unreconstructed defenders of medicare as socially unjust. They are also seen as offensive to a medicare model that produces a redistribution of income from better-off to poorer Canadians, since the better-off provide through the personal income tax system a greater share of the revenues for public health care than the costs they impose on it for their own care.

Today, the NDP, labour unions and others on what we might call the political left ferociously oppose premiums or personal payments for essential medical services. Tommy Douglas is their patron saint. But, as happens with many saints, one of his important teachings has been overlooked—that citizens should pay for at least some of their health-care needs directly or through a dedicated tax. The CCF did not impose premiums only for hospital care, it required payments for physicians' services and hospital visits: $12 for individuals, $24 for families; $1.50 per visit and $12.50 per day for a hospital stay. An NDP government in Saskatchewan subsequently eliminated both premiums and payments.

Tommy Douglas, born in Scotland, looked to Britain for intellectual inspiration. The United States in the 1940s had a private system without today's government programs for seniors and the poor and, as such, represented what Canadian health-care reformers disliked. They sought a state-run and -financed system; the United States had neither. They wanted doctors to contract their services with the state, or to become employees of the state, whereas U.S. doctors worked for themselves. Canadian public health-care advocates wanted an end to private insurance; U.S. doctors wanted more of it.

Douglas and other health-care reformers were inspired by the United Kingdom's Beveridge Report of 1942, which galvanized those in Canada who sought a postwar welfare state, including socialized health care.

Beveridge proposed a safety net of social insurance to provide a minimum standard of living for all citizens. The plan would include pensions, unemployment insurance and social security and involve "medical treatment covering all requirements ... provided for all citizens by a national health service organization under the health departments, and post-medical treatment will be provided for all persons capable of profiting by it." Beveridge declared that "restoration of a sick person to health is a duty of the State and the sick person, prior to any other consideration."

The state, he said, should provide a minimum of service, including health care, but individuals could go beyond that minimum, an idea rejected by Canadian reformers then and now. "The State," wrote Beveridge, "should offer security for service and contribution. The State in organizing security should not stifle incentive, opportunity, responsibility; in establishing a national minimum, it should leave room and encouragement for voluntary action by each individual to provide more than that minimum for himself and his family."

The Beveridge Report became the foundation, intellectually and politically, of the British welfare state and the subsequent Canadian one. Forgotten, or rejected, was his suggestion that individuals should be encouraged to add their own money to basic health benefits. The idea of minimum of coverage for all, supplemented by additional coverage for some, has been overtaken by the assumption of maximum coverage for all.

Beveridge made no recommendations about the role and payment of doctors. He did insist—and this position might have influenced Douglas's view of premiums—that his social-security scheme be financed on the insurance model, with individual contributions defraying some of the costs. Beveridge said, in words that would inspire Douglas and many others, "From the standpoint of social security, a health service providing full preventive and curative treatment of every kind, to every citizen without exceptions, with remuneration limit and without an economic barrier at any point to delay recourse to it, is the ideal plan."

Saskatchewan's doctors offered limited support for "socialized medicine," as critics called it. During the Depression, they were being paid in kind, or far less than their normal fees, or not at all. Therefore, any government plan for the poor would help the doctors, since they could be guaranteed at least some payment from those who could not afford treatment. Doctors therefore supported limited public health care and eagerly signed on when the Douglas government, as one of its first acts, proposed health care for the poor. As the government extended public coverage to other health-care services, tensions and suspicions grew among doctors that the CCF really intended to introduce full-blown "socialized medicine," starting with hospitals and eventually to all physician services. Initially courteous relations between the CCF government and the doctors' associations deteriorated into formality, suspicion and, finally, confrontation.

The province's doctors considered themselves a hardy breed. They practised in a poor province, battled the elements of wind and snow, drove long distances between patients and earned what they considered to be low incomes. They saw themselves as pioneering types, individualistic, proud and professional. Up to thirty-five of them had signed on to the first regional health plan, in Swift Current in 1945, where doctors were paid a salary to serve a certain population, an extension of the old municipal doctors schemes scattered across the province. The cost of the plan was paid by premiums and property taxes. Although the plan was working in Swift Current, it alarmed doctors elsewhere who disliked payment by salary and this collectivist kind of practice. As the province's postwar population grew, immigrant doctors from the United Kingdom arrived, many of them claiming to be "fleeing" British socialized medicine. These self-described refugees from the National Health Service could be counted on to oppose anything inspired by the system they had fled. By 1960, one-third of Saskatchewan's 750 doctors were British immigrants.

As the CCF government slowly unveiled its intentions for health care, the chasm between it and the doctors became evident. For starters, the doctors insisted that any plan must be administered by a commission, at arm's length from the government with a majority of physicians as members, whereas the government argued that public health care ultimately had to be, in a democracy, the responsibility of the government. Government financing for all health care, insisted the doctors, meant government/political control, which in turn would lead to doctors becoming bureaucrats. As such, they would be forced to conduct their practices according to the dictates of government, not professional guidelines. People who knew little or nothing about health, they feared, would be telling trained medical professionals how to practise, perhaps even where to practise, and at what remuneration. The end would be nigh for physicians being a self-regulating body of independent practitioners, who enjoyed direct and privileged relationships with individual patients, and were paid by those patients, except for limited government subsidies for the poor and perhaps pensioners. Government health care threatened a patient's right to select his or her doctor, they argued. It represented a twin assault on the doctors' status as professionals and their incomes.

Medical associations could not just oppose the CCF plans. They needed an alternative that would work better for patients, cost taxpayers less and guard the profession's prerogatives. What might be called the doctors' blended system of coverage consisted of accepting that the government could and should offer subsidized care for certain segments of the population, and perhaps even subsidies for hospitalization. This subsidized scheme had to be administered by a commission controlled by the profession to keep politicians and civil servants, some of whom in those days were patronage appointments rather than professionals, as far from medical administration and policy as possible. For the remainder of the population, there would be private insurance or, as time went on, insurance plans developed by the doctors themselves. Citizens without insurance could pay doctors directly according to fee schedules established by the profession, since fee-for-service was a bedrock principle of payment for the medical professionals.

By 1955, doctors' prepaid insurance plans had signed up 185,000 Saskatchewan residents and had inked prepayment contracts with sixty municipalities covering tens of thousands of additional people. By 1959, when the CCF government moved irrevocably for comprehensive public health care, the doctors could boast insurance coverage for 280,000 residents under their insurance plans, with the prospect of continuing growth.

Then there was the question of cost. A full-scale public medical scheme would be expensive, the doctors warned. It would require higher taxes of some kind, plus premiums. No matter what assurances governments gave, costs and taxes were going to rise. Look at the CCF's Hospital Services Plan, the doctors argued. New hospitals had been built across the province, all right, and this network had greatly improved access to care. But costs had continued to rise, so that premiums were increased. Chronic-care patients occupied too many beds in the absence of less-expensive accommodation. Too many hospitals had been sprinkled across the province, sometimes to meet genuine needs, sometimes to satisfy political imperatives. Without the arrival of federal funds following the national hospital financing legislation in 1957, Saskatchewan would have been sorely stretched to finance the operation of its hospital scheme. Did taxpayers, asked the doctors, really want to take on the burden of a full-blown public health scheme after the experience of burgeoning costs and higher taxes?

The dustbin of history is where the doctors' approach resides, but in the 1950s and early '60s it commanded a fair measure of public support, in Saskatchewan and beyond. Support came because the system was what people knew and, at least in some cases, felt comfortable with. Change of any kind often evokes fears, and many patients feared the erosion of doctor-patient relations under state-run medicine. Individual doctors enjoyed status and stature in communities. When doctors spoke about medicine and health care, they were presumed to know what they were talking about and to have the public interest at heart. No government in Canada had taken on the medical profession for what seemed the very good reason that the government could not win a confrontation with such a powerful and organized group.

Tommy Douglas's CCF government, however, was unlike any other in Canada. It kept getting re-elected after that first win in 1944, and it did believe in serious social reform. Whether they called themselves social democrats, social reformers or socialists, and whether they were pragmatists or idealists or a bit of both, CCFers saw the role of government differently than Liberals and Conservatives. They had been committed to comprehensive public health care since the Regina Manifesto. Now, in April 1959, fifteen years after their first victory, Premier Douglas declared during a by-election that his government intended to implement universal and comprehensive medical insurance. The premier took pains to stress that doctors would be fully consulted. No matter. The Saskatchewan College of Physicians and Surgeons stated in a resolution passed unanimously that its members "oppose the introduction of a compulsory government-controlled, province-wide medical plan and declare our support of and the extension of health and sickness benefits through indemnity and service plans." For three subsequent years, nothing closed the gap between what Tommy Douglas had promised and what the doctors would accept.

Douglas asked a committee of civil servants to organize the administrative framework for his ideas. The principles that these civil servants articulated became the core of today's medicare: universal public coverage paid for by taxes and premiums; physician and diagnostic services, pharmaceuticals and home nursing; optical, dental and rehabilitation services; preventive health; government responsibility and accountability. Not everything they recommended could be done at once. Pharmaceuticals would have to be excluded "because of the extremely difficult question of cost control," a situation that still prevails today. A premium, or personal tax, was essential (just as Tommy Douglas had always argued) "because the public should always be aware that changes in utilization and remuneration of physicians have a concurrent [read consequential] effect on each individual's cost."

Premier Douglas announced his detailed intention to proceed in a radio address. He picked up all the themes of the civil servants' report. He said the plan "must be in a form that is acceptable both to those providing the service and those receiving it." The phrase "those providing the service" meant the doctors. His promise became their rallying cry. If a plan were not acceptable to them, there would be no plan, because medical care could not be delivered without them. For Douglas, the phrase that the plan must be "acceptable ... to those providing the service" meant consultations and negotiations with the doctors, not a veto. The CCF, with its health-care plan squarely in the political window, won the subsequent election.

The government then approached the profession to participate in a committee to work out the details of the plan. By then the doctors were so angry that their association refused for three months to appoint any members to the committee, and demanded all sorts of fundamental changes in the committee's terms of reference. When the doctors' representatives did take their places, it quickly became clear that their participation was not directed to shaping a government-run health scheme but to sabotaging it. Election or no election, olive branch or otherwise from the government, this would be a fight, and a very nasty one at that, with the anti-CCF Sifton newspapers across the province offering doctors tub-thumping support.

Medical associations began to raise money from their members for the fight. Warnings were directed at patients and taxpayers about an exodus of physicians from the province, a dilution in the quality of care, the certainty of soaring costs, a decline in medical school enrolments. The committee received briefs and visited other countries. But it was split from inception and ended with a majority report recommending essentially what the civil servants' committee had proposed, and a minority report from the doctors and the representatives of the chamber of commerce recommending the blended system. Nothing had closed the chasm between the two sides.

With a fresh electoral mandate—the CCF won thirty-eight of fifty-four seats and 41 percent of the votes cast in the 1960 election—Tommy Douglas's government introduced legislation to give effect to public health care. The legislation received royal assent in November 1961.

Democracy had spoken, the CCF argued, but the doctors were not listening or did not hear. For them, the fact that Douglas, having won the 1960 election, heard the call to assume the leadership of the freshly created federal New Democratic Party, thereby leaving provincial political politics, demonstrated the crassness of his ambitions. Government-run health care had merely provided a stepping stone to bigger things for someone who put personal ambition ahead of the public interest. He had given birth, politically, to a mess and was now departing, said the doctors' spokesmen. For three months after the election, the doctors' representatives refused to meet with government officials. When finally the two sides did gather, the doctors insisted that talks could be based only on the government's scrapping its scheme, which of course the CCF would not do. The government offered compromises to and clarifications of its plan to assuage doctors' concerns to no avail.

Talks broke down in April. Doctors across the province were summoned to an emergency meeting in Regina on May 3 and 4 to plan further steps. Two-thirds of them showed up, loaded for bear, their offices temporarily closed. Premier Woodrow Lloyd, who had replaced Tommy Douglas, asked for a chance to address the doctors. He spoke calmly and at length, explaining the reasons for the government's policy. Hisses, boos and occasional jeers greeted some of his remarks. When the premier finished speaking but while he remained on the platform, he witnessed the president of the doctors' association ask those attending to stand if they opposed the government's legislation and would refuse to practise under it. All but 5 of the 550 doctors stood, applauding loudly. The assembly then voted to prepare for "emergency measures" on July 1, the day the legislation would enter into force. Those "measures" meant a strike.

Letters were exchanged between the two sides, as the government desperately tried to accommodate some of the doctors' concerns, especially about method of payment and freedom to practise as professionals. Face-to-face discussions resumed between the government and the doctors eight days before the strike deadline. They lasted four days and ended, again, in impasse.

The doctors allowed themselves to be buoyed by developments that they interpreted as favourable to their cause, the most important involving Tommy Douglas, their *bête noire*. A federal election had been called for June 18, 1962. Douglas, the new NDP leader, had chosen a Regina constituency, but the constituency did not choose him. Instead, Douglas was washed away in another landslide across Saskatchewan for the native son Progressive Conservative Prime Minister John Diefenbaker. Doctors were trained in medicine, not political science, so many of them wrongly interpreted Douglas's third-place finish as a statement about the health-care plan he had left behind, whereas the election throughout Saskatchewan was mostly about Diefenbaker. If anything, the PCs benefited from the tensions over health care, since they had taken no position on provincial medicare, while the provincial CCF and Liberals had quarrelled incessantly over it. Having no defined position, in this case, seemed better politically than having one.

Douglas's defeat heartened the doctors, as did other manifestations of what they chose to believe was public support for their cause. Four Regina women, or so legend has it, met over coffee, fretted over the possible loss of doctors' services and decided to do something. They began organizing a movement that quickly mushroomed with the support of the provincial Liberals, business interests, pharmacists, dentists, people with whatever grievance against the government and, of course, doctors. What became known as the Keep Our Doctors (KOD) committees took out newspaper ads, circulated petitions, held meetings and organized cavalcades, including one bringing about nine hundred people to Regina. The Sifton press kept up a steady drumbeat of editorials supportive of the doctors. The professional association sent doctors two copies of a sign to be posted on their offices:

TO OUR PATIENTS

This Office Will be Closed After
July 1, 1962
We Do Not Intend to Carry on Practice
Under
The Saskatchewan Medical Care

Doctors also received a letter from the association to give to their patients explaining that "you will appreciate that I am deeply concerned about taking what must seem to you a drastic step. Unfortunately, the attitude of the government leaves me with no other choice ... I support medical insurance. I am willing to accept an arrangement which is purely insurance and which does not attempt to control your doctor or tell your doctor how to treat you." With the press supportive, the KOD committees active, Douglas defeated, patients alarmed and their own forces mobilized but for a dissident handful of doctors who supported medicare, it seemed reasonable, or at least possible, for the doctors to believe that the government would retreat once they went on strike.

When the strike began, emotions among the governments' opponents intensified and rhetoric became even more incandescent. At one meeting, the controversial Catholic priest Father Athol Murray laid aside his coat, tore off his clerical collar and, with a province-wide audience listening on the radio, declared that "a 'wave of hatred' was sweeping Saskatchewan. There has been death, there will be violence, and there could be bloodshed. There are Reds here. I can't see them. I can smell them. You Communists may think we're naive and hollow-chested but we gave a hundred thousand boys fighting for freedom you're fighting against. You Reds, I want you to know that we're as proud as hell to be Canadians." He wasn't finished. "Tell those bloody Commies to go to hell when it comes to Canada. I loathe the welfare state and I love free-swinging freedom. I am seventy and I'll never ask you for the Old Age Pension. To hell with it. I want to be free."

The priest showed that the medicare debate was about more than health care. The fight was rather about two visions of society, of which a public health-care system was one manifestation. Although housewives and mothers offered the benign, concerned face of the KOD movement, the business community, the doctors and the government's political opponents were the financiers and strategists. The KODs did mobilize part of the population, and they did receive extensive media coverage. For a while, it appeared that KODs might reflect a majority of public opinion.

The doctors read too many press clippings. The CCF

government was not for turning. Premier Lloyd made a strategic-
ally shrewd move by ordering his supporters not to attack the
doctors, organize counter-demonstrations or mobilize politically.
He just kept repeating that the will of the people, as expressed
in the election, must be respected. The issue evolved into one
of democracy. Who would govern? The duly elected government
or a powerful set of interest groups? That refrain poured into
the province from outside its borders, echoed by almost all the
national media, whose reporters hurried to the province to cover
the strike and whose editorial writers commented on developments. The strike itself, rather than the government's proposed
legislation, became the focus of media attention, most of it
negative. What the doctors missed was the generalized support
that previous extensions of public health care—to seniors and
hospital care in particular—had earned among the majority of
the people. Yes, people of Saskatchewan had been taxed to pay for
these extensions, and, yes, these taxes had risen, but the largest
number of people thought the trade-off a reasonable one. If there
were such a thing as a silent majority, it stood with the government on the principles involved, much as individuals might
admire their doctors as friends and practitioners.

As the strike loomed, it garnered attention outside Canada.
U.S. newspapers found the story intriguing: socialized medicine,
a foreign concept for their country; doctors on strike, another
bizarre development. In Britain, home to the NHS, the story
received widespread attention, in no small measure because
the CCF government began recruiting British doctors to supply
services in the event of a strike. Once the strike commenced, 110
doctors arrived from outside the province, mostly from Britain.
"Foreign scabs" they were called by militant members of the
KODs; welcome healers they were thought of by residents who
needed their skills. In some communities, co-operative health

arrangements sprang up, but in others emergency services were stretched exceedingly thin. It was one thing for doctors to be unhappy; it was another to leave so many patients without care. As the strike moved into its second week, with most doctors' offices shut and some of them out of the province on vacation, support for their cause was waning. They were seen increasingly to have overplayed their hand and to have engaged in rhetorical overkill of the kind used by Father Murray.

The doctors and KODs promised a mammoth rally in front on the legislature on the eleventh day of the strike. They intended to present a petition to the legislature, then not in session. The Liberal opposition was out in full force to greet and encourage them. Liberal leader Ross Thatcher even went so far as to try to kick down the door of the legislature for the television cameras, while comparing the refusal of the government to convene the legislature to something likely to occur in the Soviet Union or China. It was splendidly prepared theatre, except that most of the actors did not appear. Whereas organizers had promised thirty thousand, the Canadian Press estimated four thousand protestors. The paltry turnout deflated the doctors, or at least began persuading their leaders that perhaps the strike was fizzling. Doctors were arriving from elsewhere; the out-of-province press was pounding them; the government was not budging; their rallies were dwindling; some of their members were drifting back to work. White flags of surrender began to go up in the form of letters from the doctors' association to the government, each one demanding less to resume negotiations. When the head of the association asked to address the CCF convention—a sort of reciprocal visit for the one Premier Lloyd had paid the angry doctors—and offered a resumption of talks if the government accepted that doctors could work outside the medicare act and have payment routed through agencies rather than the government, the premier agreed, noting that the doctors no longer demanded withdrawal or repeal of the act.

Into the drama stepped Lord Taylor from Britain, whom the Saskatchewan government had consulted while recruiting doctors in Britain and who had visited the province in 1946. He was a doctor by profession and a Labour Lord, having been involved in the establishment of the National Health Service. The CCF government asked him to come to the province to mediate the dispute. He agreed to work for no pay, provided that the government paid for a week's fishing trip afterwards. Within a day of arriving he was shuttling between the cabinet ministers and the doctors' representatives, leaning on both, cursing where appropriate, nagging constantly, pleading and cajoling, breaking down barriers. He was, in one description, "histrionic, colorful, hyperactive, tall and shaggy-browed." He was also effective. Some thawing had occurred before he arrived, but much more was needed before a settlement. As Lord Taylor recalled later, his shuttling and exchanging of drafts often produced minimal progress. "I told the doctors I'm fed up with this. I'm utterly fed up to the teeth. I cannot take any more. Either you agree or I'm off. They begged me to stay ... we had a frightful struggle over certain phrases and certain words ... I lost my temper. I swore and raved." After exhausting days, the Saskatoon Agreement was signed.

The doctors capitulated on principles but won on details, none of which mattered over time. Doctors had always hated the idea of being paid by the government. So the Saskatoon Agreement offered four methods for doctors' payment: private payment by patients; payment by the patient after he or she received reimbursement from a medical insurance fund; payment by the doctors' insurance plans; payment by the doctors' own medical insurance agencies, which in turn would be paid by the state.

Here, thought the doctors, was what they had been seeking all along: no payment by the state.

Except that it turned out that patients did not want to pay directly compared with other alternatives. Most of them preferred to send their bills to the medical insurance agencies that were, in turn, simply reimbursed by the state. In time, it became clear that these agencies made payment messier and involved more bureaucracy. Doctors began to be paid directly for their services by the state, something they had fought against up to and including going on strike. Eight years after their apparent victory, half of them were billing the government directly for their services, bypassing their own agencies. They won a fleeting victory on payment methods, but they conceded on the essential principles that Saskatchewan would have a government-administered, publicly financed health insurance plan for all.

That model, developed in a small, relatively poor province, became the template for Canada. Saskatchewan doctors' incomes rose, helping reconcile them over time to their fate. Medicare in Saskatchewan produced the most bruising fight in the history of health care in Canada. Woodrow Lloyd, Douglas's successor who endured the strike, confided to his diary, "I doubt if anyone can go through a period of being lied about, hated, misrepresented and ever be the same."

FOUR

The Father of Medicare

Medicare's triumph in Saskatchewan encouraged those who wanted something similar for Canada. A Gallup poll as far back as 1944 had found 80 percent of Canadians willing to pay for a comprehensive public health-care system. So many obstacles had slowed down the fight in Saskatchewan, however, that nothing guaranteed a straight line from medicare in Saskatchewan to a national program.

No greater example of unintended consequences in the history of medicare occurred than on December 12, 1960, when the Canadian Medical Association sent a letter to Progressive Conservative Prime Minister John Diefenbaker. The CMA noted mounting public interest in "socialized medicine" of the kind being introduced in Saskatchewan. That province, the CMA believed, had made a terrible mistake that the rest of Canada should avoid. A disinterested, independent inquiry, argued the CMA, would underscore the cost, the threat to patient-doctor relations and the increased bureaucracy of the Saskatchewan model. The rest of Canada would surely wish to avoid the divisions that had roiled Saskatchewan. Removed from what the CMA called the "hauling and pulling" of politics, an inquiry would recognize and build on the existing voluntary medical insurance plans. A Royal Commission, the CMA advised the prime minister, would "take account of the quickening of public interest in the whole area of health services," but arrive at conclusions "wisely and objectively."

The CMA's request for an inquiry seemed like smart politics. The Progressive Conservative Party had long offered a blank sheet on health-care policy. John Bracken, a previous PC leader, had commissioned Charlotte Whitton's study in 1943 recommending a public system financed from general revenues. Bracken had done nothing with the Whitton study. Many doctors, as small businessmen, were among the party's staunchest supporters. The PCs were the party of small government, low taxes and Bay Street. Ontario's Progressive Conservative Party strongly supported doctor-run insurance programs. As for John Diefenbaker, he had never in public manifested much interest in health-care issues. He had not campaigned on health care, nor had he spoken much about the issue, despite his Saskatchewan background. With the CCF committed to "socialized" medicine," and a few Liberals inclining in that direction, the CMA sensed a chance with a Progressive Conservative prime minister to draw a line in the sand. If a Royal Commission sided with organized medicine, as the CMA believed it would, political pressure for government-run health care would dissipate.

Diefenbaker mulled over the request for only eight days before announcing a Royal Commission, although the appointment of all the commissioners took another six months. He could sense the budding interest in public health care but knew his party's general aversion to it. The Royal Commission's creation would not commit the government to any particular course of action. It would allow time to study the public mood, avoid federal–provincial disputes and keep his party united while indicating an interest in the issue to the public. Not for the first time, and certainly not for the last, a Royal Commission would provide a substitute for early action.

The CMA was pleased with Diefenbaker's decision and the commissioners. There was a surgeon, a dentist, a past president of the Saskatchewan Medical Association, a past president of the Canadian Medical Association and a millionaire businessman from Toronto, Wallace McCutcheon from the upper executive echelons of Argus Corporation, who later become a senator and Diefenbaker cabinet minister. By occupation and background, five commissioners appeared to be unsympathetic to public health care. With these five men forming the majority of the eight-member commission, no wonder a cynic wrote that "putting the prospects of a national medical care scheme in the hands of that commission—composed as it is of the past president of the CMA and the head of the Argus Corporation is like asking Colonel Sanders to protect your chicken farm." Another commissioner, Dr. O.J. Firestone, was a former federal civil servant and a wealthy economist known for somewhat iconoclastic views. He might lean to the political left, as might a past president of the Canadian Nurses Association. No one could predict the instincts and preferences of the chairman, Emmett Hall, chief justice of the Saskatchewan Court of Appeal, for he had said nothing about health care as a lawyer, political actor or judge.

Emmett Hall's background offered few clues to which way he would lean. He had grown up in an Irish enclave near Montreal where the nearest school was French, a language Hall mastered. Later, after the family moved to Saskatchewan, he warranted the nickname "Frenchy." His younger brother, Anthony, went into the priesthood, and there were those who suggested that his brother's vocation inspired in Hall a sense of "caring for thy neighbour." Hall was one of only two in a family of eleven children to receive a university degree, in law from the University of Saskatchewan.

There, and subsequently when both were articling students, Hall met Diefenbaker. Theirs was a relationship born in friendship, defined by lawyerly competition, shaped by political co-operation after Hall bolted the Liberals for the PCs in the early 1940s because he smarted from the provincial Liberals' refusal to name him a judge. Later in Diefenbaker's life, estrangement set in as the old, embittered politician began falling out with many who had been his friends. When Diefenbaker asked Hall to lead a Royal Commission, the prime minister was well aware of Hall's talents but knew nothing about his views on health care. Nor did Hall himself.

Hall was by then a pillar of the Saskatoon establishment. When his judicial appointment required him to move to Regina, he bought a nine-room house in the city's best neighbourhood and joined the Assiniboia Club, a refuge for the city's elite. He had run three times for public office, once for city council, once as a provincial PC and once for a federal PC nomination. He lost every time. He had spared no rhetorical effort to denounce what he considered extremist parties such as Social Credit and the CCF. In the 1948 campaign, he had warned that the CCF displayed Nazi tendencies, especially after CCF leader Tommy Douglas criticized a court decision about trade unions. "Mr. Douglas is running true to form in the pattern of National Socialism," Hall declared.

Hall had been a first-rate courtroom lawyer, with a sometimes brusque style and a get-to-the-point attitude. He said on accepting the appointment to head the Royal Commission that he had no preconceived ideas about health care. Nothing in his background or career suggested that Emmett Hall would become, with Tommy Douglas and Monique Bégin, an architect of Canadian medicare.

Hall's commission, which began hearings in 1961, could have recommended a variation on what already existed and what the CMA wanted—doctors' insurance plans for patients who could afford them, coupled with expanded social insurance and a government scheme for the poor. That approach was endorsed by nine of the ten provinces and by a sizeable share of the national Progressive Conservative Party.

Various options existed between what the CMA sought and what the commission eventually endorsed. There could have been co-payments, or user fees, for basic medical services; a mixed public–private system with a larger role for the public sector than the CMA wished but less than full public coverage; a social insurance model of the kind developed in certain continental European countries; special health taxes; doctors on salary. When the Royal Commission began, some interest groups (farm organizations, unions, social activists, the CCF) argued for public health care, but just as many opposed the idea (business organizations, provincial governments, medical associations).

Saskatchewan's experiment with public health care reflected the political culture of just one province. That province had a particular take on government's role in society, shaped by its fragile, agricultural economy that had collapsed during the Great Depression. Just because a somewhat eccentric (by the standards of the time) province had endorsed public health care, and only after a prolonged and bitter fight, by no means meant that the other nine would follow. It took Emmett Hall's Royal Commission to turn one province's approach into a national cause.

That the commissioners should have endorsed this cause without a dissenting vote would have been astonishing, and in fact one of them vocally did not agree. Wallace McCutcheon left the commission on becoming a member of Diefenbaker's cabinet as a senator, the prime minister being by then desperate to repair frayed relations with the business community. When the bill creating medicare years later arrived in the Senate for final consideration, McCutcheon denounced it as "one more evidence of the new socialism ... based on the philosophy that government—and it seems particularly true of the federal government—knows better what should be done for the people than the people know themselves."

The doctors on the commission who eventually signed on to the commission's report were regarded as traitors by their medical colleagues. One of them, David Baltzan of Saskatoon, held out until the last minute, fighting for fee-for-service payments for doctors. Hall pounded away at Baltzan, eventually wearing him down. Baltzan threatened to write a minority report, bargaining to the end for fee-for-service payment as an unalterable bottom line. For Hall, who had become convinced of the virtues of public health care during the hearings, yielding to Baltzan (and through him to the medical profession) on fee-for-service represented the commission's key compromise. That compromise, and the previous commitment in Saskatchewan for fee-for-service, established that payment model for medicare nationally, then and today.

What would have happened if McCutcheon had not been appointed to the Senate? Had he stayed a commissioner instead of going to the Senate, this crusty, forceful businessman would never have signed the final report. He might well have persuaded Baltzan and the other two medical professionals to sign a majority report proposing a very different health-care model, consigning Hall and the other two commissioners to a minority report. Firestone, a forceful advocate of public health care, later remarked, "Politics saved the day when Diefenbaker chose McCutcheon as a senator."

Strict geographic determinism has no place in historical analysis, but Emmett Hall's origins in Saskatchewan likely influenced how he saw health care. He had witnessed the debates around public health care from the CCF's election in 1944 to the introduction of universal hospital insurance in 1947 to universal medical care insurance in the teeth of the doctors' strike in 1962. What might have seemed radical, even unthinkable, elsewhere in Canada had come to be accepted in Saskatchewan. Hall knew that the provincial Liberal Party, having railed against universal health care while in opposition, kept the system intact on forming the government in 1964 because a majority of Saskatchewan citizens approved of public health care.

Who knows what attitudes a chairman might have brought to the commission from, say, Quebec, where medical associations remained opposed to public health care and the provincial government rejected any federal intrusion into what it considered provincial jurisdiction? Or Ontario, where private insurance had sunk deep roots and was supported by the business community and most of the political elites? Or Alberta, where another form of populism (Social Credit) had produced a highly individualistic political culture in which episodic flirtations with public medicine had been swept aside by a preference for people taking care of themselves? No one is entirely a creature of the environment in which he or she grows up and knows best, but Emmett Hall's roots in Saskatchewan could not have helped but influence how he sifted through the 406 briefs, twenty-six research reports, testimony at public hearings, debates with staff and, of course, other commissioners.

The Canadian Medical Association, the body that had asked for an inquiry, naturally tried to influence the commissioners' thinking. In its longest submission, the CMA argued that "the development of voluntary forms of coverage is making steady progress and the prospect of availability of insurance to every Canadian who needs and wants it is in sight." Fifty-six percent of Canadians already enjoyed private medical insurance coverage, the CMA pointed out. That share of the population would increase to 70 percent by 1970. With expanding private coverage and the public plans proposed for poor people, the CMA reckoned that over time almost all Canadians would have insurance of one sort or another. Physicians were willingly treating those in "poor economic circumstances," so "it cannot be maintained that necessary medical care is lacking to any demonstrable degree." The CMA saw nothing wrong with using means tests to determine who was on welfare, indigent or otherwise unable to pay. Governments used a means test in other areas, and "the humiliation and embarrassment which is said to accompany its application seems to us to be more theoretical than real."

The CMA categorically rejected "universal, compulsory, tax-supported comprehensive medical services insurance under government auspices and we feel that public funds should not be applied to the self-supporting in the area of medical insurance." Already, the CMA argued, "in many provinces the limits of taxation appear to have been reached and in some provinces difficulty is being experienced in the financing of existing health services." Instead of necessary tax increases to pay for comprehensive public health care, the government should devise public protection for only two groups: the approximately 8 percent of the population that the CMA thought "medically indigent," and for "persons just superior to the identifiable indigent." With the support of many provinces, including British Columbia, Alberta and Ontario, of business associations, and indeed of many citizens adequately covered by private insurance, the CMA remained confident that the Royal Commission would see things its way.

This major CMA submission, one of the most substantive at almost two inches thick, came at about the mid-point of the Royal Commission's public hearings, by which time there were already indications that perhaps the chairman was drifting toward the comprehensive public approach.

Submissions by medical groups were being met with increasingly testy, argumentative questions from Hall and Firestone in particular. An adviser to the commission later recalled Hall's muttering, "Those damned doctors. They think they know everything. All I hear is propaganda and not a shred of evidence to support their opposition to my question."

Malcolm Taylor, the commission adviser, later recalled the defining moment when Hall opted for a public system. He had asked the staff to analyze organized medicine's proposal for private insurance schemes, such as the ones doctors' associations had organized. He wanted a calculation for government subsidies of premiums beyond 5 percent of family income for a full range of medical services. The calculation revealed means testing for 10 to 15 million people. Hall concluded that it would be more socially just and economically efficient to subsidize ten provincial health plans with federal money, the germ of medicare. Once his mind turned, he drove the group (except McCutcheon) toward its final destination. Hall was the intellectual piledriver (along with Firestone), the master of all briefs, the inquisitor at hearings.

Hall is said to have written all of the proposed healthcare charter that the commission recommended, and was very hands-on with the rest of the 941-page first volume. Hall, appointed a Supreme Court judge in Ottawa during the commission's deliberations, threw off his judicial robes and argued forcefully and publicly in favour of the recommendations while still on the bench.

The commission earnestly declared that "as a nation we now take the necessary legislative, organizational and financial decisions to make all the fruits of the health sciences available to all our residents without hindrance of any kind. All our recommendations are directed toward this objective."

In recent years, various Canadian studies recommended enshrining medicare's principles in something loftier than mere legislation. Roy Romanow, leading a federal commission in 2002, proposed a health-care covenant, having rejected a charter on the grounds that it might lead to an explosion of legal cases. An Alberta legislative committee in 2010 recommended a health-care charter for the province. Hall's commission beat all subsequent comers by at least four decades. It recommended a health charter with a commitment to "comprehensive" and "universal" health services, freedom of choice for patients, improvements in public health, the development of representative health agencies. No such charter has ever been enacted, but the commission's recommendations anticipated many of the debates that surround medicare today, including "quick action" in the field of mental illness, a "program to help the aged and infirm," a "crash program" to train more medical professionals, programs to face "the burden of drug costs" and improved medical-research facilities. In style, sweep and depth of analysis, the Hall Royal Commission was the most consequential of the multitude of studies of Canadian health care. It established a mould for medicare that has never been broken, although it is now cracking.

At the opening of the first volume, the commission left dangling an analytical thread that it never subsequently developed and still remains at the margin of debates about health care: individual responsibility for health. The commission said a public health-care system would guarantee rights to all citizens—a right of free access to all medically necessary services. But what of the individual's responsibility not to abuse the exercise of that right? "The individual's responsibility for his personal health and that of the members of his or her family is paramount to the extent of the individual's capacities," wrote the commission. An individual, Hall and his colleagues affirmed, has a "wide scope for the determination of his own health and well-being." A person must "be prepared to assign a reasonable part of his income by taxes, premiums or both to meet the costs of health services which will be faced by every person during the course of his lifetime." Then the commission offered three sentences that remain central to contemporary debates about the sustainability of medicare: "The wise use of available health services cannot be over-stressed. Much serious illness and unhappiness would be avoided if this were done. It goes without saying that since all such resources are scarce, it is the duty of the individual, as well as of the practitioner prescribing them, to see that the services are used with prudence and economy."

What did the commission mean by the "duty of the individual"? What constituted "wise use"? The system of universal free medical care that it proposed provided no impediment or caution in the form of a monetary payment that would shape "wise use," with the result that as with all "free goods," the possibility arose for overuse or even abuse.

Hall seemed to understand the tensions among free access, the state's scarce resources and the possibility of overuse. His slightly contradictory answer to the dilemma, however, remains a characteristic of medicare. For hospital and doctors' services, he argued that access should be free, but for drugs he suggested some form of financial contribution by the user, or co-payment.

The commission recommended a $1 contribution by patients for every pharmaceutical prescription, except those required for long-term therapy, since such payments were the norm in other countries with public health systems. The same principle applied for eyeglasses: the patient should pay a portion of the cost, since the commission recommended full inclusion of optometry in the new health-care system, a recommendation never acted on. Nor did any federal government ever act on another proposal: dental services for children under eighteen years of age, expectant mothers and those on welfare as part of the public health care.

Hall had wanted a much wider public health-care system than the one that governments subsequently organized. What emerged instead was a narrower system with public coverage for hospitals and doctors, some public coverage for drugs depending on age and provincial residence, patchy public coverage for home care and none at all for dentistry and eye care.

Today, from the distance of half a century, who cannot admire Hall's prescience in recommending an expansion of home care, a need that grows more urgent with each passing year? Canada would now be better prepared for the increase of the elderly population had governments followed his commission's advice that every hospital with more than one hundred beds develop a home-care program either independently or with other hospitals. And how much better off would provincial budgets be with a national drug formulary, instead of the absurd situation in which each province devises its own formulary and then negotiates individually with the powerful pharmaceutical companies?

The Hall commission's recommendations, had they been completely followed, would have created a somewhat different health-care system than what eventually emerged. It would have offered a wider variety of basic public services, but it would have incorporated some payments by patients across a range of services to help alleviate the burden on the public treasury. Instead, the issue of patient payment became so politically toxic in Canada that what emerged was a system with no payments for some of the system and patient payments in whole or in part for the rest, a rather uneven arrangement that defied the notion of public coverage for care along a continuum of health-care needs.

The Hall commission could not avoid a central issue facing all health-care systems: how to pay doctors. Fee-for-service had been the medical profession's preferred method of payment from the earliest days of health-care delivery. It was central to the compromises that shaped the Saskatchewan system, and it was the payment method recommended by the Hall commission. Salaries for doctors, or a blended system of salary and fee-for-service, had been used in a few instances in Canada and overseas, but because fee-for-service was so deeply embedded in Canadian practice, the commission saw no point in trying to change it. The fees should be negotiated between the medical professions and the government. But, wrote Hall about a subject that a decade later would flare into one of medicare's most intense debates, "Extra billing would not be permitted."

Then there was the necessary business of financing a comprehensive public health-care system. Public-opinion polls, then in their infancy, and testimony at the commission's hearings suggested that the public was indeed willing to pay in the form of taxes and premiums for health care. The commission recommended both methods. The commission also wanted both levels of government involved in financing the new scheme. Provinces could decide how to finance their programs, and Ottawa would pay approximately 50 percent of the cost. It should also chip in 5 percent for administrative expenses and offer special grants to poorer provinces. These proposals did not stand the test of time. Nor did any government follow the commission's recommendation that money transferred by Ottawa to provinces for health care be designated so that taxpayers understood where the money was coming from and for what purpose. As a result, taxpayers today remain either dimly aware or utterly ignorant of the federal contribution to health care.

In an uncannily prescient aside, the commission suggested that a province could ask Ottawa for permission to establish a lottery to help fund health care. In 1979, Prime Minister Joe

Clark's PC government unilaterally ceded Ottawa's power to organize lotteries, a windfall for provinces. They launched their own lotteries, with proceeds intended for culture and recreation. Instead, the pressure of rising health-care costs diverted many or all of these lottery proceeds into the health-care system, as the Hall commission had believed might be necessary many decades before.

With the best will in the world, and the most excellent forecasting models, intelligent people peer through a glass darkly in predicting the future. So it was for the Hall commission's financial projections. They were accurate for the early decades of medicare but grew increasingly useless because they hugely underestimated the costs of the commission's proposals. Canada's population reached about 35 million in 2012, for example, whereas the commission had predicted that level in 1991. Hall and his colleagues had not foreseen the decline in the fertility rate, and that miscalculation threw off the commission's cost projections.

When the commission reported in 1964, Canada was spending 5.4 percent of its gross domestic product on health care. Without any change to the basic system, the commission thought the share of GDP would nudge up to only 5.5 percent in 1971. The implementation of its proposals, the commission forecast, would push health care to 6.4 percent of GDP in 1971 and 7.4 percent in 1991. Additional revenues would come from higher personal income taxes, premiums, sales taxes or whatever revenue-raising methods provinces chose. Such an increase, Hall asserted, could be accommodated "without affecting detrimentally the requirement of the Canadian people for other goods and services." Instead, health-care costs blew past what Hall had predicted, and other "goods and services" desired by Canadians did suffer as health care squeezed the budgets for other programs.

Hall's predictions were wobbly from the start. In 1971, health care took 7 percent of GDP, not 6.4 percent; by 1991 it consumed 9 percent of GDP, not 7.4 percent. Two decades later, it used 11.7 percent of GDP, an increase of about 70 percent in the share of GDP since medicare began. Remember that the commission proposed a considerably wider public health-care model than the one that governments subsequently negotiated. Even the narrower system that emerged from federal–provincial negotiations soon outstripped the costs of the wider one that the commission had recommended. Higher costs than anticipated, plus an aversion to higher taxes, shattered any hopes that the commission's more comprehensive model might have been implemented.

In fairness, how could the Hall commission have predicted the OPEC crisis of the early 1970s that dramatically slowed economic growth and caused soaring inflation and high unemployment? How could it have known that the future would mock its optimistic projection of only 4 percent unemployment and strong productivity growth? How could it have predicted, decades ahead, the surges in expensive medical technology and drug costs, the feminization of medical schools, the ever-increasing demand for health-care services with little concern for their "wise use," the confrontations between unionized employees within the health-care sector and provincial governments, the aggressive pursuit of self-interest by doctors' organizations in fee bargaining, the massive health-care bureaucracies, the radically changed demography of Canada and a host of other changes?

When Canadians embraced Hall's dream, they wedded themselves with such passion to its nobility of purpose, its humanitarian and nation-building impulses and its egalitarian values that no politician of any stripe dared to tear the marriage asunder. Hall's dream prevails today, and Emmett Hall deserves to be called the "father of medicare." He, arguably more than any other Canadian with the exception of Tommy Douglas, laid the foundation and built the intellectual superstructure for Canada's unique system. Within a few short years of its start, however, medicare began to be rocked by events far from home that produced renewed domestic battles over health care.

FIVE

The Liberals and Medicare

It took almost half a century from promise to realization, but the Liberal Party finally delivered on public health care on July 1, 1968. Many reasons explain why public health care took so long to arrive, but one was the nature of the Liberal Party, which often prided itself on being more progressive than it actually was.

Mackenzie King, the prince of caution, first inscribed a commitment to public health care in the party program in 1919 at the convention that made him Liberal leader and prime minister. Canada needed an "adequate" sickness-insurance program, read the program that King himself largely wrote, with four conditions: co-operation with the provinces, financial capacity, scope of the program and timing. Each condition was enough to slow down progress; together they stymied public health care for a very long time. As one Liberal government yielded to another, the original promise flickered in the party's mind. Those who wanted action pointed to the promise, but the timing, circumstances and cost never seemed to align until the mid-1960s. Saskatchewan had implemented medicare in 1962, the Hall Royal Commission had reported, and the party had re-committed itself to public health care at a policy conference in 1961. The stars, it seemed, had finally aligned, so the government of Prime Minister Lester Pearson decided that the party was willing and the country was ready for what became known as the Medical Care Insurance Act, or medicare, as it became popularly known. When the parliamentary vote came on December 8, 1966, to begin medicare about eighteen months later, the vote was 177 to 2, the only dissenters being a pair of Social Credit MPs.

The overwhelming parliamentary majorities for public coverage of hospitalization costs in 1957, medicare in 1966 and the Canada Health Act in 1984 illustrated that public health care enjoyed substantial citizen support. Still, it took a very long time for Mackenzie King's 1919 promise to become reality. King, periodically enjoined by Liberal ministers to act on the promise, recoiled at the cost during the decades of Depression and war. The notion of a welfare state that included health insurance took hold only, and then just among some Canadians, during the Second World War, the privations and tragedies of which made a few policy thinkers believe that such sacrifices demanded a compassionate postwar response from government. Ian Mackenzie, a King minister and a much-neglected figure in the fight for public health care, argued in 1943, "Few today can regard war as an adventure and therefore it only becomes tolerable as a crusade with social and economic reform as a banner under which we fight."

Mackenzie, more than any other minister, prodded King into realizing that the government had to respond to legitimate desires for social protection, as the Beveridge Report had outlined in Britain. While King delayed action for the first half of the war, Mackenzie, the minister of pensions and health, managed to get cabinet approval for what seemed like an innocuous-enough request: a group of civil servants and outsiders to examine the state of the country's health and recommend ways of improving it. A dirty secret of the war, as during the First World War, was how many Canadians who volunteered for military duty were deemed physically unfit or barely fit to serve.

The first blueprint for national health insurance in Canada emerged from this innocuous initiative. Published in late 1942, after only nine months of work, the so-called Heagerty report (named after the chairman, J.J. Heagerty, director of public health services) outlined something uncannily similar to today's medicare. The report insisted that a health-care plan should embrace everyone, be paid for by compulsory contributions and be national. The constitution prevented Ottawa from acting unilaterally, but Ottawa could finance the program by giving grants to the provinces. MacKenzie met two immovable obstacles in cabinet: the prime minister's innate caution and the department of finance's analysis that the scheme would be too costly.

The report did go to a parliamentary committee that heard from a parade of witnesses, including the famous Sir William Beveridge himself. Sir William heartily endorsed the principles of the report. He spoke passionately about the need for social insurance of all kinds, including health, but added something since forgotten in Canadian medicare: "Every insured person should make a flat contribution of about one-quarter of the cost ... [because] it adds to their sense of self-respect to make a contribution irrespective of means. If you have such a system people will realize that they cannot get unlimited benefits without paying for them, and I believe that is an element of sound finance." Buoyed by favourable testimony from the majority of witnesses, the committee approved a bill authorizing federal payments to provinces for health insurance. The government did give the committee a commitment that it would convene a dominion–provincial conference after the 1945 federal election that returned King's Liberals to office with a reduced majority.

That conference produced disagreements that could not be overcome. When it adjourned, the idea of a national public health-care program was shelved, never to return in Mackenzie King's time. He departed office in 1949 with nothing to show for his limited efforts, except many diary entries of self-congratulation.

The public health-care idea lived on for true believers who could point to the Canadian population's poor health as urgent evidence for the need to act. Their case was buttressed by one of those reports of door-stopping size that punctuate the history of Canadian health care. The Canadian Sickness Survey of May 1953, compiled under the auspices of the Dominion Bureau of Statistics and the Department of National Health and Welfare, recommended nothing but uncovered much. It provided for the first time a comprehensive examination of the state of Canadians' health and their financial preparedness for illness. Accidents of all kinds were many; absenteeism for reasons of ill health was rampant. Almost 60 percent of Canadians were disabled at least once a year, and almost half the population was ill in bed during the year. An unmistakable pattern showed that many Canadians, especially low-income Canadians, were without any medical or hospital insurance. Wide disparities existed among provinces in availability of doctors and hospital beds, and the per capita amounts spent on health, with spending in British Columbia and Saskatchewan being roughly two and a half times that of the Maritime provinces, and more than twice that of Ontario.

Of the $373 million that Canadians spent on health care, 76 percent of it came from their pockets. Prepaid insurance plans covered only 24 percent. More people were covered for hospital expenses than for seeing a physician, which was too bad for most, who saw physicians far more than hospitals. The report estimated that more than half the population needed to see a doctor, but very few Canadians had insurance to cover such a cost.

The richer you were, the more you spent on health care, in

part because richer Canadians more likely had prepaid insurance. Low-income people used health services less, even though their overall health was worse, a clear indication that lack of coverage inhibited some low-income people from seeing a doctor or visiting a hospital. The survey concluded, "The income group distribution of persons with any health-care needs indicated that, generally, the low-income group received the least care."

Private insurers and doctors insisted that low-income people, or the "indigent," as they were sometimes called, could receive free coverage from doctors willing to assist. The quid pro quo for this free coverage, a kind of medical noblesse oblige, came from the direct payments and insurance coverage of high-income earners. The trouble was that too many low-income people fell through the yawning cracks in the system. There was no avoiding that the Canadian population was unhealthy, or at least much less healthy than the country's wealth could provide.

Prime Minister Louis St. Laurent, King's successor, had no inclination to move on health care. Any health-care proposal, he feared, would lead into the swamps of federal–provincial relations, as the King government had discovered. The postwar economy was booming, which seemed to mean that more people would be able to afford health insurance provided by private companies and the doctors' insurance plans. The federal Progressive Conservatives had lost what little appetite they had occasionally displayed for public health care. The CCF, enthusiastic boosters of British-style public health insurance, had just thirteen MPs. The Canadian Medical Association in the war years had philosophically warmed to the idea of universal coverage, perhaps even publicly provided. After the war, the CMA resumed its traditional opposition to universal public health care, offering instead a blended system of government subsidies for the poor and private insurance for everyone else.

Yet there was no contesting the findings of the Canadian Sickness Survey. And there were Liberals in cabinet and caucus, especially Paul Martin Sr., who remembered the party's 1919 promise. Without Martin, the first major national step toward medicare might never have been taken, at least when it did. When Martin became health minister in 1946, he resolved not to allow the disappointing results of the 1945 federal–provincial conference to deter further efforts to get something done in health care. Martin knew what he was up against when King asked him to become minister of health and welfare. As Martin wrote in his memoirs, "Although my enthusiasm was great, I also worried because I knew that I would run into all kinds of opposition from within the cabinet, starting with Mackenzie King himself. Health and welfare programs cost money, and King always considered himself the guardian of the privy purse." The best Martin could pry from cabinet before the 1953 election was more federal money to the provinces for hospital construction. A few of them wanted some form of expanded health care.

St. Laurent replied that the country had other priorities. Health care would drag Ottawa into an acrimonious, lengthy struggle with the provinces. Any plan would cost too much money. It was best to tackle other matters and wait for a more propitious moment to proceed. Martin would have none of it. If the party abandoned its 1919 commitment, said Martin directly to the prime minister, he would resign.

Ministers do not threaten resignation lightly, nor do prime ministers generally brush off such a threat from a senior minister. With a ministerial resignation in the offing and pressure from some provinces to put health care on the agenda, St. Laurent relented. The question of "health and welfare services" would be on the agenda, after all, when he and the premiers next gathered. Paul Martin Sr. had won the showdown. Now he would try to secure the objective for which he had threatened resignation.

Toward the end of his political career, Martin seemed like an aging windbag about whom more jokes were told than accolades offered. He had developed the art, if that is the proper word, of talking up and down and around issues at considerable length, so listeners were certain they had heard many words but remained uncertain just what had been said. It was accepted that his memory for names was elephantine but that just in case his memory slipped, he had the largest filing system for names and people in the country, second only to the revenue department's. This attention to the personal minutiae of politics—letters, cards, thank-you notes—plus his own dedication to the people of Windsor made him unbeatable there. Martin lived the political truism that all politics is local, and Windsor admired him for it.

Martin to the end of his career saw himself as a progressive in the Liberal pantheon. Whether his record justifies such a label is beside the point. As minister of health, he was determined that on his watch something big would happen in the health-care field. A full-blown public health-care system, such as the British Labour government had introduced after the war, inspired social reformers in Canada. But Canada was a federation, unlike centralized Britain. No Canadian government could implement a health-care scheme without the co-operation and consent of the provinces. When Martin began canvassing provinces about what might be accomplished, public coverage for physicians' services was to be found nowhere in Canada, whereas the idea of public money for hospitals was well established. He would work, then, on a national scheme of public hospital care.

Two camps tussled within cabinet: those who wanted a minimal offer and those who sought a grander program. Martin obviously was in the latter camp. He worked with all his energy to bring around the hesitating ministers, inviting some of them to sit in meetings with the provinces to better understand the issues, or simply to wear them down. Eventually, he convinced the prime minister, who offered the provinces half the cost of diagnostic services and hospital care. This carrot of federal money, justified by the federal government's spending power, came with conditions that became central to medicare. Ottawa would finance provincial plans instead of insisting on a uniform hospitalization scheme across the country—just as today there is no national medicare scheme but rather a series of plans that conform very loosely to national standards. Provincial plans had to offer universal coverage, just as today. Provinces had to "limit" but not abolish co-insurance, or what Canadians today call "user pay" provisions, which provincial plans featured before the Martin proposal.

The usual provincial wrangling thus began, over money, terms and phase-in of the program. The federal money certainly provided an inducement to provinces, but only three of the minimum of six (British Columbia, Alberta and Saskatchewan) immediately accepted the offer. Others balked or hesitated or wanted further negotiations. Martin, indefatigable throughout, went to see the Ontario premier, Leslie Frost, who greeted him with seven conditions—one of which resonates today: home care. Frost wanted home care included in hospitalization, which is what many reformers want today. Frost was therefore well ahead of his time, but he was also too late to convince Paul Martin, who had extracted all the leverage possible from a cautious prime minister and recalcitrant cabinet colleagues. It was time to act now or not for a long time, Martin told Frost, who agreed to cogitate on the matter. Which the premier did for some time, before coming around.

Martin, sensing that Ontario was swinging onside and having cajoled other reluctant provincial governments, presented the Hospital Insurance and Diagnostic Services Act to Parliament, both because he believed passionately in it and because its appearance there would force provincial hands. In the House, the CCF of course expressed delight. The Progressive Conservatives, too, thought the time had come for public hospitalization. The House passed the bill unanimously. So did the Senate. A giant step toward full public health care was taken. One by one the provinces came onside. In 1957, when the hospital bill passed, provinces were much weaker than they later became. They accepted conditions that today's provinces would never allow in a more decentralized federation. In exchange for the federal cash, they accepted detailed reporting to Ottawa about how they were spending the money, and whether they were adhering to the principle of "uniform terms and conditions" for all citizens, which accounted for everything from hospital construction to the tables and chairs inside. The number of hospital beds more than doubled from the time before the bill to when medicare was extended to physicians' services. Patients who might have been financially hurt without public hospital care were spared the burden and fear.

Leslie Frost had raised the important issue of home care. By excluding federal funding for home care, provincial governments rushed to build more hospitals, thereby designing a health-care delivery system top-heavy with hospitals but light on less expensive ways of providing care, which is exactly where Canada remains more than half a century later. As for Paul Martin Sr., he enjoyed the justified satisfaction of seeing what he had worked so hard to achieve in law spread in practice across the country. While the provinces were signing on to his hospitalization program, however, the Liberal government was defeated in the 1957 election. Martin could only watch from the opposition as the Diefenbaker government rolled out his program. Martin did many other things in public life as an opposition MP and cabinet minister, winding up in the early 1980s as Canada's high commissioner to Great Britain. It is doubtful that anything he did touched more people than public hospitalization.

It was shocking enough for the Liberals to yield to a Diefenbaker minority in 1957. Less than a year later, Diefenbaker's Progressive Conservatives flattened them en route to the then-largest majority in Canadian history. The Liberals had been in power for twenty-two uninterrupted years. Opposition was for others; now it was for them. Opposition turned out, somewhat unexpectedly, to be a particularly productive time for the Liberals. Of course, they harried the PCs in the House, as opposition parties are supposed to do. But they spent creative time reflecting on what they would do when in power again. They had a new leader, Lester Pearson, a neophyte in electoral politics pulled from the diplomatic service, with a Nobel Prize to his name. They had new blood: Tom Kent, the British immigrant-cum-newspaper editor who brought his *Manchester Guardian* liberalism to the prime minister's office as policy adviser; Walter Gordon, the nationalist businessman from Toronto; Keith Davey, the ebullient radio man and dedicated progressive whose credo was always that the Liberals would win elections by running from the left; the flamboyant Judy LaMarsh breaking a path for women.

John F. Kennedy had defeated Richard Nixon in the 1960 U.S. presidential election. That victory encouraged Liberals to dream that perhaps something similar might happen in Canada, especially since the Diefenbaker government, led by its mercurial, bombastic prime minister, was beginning its slow implosion. If modern liberalism was to have political meaning in the 1960s, the new crop of Liberals believed, it could not just be by the managerial politics that the party had long practised but by an expanded state giving more opportunity to more citizens.

The Liberals who gathered at the Kingston conference of 1960 held many ambitions for social reform, including health care. Kingston was not a party conference at which policy resolutions were adopted; it was, rather, a kind of gathering of people interested in policy. Tom Kent, the intellectual journalist and policy adviser, was instrumental in organizing the conference. He had recommended that the party take the next logical step—logical to him, anyway—of expanding the hospitalization scheme to include doctors so that a British-style public health system would come to Canada. The next year, in 1961, the deliberations at Kingston became the focused policy debates and resolutions at the much bigger and more authoritative National Liberal Rally. It was there, with more than two thousand Liberals in attendance, that the party formally endorsed what it would finally accomplish seven years later: medicare.

The "Plan for Health" that delegates accepted promised comprehensive medical care, including drugs, financed by general taxation, not premiums, which Liberals considered regressive. At the instigation of Tom Kent, the party adopted a proposal for how to pay for the new program that, had it been adopted, would have set medicare on a very different course. Kent explained his idea in his memoirs: "Government would pay all the doctors' and druggists' bills but would make a return of the total, for each individual, which would then be included on his or her tax form as an item of income. The effect would be, of course, that people with low incomes—below the taxable level—would get all their medical attention without cost while richer people would pay the proportion that is 'fair' by the standards embodied in marginal tax rates."

Provided that the tax system was steeply progressive and people could forward-average medical expenses, should they be quite high in one year, this method of payment, he reasoned, would raise a lot of money to pay for medicare. It would, in effect, be a double burden for the better-off, since they were already paying through the income tax system for medicare; Kent's system would have had them pay again once they used the system themselves. The Rally conference endorsed this method of payment, but the party platform did not, nor did provinces when they came to negotiate medicare. The burden on middle-class earners of paying at their marginal tax rate for unexpected, expensive treatment scared plenty of Liberals, as did the complications of the idea. Kent's proposal never made it into Liberal doctrine, and therefore never became part of Canada's medicare system.

When the Liberals returned to office with a minority government in 1963, the party had become wedded to full-scale public health care. By all accounts, the Saskatchewan plan seemed to be working satisfactorily. In 1964, the first volume of the Hall Royal Commission recommended a medicare plan. Public-opinion polls suggested that Canadians were ready for the next step.

In the summer of 1965, therefore, Pearson announced at a federal–provincial conference that Ottawa would provide half the financing of provincial health plans that met four conditions. Benefits were to be for all physicians' services as a first step toward a more comprehensive health plan that would include dentistry and drugs. (Here was the dream, never realized, of a much more comprehensive public health-care model that would go beyond hospitals and physicians.) Coverage had to be universal, although provinces could decide how to reach that objective. Provincial governments would be responsible for administering the plan. (Here, again, was the seed of much future confusion, since provincial administration need not have been equated with delivery of service by provincial governments or agencies.) Benefits had to be portable—that is, transferable from one province to the next. Comprehensive, universal, government-administered, portable. Here were four of what were to become in the Canada Health Act of 1984 the five iconic principles of Canadian medicare, the fifth being accessibility or free access.

Most premiers reacted cautiously but favourably to Pearson's proposal, the exception being Social Credit Premier Ernest Manning of Alberta, who vigorously attacked the idea as socialism by another name. The 1965 election, which the Liberals won with another disappointing minority, forestalled immediate action. When health-care debates resumed, those inside the Liberal Party were as intense as those between Ottawa and the provinces.

The Pearson minority governments were immensely creative, despite Progressive Conservatives' harrying over real or imagined scandals, internal recriminations about not having won a majority, tempestuous relations with provinces, the upsurge of Quebec nationalism and the federal caucus's own internal divisions. These divisions were presided over with diplomatic skills but a sometimes-unsteady hand by Pearson. After the 1965 election, Walter Gordon resigned from cabinet as finance minister, rather melodramatically accepting responsibility for having advised Pearson to call a precipitate election that the Liberals did not win with a majority. His replacement, Mitchell Sharp, shared neither Gordon's preference for economic nationalism nor his commitment to expanding social programs. When Gordon left the finance portfolio, and Judy LaMarsh was transferred from health and welfare, the cabinet lost two of its most ardent pro-medicare supporters. After the government settled into the post-election period, there were different players in key portfolios as cabinet and caucus debate resumed about medicare.

Provinces, too, had been given time to consider their positions. Ontario's PC government moved into steadfast opposition, and the Quebec government balked because that province intended to create its own public health-care system.

The original hope of those Liberals who wanted fast action was to push legislation through Parliament so the law would come into force on July 1, 1967, thus draping the health-care plan in the new Canadian flag. But Mitchell Sharp began fretting about the costs, the potential nervousness of foreign investors over the additional government spending and the threat of inflation. He suggested that given economic uncertainty, perhaps the whole scheme should be delayed. He said so to the press, creating headlines and shocking colleagues. Judy LaMarsh, for one, was furious. She had always believed that Sharp opposed medicare. "During the whole of Walter Gordon's term as Finance minister, there was subtle opposition from Sharp ...," she wrote later. "He always prefaced his arguments against proceeding with the caveat that he was really in favour of Medicare himself. No one ever believed him." In her acid portrait, LaMarsh added that Sharp was "probably the worst finance minister of recent years." Allan MacEachen, LaMarsh's successor at health and welfare, talked of resigning, as did Jean Marchand, a new minister from Quebec. For MacEachen, medicare had been a personal cause since 1950, when, at St. Francis Xavier University in Nova Scotia, he had participated in a broadcast debate in favour of public health insurance against the head of the Canadian Medical Association. When he took the health portfolio, it seemed a good fit, although as he reflected in his memoirs, "What I did not foresee was what a 'hot potato' I had been handed, and the anger, frustration and disappointment I would experience along the way."

Walter Gordon, freed from the conventions of cabinet solidarity, undertook a speaking tour, saying publicly, "I am not happy about the decision to postpone Medicare. The argument that Medicare should be put off in order to combat inflation will not stand up upon reflection." Sharp, for his part, later recalled that "it was only the timing of the introduction of Medicare that concerned me as minister of finance. I believed in a federal-provincial system of Medicare and I wanted to see it in effect throughout the country." It was just that adding "hundreds of millions of dollars" would be inflationary and might shake international investors' confidence in the Canadian economy. The debate around his proposal for delay, according to his recollection, was "bitter and divisive."

To this internal disarray, compounded by incessant leaks to the press by different factions, was added federal–provincial confusion. The federal government had said it would provide half the money for provincial programs that met the four conditions, but what if provinces decided against participating? Ontario, Alberta and Quebec appeared determined not to participate. All provinces, as is their wont, demanded more money and assurances of future payment from Ottawa. The economy was softening, too, with the actual deficit for 1966–67 being three times higher than had been forecast, and the one for 1967–68 five times greater than had been predicted. Angry provinces, dissident Liberals and a softening economy brought matters to a head inside the Liberal caucus. To delay or not to delay became the issue, and it was resolved, sort of, by Pearson, who sided with those wishing to proceed. Find someone else to be your leader, he told the caucus, if you want medicare delayed indefinitely. He could accept a one-year delay, given the economic circumstances, but that was all. And that was it, a compromise of sorts between the prime minister and his minister of finance that a delay would occur but only for one year.

Allan MacEachen was unimpressed. He felt that Pearson had been altogether too passive in advancing medicare. He had been given a meeting with Pearson during which he urged no delay, and had followed up with a letter at the end of which he threatened that if the bill were abandoned "it would be almost impossible for me to continue in this job and put myself forward as a believable Minister of National Health and Welfare." Years earlier, Paul Martin Sr. had threatened to resign because of Liberal shilly-shallying over health care. Now, another minister was doing the same.

Cabinet meetings were acrimonious, but the decision was finally reached to delay implementation until July 1, 1968, without the cabinet splitting publicly. MacEachen did not resign but steered the act through the House, after an amendment from the NDP to retain the original July 1, 1967, starting date was defeated.

Provinces, eagerly or reluctantly, joined the scheme, the lure of federal cash proving irresistible even to the recalcitrant. Saskatchewan (naturally) and British Columbia joined right away and began receiving their federal payments. Between 1969 and 1972, Newfoundland, Nova Scotia, Manitoba, Alberta, Ontario, Quebec, Prince Edward Island, New Brunswick, the Northwest Territories and Yukon signed up in that order. An inspiring and noble scheme of public health care for all had taken shape in a decade when Canada seemed to have come alive as a country. Medicare was part of the energetic, all-things-are possible zeit-geist. Its opponents were vanquished: the medical professions and insurance companies, the provincial governments with their aversions to public health care, the business community with its

worries, the critics of socialism. Set aloft on the highest of expectations, medicare would be supported financially by revenues
from an economy whose strong growth would go on forever and
a new tax that the Pearson government introduced on incomes.
These confident assumptions were soon shattered.

SIX

The Canada Health Act

Canadians wanted what Emmett Hall called his "medicare baby," even if the medical profession and some provincial premiers did not. Ontario's premier, John Robarts, for example, had declared that "medicare is a glowing example of a Machiavellian scheme that is in my humble opinion one of the greatest political frauds that has been perpetrated on the people of this country." But when Yukon joined medicare in April 1972, Canada finally had a universal health-care system for "all essential services," those delivered by doctors and in hospitals. The medicare idea had triumphed over private insurance supplemented by public coverage, social insurance, direct patient payment of all or some costs, a parallel private system.

Each of the three political parties could claim parentage of medicare. The NDP pointed to the introduction of medicare in Saskatchewan by its precursor party, the CCF. The Liberals boasted that they had introduced medicare under the Pearson government. The Progressive Conservatives noted that their prime minister, John Diefenbaker, had appointed Emmett Hall's Royal Commission. All-party parentage has contributed to medicare's enduring grip.

Medicare's parliamentary birth was easy—all-party approval, followed by provincial and territorial acceptance. The postpartum period, however, proved unexpectedly acrimonious. The "baby" had barely arrived when squabbling erupted among those charged with caring for it.

Medicare emerged in the 1960s as part of a series of impressive social programs that included the Canada and Quebec Pension Plans and the Canada Assistance Plan for social welfare. With medicare, they formed a trio of social policy accomplishments. Those who negotiated the programs, and the citizens who wanted them, assumed that the economic conditions of the time would continue — strong growth, low unemployment and inflation, a solid fiscal position for governments. The Great Depression was a fading memory. People remembered the boom decade of the 1950s and national accomplishments of the 1960s: the Canadian flag, Expo 67, Pierre Trudeau's arrival as prime minister in 1968. The future, it was assumed, would be much like the recent past, bright and munificent, so new revenues from economic growth would cover the additional spending that governments incurred for these new programs. That assumption had underpinned the Hall Royal Commission's projections about the financing of medicare. Events many thousands of kilometres away soon blasted that assumption.

Egyptian and Syrian armies simultaneously attacked Israel on Saturday, October 6, 1973, thereby launching what became known as the Yom Kippur War. Ten days into the war, buoyed by early Israeli setbacks, and angry at U.S. resupplies of armaments to Israel, Arab oil ministers imposed an immediate 17 percent increase in the price of oil. The next day, they announced production cuts and embargoes against countries that "demonstrate moral and material support to the Israeli enemy." One by one, Arab states with oil imposed a complete embargo on the United

States. Two months after the war, the price of oil had quadrupled. Oil prices never returned to their pre-war levels.

The Yom Kippur War and its consequences turned the 1970s upside down economically. A prolonged period of "stagflation" arrived, a previously unknown and deadening combination of skyrocketing inflation, slow growth and high unemployment. By 1975, the federal budget had moved from surplus to deficit. The deficit began modestly but kept growing, then exploded in the recession of 1981–82 and remained extremely large throughout the 1980s. Deficits were eliminated only in the mid-1990s, two decades after they began. Almost as soon as medicare arrived, therefore, the assumptions about how to pay for it were shattered. The creators of medicare had not anticipated, nor had anyone, stagflation.

The federal budget was balanced when the Liberals first planned medicare in the late 1960s. Inflation stood at 2.4 percent and unemployment at 3 percent in 1968. In the 1972–82 period, by contrast, the federal deficit exploded from $2 billion to $30 billion, or from 1.7 percent of gross domestic product to 7.6 percent. Inflation jumped from 4.8 percent to 10.9 percent, unemployment from 6 percent to 11 percent. By 1975, health-care costs were rising 15 percent a year. By 1980, health-care budgets were still soaring 16 percent a year. From 1981 to 1984, they rose 9 to 10 percent a year. Put another way, health care (public and private) consumed $12 billion in 1975, but $36 billion in 1984—of which the public share rose from $9 billion to $27 billion.

Health-care costs were rising faster than government revenues. Burdened with swelling deficits, Ottawa and the provinces faced fiscal circumstances that they had not imagined at the birth of medicare. They were being forced, and not just for health care, to find economies in this nasty world of stagflation. Doctors had been dragged into medicare, and at least some practitioners longed for bygone days. The three attendants of the medicare baby—two levels of government and the medical professions—began quarrelling over money, or the lack of it. Their quarrels included acrimonious ministerial meetings, accusations of bad faith, new financial arrangements, threatened or actual withdrawal of services by doctors and a national debate over user fees and extra-billing that would ultimately produce the Canada Health Act. That act would become the brightest of all the health-care icons; untouchable yet widely misunderstood, of limited practical use yet possessed of immense political significance, a straitjacket and an inspiration.

The Canada Health Act might not have happened without the persistence and passion of Monique Bégin. She made many contributions to Canadian public life, but Bégin will be most remembered as the architect of an act of immense symbolism but limited effect.

Monique Bégin had never considered entering politics. She was born to a family of modest means but developed a passion for reading, managed to get a bachelor's degree and eventually completed most of a doctorate in sociology at the Sorbonne in Paris. She didn't have the money, however, to finish the degree, so she returned to Montreal, where she worked at a research institute and became first president of the Quebec Federation of Women. She was attractive, brainy and personable.

At this stage of her busy life, to her complete surprise, she received a call from Marc Lalonde, then a senior adviser to Prime Minister Lester Pearson, asking her to become a commissioner on the Royal Commission on the Status of Women. She declined but did inquire about the chief staff job at the commission. Months passed, during which dozens of men were interviewed for the

Health care had never been her specialty. Pensions, the role of women and income support animated her. She had served four years of apprenticeship on the backbenches before becoming minister of national revenue for a year, and then she became minister of health and welfare. Even then, she was preoccupied not with health care but with welfare policy, pensions and income support. In the late 1970s, events changed her priorities. Medicare was under assault.

With inflation rising and deficits increasing, provincial governments faced a health-care dilemma for the first but by no means final time. They could raise taxes to pay for the unexpectedly higher costs of health care, but they balked in the face of likely public wrath and a sluggish economy. They could let health-care costs rise faster than inflation and watch their deficits expand. Or, since hospitals and doctors were by far the largest cost drivers in health care, they could restrict increases for both.

Doctors' incomes had declined against inflation. Their medical associations complained that if governments were not going to fund medicare so that doctors' remuneration at least kept pace with inflation, incomes would have to be augmented by additional means. Some provinces complained that if Ottawa would not keep its transfers at least at the rate of inflation, then they would allow, even encourage, patients other than the poor and the elderly to pay a small share of their medical costs.

Premier Ross Thatcher's Liberal government of Saskatchewan in 1964 had experimented with user fees. When the NDP returned to office in 1971, the experiment ended. One solitary academic study, frequently referred to thereafter by critics of user fees, suggested that they had deterred poor people from using the system. Could user fees be brought back at a time of soaring government deficits? After the Trudeau government lifted its anti-inflation ceiling on wage increases of 6 and 5 percent, pressure intensified among doctors to recover lost income through new revenue streams, including user fees for patients. Thus began the decade-long squabble over user fees and extra-billing.

Monique Bégin passed briefly into opposition with the rest of the Liberals in 1979. In that year, 15.8 percent of doctors opted out of the Ontario Health Insurance Plan. A doctor who opted out of OHIP billed his patients at the Ontario Medical Association rate, well above government rates. They were reimbursed by the government at OHIP rates, then doctors charged patients the difference, a method called "balance billing." In Alberta, up to a quarter of the province's doctors used balance billing. In Saskatchewan, egged on by the discrepancy between rates there compared with Alberta's, up to 30 percent of doctors were making some claims for direct billing of patients.

When Bégin's Liberals returned to power in 1980, extra-billing and user fees had become part of medicare in some, but not all, provinces. These practices were strongly supported by the medical associations. Dr. Lawrence Wilson, head of the Canadian Medical Association, put the physicians' case, saying, "As long as governments choose to underfund medicare, a transfusion of money from patients will be needed to pay a part of the costs for the services of physicians and hospitals." User fees, he said, rationed care by acting as a sensible deterrent against those who would abuse the system, as well as providing doctors with a way to make up for lost income. The CMA asserted that since only 2 percent of Canada's fifty-five thousand doctors extra-billed in 1980, the impact on patients was minimal. Without better pay, by whatever means, doctors would leave Canada. The number of doctors emigrating, overwhelmingly to the United States, rose from 242 in 1975 to 363 in 1976, 549 in 1977, 663 in 1978, although the civil servant responsible for compiling the data suggested to the press that about 800 had probably left in that year. In 1978, Canada graduated 1700 new doctors, but the net gain was only about 1160 because so many were leaving.

With inflation soaring above 10 percent, Saskatchewan doctors in 1981 sought a one-year 17.5 percent increase in their fee schedule. In Alberta, doctors rejected the province's offer of a 17 percent raise and demanded 30.5 percent. The province then imposed a 21 percent increase. British Columbia doctors demanded a 41 percent increase, with improved fringe benefits and supplemental fees for work performed outside the 37.5-hour week. The B.C. government offered 15 percent. Yielding to the doctors' demands, said the government, would cost $294 million, money the government did not have. The two sides eventually settled for 40 percent over two years. In Quebec, family physicians demanded a 42 percent increase. In Ontario, the government legislated a 14.75 percent increase, a payment that a provincial arbitrator said was at the "outer limit" of the government's fiscal capacity.

By the early 1980s, the majority of physicians—and in a few cases all physicians—in certain towns or medical specialties were extra-billing. What was the big fuss about, wondered some doctors with a sense of history? In Saskatchewan, the CCF government at the advent of provincial medicare allowed what was called Mode Three Billing. It allowed doctors to practise outside the government plan and charge what they wanted. Patients could then get 85 percent of the charge back from the government plan. Could not the difference be called a form of extra-billing? If the CCF in Saskatchewan permitted this practice, why should it not exist elsewhere? And why not now, when doctors' incomes were falling?

Monique Bégin faced angry provinces and doctors when she returned to the health portfolio in 1980. She was convinced that user fees and extra-billing put some of medicare's principles at risk. Prime Minister Trudeau, unexpectedly returned to power in 1980 with a majority, had constitutional priorities that would provoke many provinces. Did the government need to pick another fight? The federalists had won the bruising referendum in Quebec in 1980 over sovereignty-association. Did they really want Ottawa to push itself back into medicare, an area of provincial jurisdiction, thereby giving the secessionists a stick with which to beat Ottawa for interfering again in provincial affairs? What authority did Ottawa have anyway over how provinces operated their health-care systems? Ottawa transferred lots of money but had limited ability to direct how provinces spent the money. Provinces guarded their jurisdiction over health (and other matters) the way dogs protect bones. It was easier to argue in theory that Ottawa should enforce national standards than to do so in practice.

At the beginning of medicare, Ottawa and the provinces had agreed to a fifty-fifty split in financing, just as they had with hospital insurance. With stagflation eroding revenues, Ottawa began to chafe at this commitment. The provinces spent what they wanted for health, hospitals (and post-secondary education), then sent a bill to Ottawa for half the amount. The Trudeau government, watching its fiscal situation deteriorate, unilaterally limited the growth in transfers to 14 percent per capita in 1976–77, 12 percent in 1977–78 and 8 percent in 1978–79—below the yearly rates of inflation.

Arduous negotiations climaxed with a new deal that satisfied each side. Ottawa would no longer pay fifty cents on the dollar. Instead, it yielded "tax points" on personal and business income taxes to the provinces, along with a smaller yearly cash transfer adjusted for provinces' ability to raise their own revenues. Ottawa disengaged itself from monitoring provincial spending, since the provinces were now raising most of the money for health care. A greater degree of predictability would be introduced into federal finances, and the provinces would get Ottawa out of their hair. If the provinces were responsible for raising more of the revenue for health care, they would be more vigorous in restraining costs. That was the theory. Predictably, the ink had barely dried on the Established Programs Financing Act (EPF) of 1978 when the two levels of government resumed squabbling.

Ottawa had agreed not to change the EPF formula for five years. But with deficits accumulating, the Trudeau government began unilaterally reducing its transfers under the EPF, beginning in the 1982 budget. (Further reductions occurred in the Mulroney government budgets of 1986, 1989, 1990 and 1991.)

The EPF negotiations had been stickhandled by the prime minister and the finance minister, Marc Lalonde, Bégin's mentor and predecessor as health minister. Although extra-billing and user fees had appeared, the new act seemed to hand dealing with them to the provinces. While in opposition in 1979, however, Bégin had joined health- and social-policy activists at conferences to "save medicare." She participated in the SOS Medicare Conference in early November 1979 that spawned the pro-medicare lobby group, the Canadian Health Coalition. A month later, the utterly unexpected happened. The Clark government, elected in June 1979, lost a parliamentary vote of confidence and the subsequent election in 1980. Bégin's Liberals were back in power, she again as health and welfare minister.

As Bégin pondered her strategy, she received a huge boost from an old warrior. While the party was briefly in power, PC health minister David Crombie had been pestered by critics who insisted that the government had ignored the erosion of medicare. Bégin herself had accused Crombie of lacking "guts" by refusing to withdraw federal money from provinces that did not abide by the principles of medicare. She claimed (wrongly, as she later discovered) that the provinces were diverting federal funds for health to other purposes. Crombie, therefore, reached for an old tactic when uncertain how to act: ask for another study. Crombie chose as commissioner none other than Emmett Hall, then eighty-one years old, whose national eminence as the "father of medicare" was such that even the provinces had to mute their habitual mewling. Crombie asked Hall to review the state of the system, whether any changes were required and if the principles he had outlined in his 1964 Royal Commission were being upheld— portability, reasonable access, universal coverage, comprehensive coverage, reasonable compensation. Ottawa specifically wanted his answer to two questions. Were provinces diverting federal transfers from health care toward other priorities? Did extra-billing by physicians and user charges violate the principle of "reasonable access"?

Hall held hearings across the country and received a staggering 450 briefs. Hall's answer to Ottawa's first specific question was, no, the provinces were not diverting money, despite Bégin's insistence to the contrary. His second answer was, yes, extra-billing and user fees did threaten medicare. Asking Emmett Hall about such practices was akin to asking the Almighty if sin without remorse and atonement were acceptable, because Hall had declared himself firmly on the subject in his Royal Commission. There, he had written that doctors should largely be paid on a fee-for-service basis, "but extra-billing would not be permitted." He repeated the argument in this 1980 review, stating that "if extra-billing is permitted as a right and practiced by physicians in their sole discretion, it will, over the years, destroy the program, creating in that downward path a two-tier system incompatible with the societal level which Canadians have attained."

"Two-tier." That expression would wind through all subsequent debates about medicare. Two-tier suggested that any deviation from the established practices of medicare would lead toward the abandonment of universal access and social equality and, worse, U.S.-style health care. A doctor, Hall wrote, could opt entirely out of medicare and practice privately but would not be eligible for any public payments—the model Quebec had adopted from the start for its health-care system. Doctors, in losing the right to extra-bill, nonetheless deserved compensation compatible with their years of training and skills. This was what Hall called a Gordian knot. It remains tied today: How much should physicians receive from the public purse commensurate with their training and skills?

Monique Bégin could have asked for no more powerful voice than Emmett Hall's. David Crombie, catapulted back into opposition, said he would accept Hall's recommendations, although not all PC MPs agreed with him. The NDP were all smiles, of course. Initial provincial reaction was muted, perhaps in deference to Hall's status. Medical associations, however, held nothing back. The head of the Ontario Medical Association said a ban on extra-billing would be the "total conscription of the profession." Doctors would be come "civil servants working for the government, not their patients." The head of the B.C. Medical Association dismissed Hall's concerns that extra-billing would discriminate between rich and poor as a "socialist concept that comes through in a socialist report ... Hospitals treat people equally more than any other segment of society. Just look at the hospitals. We have the low-class people who aren't taking care of themselves." Marc Baltzan, head of the CMA and son of a physician-member of the Hall Royal Commission, responded, "Doctors will be part of a monolithic state enterprise. Bureaucrats will dictate how medicine ought to be practiced." The Medical Reform Group of Ontario, representing about 250 doctors committed to defending medicare, praised the report for recommending the end to extra-billing.

This medical group aside, Hall's report did not persuade medical associations or provincial governments that allowed or were contemplating extra-billing and user fees. Nor did Bégin find enthusiasm for action inside the civil service. The finance department, having negotiated the EPF, opposed stirring up federal–provincial tensions. Her own department dreaded more provincial confrontations. No longer in the business of closely monitoring provincial spending on health care, the department was not keen to resume the job.

The Trudeau government found itself beset by problems on all sides in 1981. The country was in a foul mood. Constitutional negotiations were acrimonious. The National Energy Program inflamed Alberta–Ottawa relations. A postal strike dragged on. Interest rates exceeded 20 percent. René Lévesque and the Parti Québécois lost the 1980 referendum but were re-elected in 1981, meaning more endemic tension between Quebec City and Ottawa. The Ottawa elixir of more money to soothe provincial discontent was unavailable, because the federal deficit exploded in recessionary times. Every time Bégin criticized extra-billing and user fees, a volley of denunciations came back from the medical associations and some of the provinces. The NDP in Parliament, the trade unions and other ardent defenders of medicare accused her of waffling and inaction; the defenders of user fees and extra-billing accused her of planning draconian changes. Bégin admits in her book about the Canada Health Act, "I did not know what to do about Medicare." Throughout 1982, the Liberals' popularity skidded ten points. She admits, "The year 1982 ended in

a muddle, a quasi-fiasco." Despite the troubles, she was determined to proceed. But how?

Federal–provincial meetings were especially difficult. "The
finance ministers of Canada called me in and blasted me," she
recalls. "How can I fight the finance ministers? I am the only
woman, and I'm a French Canadian, which doesn't help. The
premiers called me in at an awful meeting. So from a political
point of view, it was very, very, very disagreeable." When she
tried to be strong, it emboldened one group of adversaries; when
she tried to be accommodating, the NDP leader, Ed Broadbent,
demanded in the Commons that she resign. All this verbal conflict
unfolded in a media full of stories about the "crisis" in medicare.

Monique Bégin decided to take her case on the road. She
assembled a trio of advisers in the department whom she
called the "three musketeers," created a pool of departmental
money and offered funding to any organization that wanted to
hold a public discussion about medicare. Meetings sprang up
across the country. Bégin attended as many of them as possible,
following Trudeau's strategy of appealing over the heads of the
premiers and interest groups directly to the Canadian people.
After months on the road, and interminable meetings with the
recalcitrant health ministers, Bégin again felt that she needed
prime-ministerial guidance. She asked her officials for a breakdown of where every provincial health minister stood on every
aspect of the issue. She wanted a list of which groups favoured
extra-billing and user fees and which did not. A civil servant who
helped prepare the list called it a "stoplight chart," all red, yellow
and green, depending on the group and its attitude. Many of the
provinces and medical associations were a red or red and yellow;
the consumer groups, nurses unions, health activists were green.

Armed with this information, Bégin remembers that "one day I went to Trudeau's desk after Question Period. I got down on one knee beside him and I said, 'Prime Minister, I just don't know where to go with Medicare any more.' He asked, 'Who is in favour and who is against?' I said all the provinces are against. All of organized medicine. He asked, 'Where is the public?' I said the public was in favour. He said, 'Then it's a sure win.' It gave me the signal that the Boss was in favour."

For Trudeau, federal action would offer another example of Ottawa asserting its constitutional authority, instead of allowing the federal government to become, as he once said of Progressive Conservative leader Joe Clark's view of Ottawa, a "head waiter" to the premiers. Not for him a "community of communities" Canada but a country with a strong federal government. Bégin needed the prime minister's "signal" to move the bureaucracy and influence cabinet in order to continue her appeal past the premiers to their citizens who rallied to the call to "save" medicare. An additional push came from legal opinions from the justice department and from three outside legal experts that the legislation Ottawa contemplated would be within the federal government's constitutional "spending power." A parliamentary committee under Liberal MP Herb Breau from New Brunswick agreed that medicare's principles were indeed threatened, and Ottawa should act.

Federal legislation already gave Ottawa the option of withholding *all* federal transfers in the event of provincial transgressions. Bégin concluded that Ottawa needed a scalpel, not a hammer. Various formulas were examined to penalize provinces for the amounts of extra-billing and user fees they permitted—for example, $3 withdrawn by Ottawa for every $1 of extra-billing and user fees—before Bégin settled on $1 for $1. "I always had the idea," she recalls, "that it had to be very simple, and very clear. One for one."

The Canada Health Act that eventually became a Canadian legislative icon did not seem that way to a lot of Liberal ministers. It took six months for cabinet to approve the act. During that period, Bégin was often angry at the hesitations, roadblocks and demands for new "communications strategies." Trudeau said very little about the issue when it came before cabinet. Allan MacEachen, the taciturn deputy prime minister, also said little but gave the impression that he was opposed, an odd position for someone who prided himself on being among the Liberals who pushed hardest for medicare. Ministers were nervous about public opinion, given the battering the government was taking on so many fronts. Bégin's own department estimated in 1983 that extra-billing amounted to about $100 million a year, a tiny fraction of the total public spending on health care. Was that sum large enough to worry about, some ministers wondered?

Bégin asked her department to commission a massive poll of six thousand Canadians. It arrived in June 1983 and revealed that respondents rejected extra-billing and user fees and by majorities of 70 to 80 percent. The poll confirmed what political pros around the prime minister sniffed: an issue to take to the people in the next election campaign. The Liberals would portray themselves as the defenders of medicare, whereas the PCs could not be entrusted with that responsibility. A white paper was published explaining the government's intentions, further testimony to nervousness about public reaction. It argued, "We cannot preserve Medicare by charging the sick; we cannot preserve Medicare by judging who is poor and who is not; we can only preserve Medicare by ensuring its basic principles."

Furious reaction greeted the white paper. There were full-page newspaper advertisements paid for by the medical associations, verbal assaults from irate provincial ministers, cries of federal intrusion into provincial jurisdiction from the Parti

Québécois government. The proposed bill was called a "political ploy to prop up Liberal support" (Newfoundland health minister Wallace House), a "delightful piece of window dressing that will complicate the Medicare system," (B.C. health minister Jim Nielsen), "the whole thing is a sham," (Ontario finance minister Larry Grossman). At a federal–provincial meeting in the fall of 1983, Bégin was roasted by almost all the provincial health ministers.

Bégin went to see Pierre Trudeau. For only the second time in her ministerial career, she asked for a one-on-one with the prime minister. "Trudeau appointed me. He never said the times are such and such, and we should do this or avoid that," she recalls later. "Never. He was not interested. He was interested in the philosophy of it [health care]—the values but absolutely not the administration of it. He assumed that everything had been fixed with the 1977 EPF agreement. He had been sold that bill of goods ... In my abrupt way, which is my way, I said, 'Boss, are you in favour of or against Medicare'?" Trudeau said that of course he was for it, but he preferred that the money Ottawa collected for penalties against provinces be refunded directly to those who had been extra-billed or subjected to a user fee. A cheque arriving directly from Ottawa would reinforce the federal presence in the minds of citizens.

Another spoke had just been put in the grinding wheels of Ottawa machinery. Hurriedly, the health department put together a paper showing how the prime minister's idea would be cumbersome and costly to administer. Trudeau backed down, but time was spent considering this option. Finally, almost at the end of 1983, with all the legal objections canvassed, public opinion consulted by polls, departmental hesitations overcome, the last efforts to persuade provinces exhausted, the prime minister's option discarded, Bégin had her bill ready for Parliament.

In retrospect, for those who do not know the history, it seems incredible that the Canada Health Act should have been so long in gestation. Another health minister, possessed of less passion, resilience and determination, might never have pushed past the obstacles that Monique Bégin did.

In Parliament, the only political question swirled around the position of the PCs. The Liberals were all on side, as were the New Democrats. The bill would easily pass, but would the PCs agree? In their caucus lurked plenty of MPs who approved of extra-billing and user fees or who cringed at disagreeing with PC provincial governments where such practices existed. They were brought to heel by their new leader, Brian Mulroney, who saw the potential political trap yawning for his party in opposing a bill so popular with Canadians. As Mulroney recounts in his memoirs, "Doctors, who are essentially small business owners, were traditionally among our party's strongest supporters. The Liberals figured that we'd revert to our old ways and implode on this issue, to find ourselves yet again on the wrong side of a key public issue. To be sure, extra-billing was a live grenade for us." Bégin had told fellow Quebec cabinet members that Mulroney's political instincts would lead him to support the bill. She was right. The Canada Health Act passed without a dissenting vote.

For legislation subsequently imbued with such importance, the Canada Health Act is modest in size and intent. It runs to only thirteen pages, small by parliamentary standards, with several pages taken up by definitions. It's hard to imagine anyone being inspired by the formal title: "An Act relating to cash contributions by Canada in respect of insured health services provided under provincial health-care insurance plans and amounts payable by Canada in respect of extended health care services." The act outlines medicare's five principles, the ones at the centre of all debates about health care in Canada: public administration, comprehensiveness, universality, portability, accessibility. Each is subject to interpretation.

For example, public administration is defined such that the "health insurance plan of a province must be administered on a non-profit basis by a public authority or designated by the government of the province." It continues that the "public authority must be responsible to the provincial government." An agency designated by the province can "receive on its behalf any amounts payable under the provincial health plan," provided that the accounts are "subject to assessment and approval by the public authority and that the public authority shall determine the amounts paid." In other words, "public administration" can mean a public agency delivering and paying the costs of health care directly. Or, the government can "designate" another body, such as a private company or private institution or privately incorporated entity (a group of doctors in a clinic, say) to provide the service and be paid by the "public authority."

Much confusion has surrounded these words, because *public administration* has come to mean that only the government or someone directly employed by a public agency can deliver medical care, whereas what the Canada Health Act actually says is that health care has to be administered and paid for publicly, on a non-profit basis, but delivery by whom and how remains flexible. This misunderstanding has done much to choke off debate about the methods of delivery of health care, with defenders of the status quo insisting, wrongly, on a narrow definition that is not consistent with the wording of the act.

Further evidence of the correct interpretation is provided by an "interpretation manual" prepared by senior officials in Bégin's department but never made public before this book. The manual was written to provide the most comprehensive interpretation of the different clauses of the act for federal officials. Dated July 5, 1984, it says that the act "cannot be interpreted to mean that services cannot be provided on a 'for profit' basis. It simply states that the organization, commission, or agency that administers the provincial plan cannot record a profit on its operation." Later, the manual states, "The Act cannot be interpreted to mean that medical practitioners are precluded from making a profit or that hospitals providing publicly-insured health services cannot run a surplus or must be publicly owned and operated."

Put matters another way. From the beginning of medicare in Saskatchewan, doctors successfully fought for fee-for-service payment as private professionals working for themselves but within the public system and paid for by the public system. Their associations negotiated fee schedules with provincial governments, and they were paid according to the services delivered. And yet, if physicians band together in a clinic that operates privately, which then sells services to the government at standard negotiated rates, this can cause a political firestorm, as critics clamour that such a clinic dilutes medicare, pushes public health care toward private, "two-tier" (Emmett Hall's famous phrase) medicine. A misunderstanding of the Canada Health Act has become a straitjacket for medicare. The correct interpretation of the act, at least from those who wrote it and were charged with its implementation, is the one contained in the federal government's own manual, which, to repeat, has never been made public.

Or consider portability. Canadians can and do receive treatment out of province in Canada. But it is not necessarily true that provinces will pay, as required, the rates of another province. Section 10 of the act gives Quebec the power to opt out of paying rates of other plans for Quebec citizens who might need health care outside the province. The clause says the "prior consent" of Quebec must be sought before a person can reclaim from the Quebec plan the higher rates charged elsewhere. This consent will not be given if "the services in question were available on a substantially similar basis in the province." In effect, this means Quebec will not pay the higher rates of other provinces, except in cases of emergency.

The principle of accessibility is safeguarded, in theory, by giving the federal government the power of dollar-for-dollar withdrawal from federal transfers any monies collected from extra-billing and user fees. That threat of automatic penalties sufficed to stop the two practices. One after another, provinces decided they could not afford to lose any money from Ottawa. At the end of three years following the Canada Health Act, penalties of $245 million had been levied, $134 million for extra-billing, $111 million for user fees. These penalties were returned to the seven provinces when they ended these practices. The scalpel, in other words, did its work.

The act incorporated the previous federal power to withhold *all* its transfers to a province that allowed any practices that contravened the five principles of medicare. The federal minister would decide what those offending practices were, initiate negotiations with the province and, if these failed, get cabinet approval for a penalty against the province. Occasionally, federal ministers of health (Liberal mostly) threatened to use this hammer clause against a province that allowed private payment within medicare, but only small measures were ever taken after the $245 million had been returned to provinces that stopped extra-billing and user fees.

Diane Marleau, federal health minister in 1995, wrote a stern letter to provinces denouncing "facility fees" being charged by private clinics. These fees, she argued, constituted a barrier for entry into the clinics. They were a kind of user fee and, as such, offended the Canada Health Act. She gave the provinces nine months to end the practice, after which she would start deducting transfer payments. She feared that private clinics would lessen the ability of governments to control costs, scoop up "easy procedures," leaving more difficult, costly cases for the public sector and draw practitioners away from the public system. She demanded that provinces put in place "regulatory frameworks to govern the operation of private clinics." Ottawa did withhold small sums from four provinces, the largest penalty being levied against Alberta, for these private fee-paying private clinics, then the practice died out. Later, her successor as health minister, Allan Rock, hurled various threats at the provinces, but the threats melted away and no action was taken.

The Canada Health Act therefore met its goal. It dealt with certain practices that had cropped up within the first decade of medicare. It was never really intended to do more, although the act has been invested with an ambition it could not carry in practice, as Monique Bégin acknowledged long after the fact.

The Mulroney Progressive Conservatives' arrival in office in 1984 seemed to answer some provincial prayers. Alberta minister David Russell, always a hardline adversary, said he would change Bégin's mind by getting "her out of office. That's what we're going to do in Alberta." Keith Norton, his Ontario colleague, called the act "one of the darkest moments" of Confederation. He declared himself eager to talk about scrapping it with the new PC minister, Jake Epp. They were deluding themselves. Mulroney had laid down the PC line. He would not move from it during nine years as prime minister.

The Ontario Medical Association, supported by the Canadian Medical Association, launched a constitutional challenge against the Canada Health Act in 1986. It ground slowly through the courts and was abandoned by the CMA in 1991. Pockets of resistance kept fighting. In 1986, Ontario doctors went on strike against legislation that banned extra-billing. The president of the OMA vowed that he would go to jail to fight "the kind of law that would not be expected outside the Iron Curtain." The strike fizzled in the face of government's refusal to budge, widespread negative media opinion and overwhelming public opposition to the doctors' position. In 1989, David Martin, president of Toronto's Hospital for Sick Children, said user fees for hospital patients were necessary to pay for new equipment, higher salaries to nurses and to shorten wait times. "I don't see another solution out there in the long term. To many politicians, the idea of co-payments is a bitter pill, but it may be one that has to be swallowed. Provinces were spending 30 percent of their budgets on health care, and they cannot spend a higher share." He was wrong on both counts: no politician wished to swallow user fees, and the share of health-care spending in provincial budgets rose from 30 percent to more than 40 percent in the next twenty years.

The Canada Health Act solved a specific problem. It was a targeted fiscal act only, with limited application. But it reiterated the principles of medicare and so became a rallying cry for medicare's defenders. It did not prevent the trickling spread of private medical care. And it could not—nothing apparently could—stop the remorseless increase in the costs of medicare that would vex provincial governments and Ottawa, and cause both to launch yet another round of studies and commissions in the 1990s to diagnose what ailed medicare and how to fix it.

PART THREE

SEVEN

How Good Is Medicare?

How good is the Canadian health-care system four decades after medicare's arrival, and five decades after public health care came to Saskatchewan? The short answer is that the system is good, but not as good as it could be. Nor is it as good as it should be, given the amount Canadians spend, nor as good as we think it to be, nor as good as we will need it to be as the population ages.

Like a physician examining a patient, government after government created commissions or task forces over the past two decades to probe the system. They all discovered Canadians' strong commitment to public health care. One task force, in Alberta under the leadership of former Progressive Conservative deputy prime minister Don Mazankowski, recommended some private delivery of essential services outside medicare. So did a study by a former Quebec health minister, Claude Castonguay. Yet another, by Michel Clair, also a former Quebec health minister, recommended private delivery of publicly financed services. An exhaustive five-volume inquiry under Senator Michael Kirby concurred with Clair's thinking. These variations to medicare were almost completely rejected by governments. They preferred the inside-the-box mindset of making the existing system work more efficiently, a mindset that framed an inquiry in Saskatchewan under Kenneth Fyke, a former deputy minister of health in Saskatchewan and British Columbia, in 2001 and, of course, the national commission under Roy Romanow. Despite the probing and recommendations of these commissions, it is remarkable how little medicare changed.

Canadians are often told by their politicians that they have the best health-care system in the world. The Romanow commission claimed, for example, that "Canada's health system compares well with those of other wealthy industrialized countries." Alas, comparative international evidence does not support the claim.

The claim rests mostly on a comparison of the Canadian and U.S. systems that are at opposite extremes of how to organize and finance health care. No country relies as much on the private sector for health care as the United States; no country squeezes out the private sector for medically necessary services more than Canada. Using aggregate comparisons—health-care outcomes versus money spent, or value for money, if you like—the Canadian system wins the bilateral contest hands down. The United States spends about one-half more of its national income on health care than Canada—slightly less than 18 percent of GDP versus 11.7 percent—but does not get better aggregate health-care outcomes. From this Canada–U.S. comparison, Canadians derive their misplaced moral superiority about health care. Moving beyond the Canada–U.S. comparison reveals that Canadian medicare is far from being the best system in the world, in large part because medicare remains a top-down, very bureaucratic, hospital-heavy system that remains much more resistant to competition in the provision of health care than all the other largely public health-care systems.

All international comparisons have limitations. It is sometimes hard to compare one country's data with another's. Countries benchmark their systems and collect information differently. Some surveys are inevitably subjective, asking patients and providers for their impressions and opinions. Sometimes the differences in ranking among countries are extremely small. A country can be ranked, say, seventh out of ten and actually be closer to the top than the bottom in absolute outcomes, because the gap between seventh and first is less than between seventh and tenth. Ordinal rankings can sometimes mislead.

The unreconstructed defenders of medicare debunk international comparisons, pointing out all their limitations. One suspects they also debunk them because the comparisons do not put the Canadian system in a good light. The defenders therefore spend more time deflating the comparative surveys than asking why, collectively, these comparisons reveal serious shortcomings with the Canadian model. Look at it another way. If the international comparisons, with all their limitations, put Canada at or near the top, you can bet the defenders would tell us all about the surveys.

Any system that refuses to be benchmarked against others is not one that will learn much about itself. If results from a variety of surveys, each with its own limitations, tend to show a similar pattern, a portrait emerges about where a country's health-care system stacks up. And where it stacks up should take into account how much is being spent. Excluding the United States, with its very different system, Canada ranks in the top five countries for per capita spending on health care. The rank varies sometimes from year to year, depending on actual health-care spending and economic growth, but Canada is right up there among the big spenders. If a country spends among the top five, one might expect results in the top five. No such luck.

Consider the Commonwealth Fund surveys. The fund, a U.S.-based charitable foundation that promotes quality health care, has been conducting comparative studies of health-care systems for the past decade. Its latest report, in 2010, brought together

data from 2007 to 2009 in seven advanced industrial countries—
Canada, the United States, New Zealand, Australia, Germany, the
Netherlands and Britain. The fund's studies are based on surveys
from patients' and physicians' opinions blended with hard data
from a variety of international sources. The studies therefore
represent a combination of the subjective and the more objective.
In Canada, more than three thousand persons are surveyed, a
huge sample size for such a study.

Canada stood sixth of seven countries in the Commonwealth
Fund 2010 survey, with the United States last, which meant
that of the countries with largely public health-care systems,
Canada finished at the bottom for outcomes and satisfaction.
Canada, with Germany and the Netherlands, stands at the top of
the rankings for per capita spending on health care but Canada
stands at the bottom among countries with largely public health
care for results. The Netherlands, Britain and Australia had the
best overall rankings. More alarmingly, Canada has been slipping
in the Commonwealth Fund surveys. Canada stood fourth in
the 2004 survey, fifth in 2006 and 2007 and sixth in the latest
survey. These were the years, it should be remembered, when
Canada was pouring money back into its health-care system.
These surveys suggest that the money wasn't producing better
results, at least not in comparison with what was happening in
the other public health-care systems. Canada did not even fare
well in the one area that makes Canadians feel proudest—the
equity of medicare. Comparatively speaking, Canada fared
poorly because, unlike the other public systems, it does not
supply anything approximating universal coverage for pharmaceuticals, dental care and other health-care needs not provided
in hospitals and by doctors.

In another Commonwealth Fund survey, this one involving
eleven countries and reported in 2011, Canada scored worst on all

questions related to timeliness of care. Canada came last for time waiting to see a family physician and specialists, and time spent waiting in emergency rooms. Here are some of the raw results for Canada and ten other advanced industrial countries. Canada's rank for waiting six days or more to see a doctor or nurse when sick: eleventh; difficulty of getting after-hours care without going to the emergency room: tenth; use of emergency because a doctor was unavailable: first; wait time of more than four hours in emergency: first; wait time for a specialist: first; wait time for elective surgery: first; ease of contacting a doctor during regular hours: tenth; quality of care from a doctor: fourth; failure to communicate test results: third; perception of inefficient or wasteful care: first; belief that "fundamental changes are required in the health-care system": second highest, 51 percent.

The portrait of medicare that emerges from the widely cited Commonwealth Fund surveys is of an expensive, rather insensitive and inefficient system that fares poorly when tested against health-care systems in comparable countries. Another Commonwealth Fund survey, used by the Health Council of Canada in 2010, a federal–provincial body established after the First Ministers' 2003–2004 accord to monitor progress in health care, tried to measure patients' engagement in primary care. How available were doctors? How much time did they spend with patients? How clear were communications? Canada scored at the average among eleven countries.

Four other studies should worry Canadians. A 2010 Economist Intelligence Unit survey (from the United Kingdom) called the Quality of Death Index ranked countries according to their provision of end-of-life care. Canada came ninth out of forty countries. A study reported in the Royal Society of Medicine in the United Kingdom analyzed mortality rates (defined as deaths that were medically feasible to avoid in people below seventy-five years of age) against a country's health spending to find a cost-efficiency ranking. Canada ranked eleventh out of nineteen countries.

The Euro-Canada Health Consumer Index (ECHCI), a joint project of the Health Consumer Powerhouse of Sweden and the Frontier Centre for Public Policy in Western Canada (a market-oriented think tank), studied thirty-two measurements to compare health-care performance across thirty-four countries—Canada and thirty-three in Europe. The ECHCI does not espouse moving away from a largely public health-care system toward anything like the U.S. model. It tries to evaluate performance "from the perspective of the consumer." Rather than focus on inputs—how many hospital beds, MRI machines, doctors per capita—the ECHCI tries to measure outcomes of patients and "customer friendliness" by such yardsticks as wait times, patient rights and information, and the range of services covered under public-health schemes. The yardsticks are a mixture of hard data and patient surveys.

The Canadian results are bad. Canada overall ranked twenty-fifth of thirty-four countries in the 2010 survey, having finished twenty-third of thirty-two countries surveyed in 2009. Canada stood far behind countries such as the Netherlands (first) and Germany (second) that use social insurance schemes, but also well behind Sweden (ninth) and Britain (seventeenth), two other countries that use the single-payer, Beveridge-inspired health-care system. Said the ECHCI, "What makes Canada's placement in the bottom half of the rankings particularly troubling is the fact that per capita health-care spending in Canada is amongst the highest in the world … Canada is the only big-spending country that does not rank in the upper echelons of the ECHCI rankings … Canadians are paying for a world-class health-care system, but for a variety of reasons, they are not getting one." The value for money of the Canadian system is poor. As also revealed in other comparative studies, the ECHCI study showed outcomes from the Canadian system to be good, but accessing the system on a timely basis and figuring out how to navigate it posed problems.

The gold standard for health-care comparisons is provided by the Paris-based Organisation for Economic Co-operation and Development. Health-care researchers in the OECD countries mine enormous data banks and numerous cross-country comparisons. The OECD results are argued over sometimes—what survey results are not?—but governments, researchers and all those interested in international health-care comparisons consider them indispensable benchmarks. Given that Canada is among the top five spenders on health care in countries with largely public systems, it would be reasonable to assume that Canada should produce among the very best comparative results. The reverse is the case.

Out of thirty-three countries measured in 2010, Canada's life expectancy rate stood twelfth, diabetes incidence eighth, breast-cancer incidence fifteenth, prostate cancer incidence eighth, heart disease twelfth. For what is called "amenable mortality," that is, deaths preventable by timely medical intervention, Canada came twelfth of twenty-seven countries. Canada was below the OECD average for vaccination rates for children against measles, but above average for flu vaccination for seniors. Canada had the longest wait times to see a specialist, and the second-worst wait times for elective surgery. Canada used to be among the countries with the lowest infant-mortality rates but now stands twenty-sixth out of forty.

Although Canadian governments have increased spending on diagnostic testing since the 2003–2004 accords, Canada ranked nineteenth for the number of MRI machines, and twenty-second for the number of CT scanners per million of population. Not surprisingly, Canada had fewer MRI exams and CT scans than the OECD average. For hip-replacement surgeries, Canada ranked twenty-first, and for knee replacements tenth—rather low rankings considering that governments had poured money into those two surgeries. Canada's hospital discharge rate was thirty-fourth of thirty-seven. Canada had the second-highest occupancy rate for acute-care beds, reflecting in part how too many patients who should be in other institutions cannot find a spot there and so remain in hospitals.

Canada's share of the population over sixty-five years of age receiving long-term care was way below the OECD average, and the growth in public expenditure on long-term care was twentieth of twenty-five. For all the talk about the need to invest in long-term care in Canada, the 3.3 percent yearly increases in long-term care here was well below the overall increase in health-care spending. Canadian drug costs are among the highest in the OECD. So are the salaries paid Canadian doctors. Drug costs and physicians' remuneration are two of the most important drivers of health-care budgets and two of the reasons why Canada has among the world's most expensive health-care systems.

The OECD's number-crunching demonstrated that Canadian life expectancy is above average, and inequalities in health status are at the average. Canada ranks well above the OECD average in per capita spending on health but slightly below average for administrative spending. Those who blame high administrative costs for medicare's sustainability challenge are wrong, according to OECD data. The Canadian system is characterized by above-average overall costs, average health-care outcomes, less high-tech equipment and fewer acute-care beds, fewer doctors and medical students per capita, less choice among providers and patients, less regulation on prices for everything outside the basic medicare services and a weak setting of priorities by payers, namely governments. Anyone, therefore, who reads the OECD reports could never conclude that our medicare is the best in the world.

The Canadian Medical Association produced a 2010 report, under president Jeffrey Turnbull, that strongly favoured public health care. Yet the report concluded, as do these international comparative studies, that a "case can be made that Canada's health-care system is not delivering value for the money spent. Canada is one of the highest spenders of health care when compared to other industrialized countries that offer universal care ... [but] Canada's health-care system is under-performing on several key measures, such as timely access." The Canadian Nurses Association, another of medicare's strongest defenders, cited the devastating Commonwealth Fund surveys and said, "Canadians are not satisfied with the capacity of the health system to provide them with timely access to care ... The inability of Canadians to access appropriate and timely care is evidence of fundamental shortfalls in the health system."

Whether or not they understood that the Canadian system did not stack up well internationally, Canada's First Ministers entered negotiations for a new health-care accord in 2003–2004 that Prime Minister Paul Martin described as "transformative." The politicians knew that their publics valued health care and wanted more of it without paying extra taxes. At that moment, Ottawa enjoyed a handsome surplus, so there was money to throw at the health-care system, which they did in the form of the biggest public-policy bet of their generation. By virtue of Ottawa's agreeing to spend $41 billion over a decade, with transfers indexed at 6 percent yearly, they reckoned that the money would buy substantial improvements, especially a reduction in wait times.

Not only had the international studies confirmed that Canada had the worst wait times among advanced industrial countries, but also the leaders all knew that wait times stood at the top of the list of Canadians' complaints about the health-care system. Sometimes people have no cause for alarm or complaint, because waiting for a procedure neither imperils their health nor seriously inconveniences them. Sometimes people put their name on a list for a procedure, only to postpone it because the allotted time turns out not to be suitable. Sometimes, however, people get sicker while waiting, causing them more pain or psychological torment. Sometimes hospitals' budgets are such that operating times or beds are not available, so that surgeries are cancelled. As the Romanow commission put it, "Canadians need to understand that immediate service is not always available." Yes, but what about timely service? The cruel, identifiable fact was (and is) that wait times are long throughout the system, which is why a succession of politicians have pledged to reduce them.

Every country with a government-run health-care system is challenged by wait times. The challenge has vexed governments in Sweden, Britain, Australia and many others as well as in Canada, because where payment does not influence demand, health-care providers have to figure out who gets treated, when and how by other criteria. Once a patient enters the system, he or she is subject to triage, that is, figuring out whose case is most serious, which means faster treatment for those most in need. Triage can take place only when a patient touches the system. But what if it becomes difficult to touch the system in the first place — for example, if no family doctors are available for first assessment and referral, or emergency rooms are jammed? Wait times can cascade through the system, except in the most urgent cases: wait to see a family physician, wait to see a specialist, wait to see a surgeon, wait for the surgery.

The leaders who negotiated the 2003–2004 agreement

therefore allocated $5.5 billion over six years to a Wait Times Reduction Fund, not for reducing overall wait times but specifically for five procedures: cataracts, hip and knee replacements, diagnostic testing, cardiac bypass surgery and radiation therapy for cancer. The leaders could have chosen five other procedures, but these were high-volume procedures and often in the news. They were especially geared to ailments of older citizens who vote in higher numbers than younger ones and who use the health-care system most. Benchmarks were established for each of the five priority areas. Provinces resolved to put the federal cash to work providing services within those benchmarked times, although there was no penalty if they failed.

The Canadian Institute for Health Information in 2011 reported on the results of the previous three years. The good news was that the money had bought improvement. Wait times were generally down for the five priorities. Eight out of ten patients across Canada received treatment within the benchmarked times. The bad news was that the provinces had set a goal of nine out of ten patients being treated within the benchmarked times. None came close to meeting that objective. The benchmarks themselves were generous to the provinces: a month for cancer radiation, twenty-six weeks for hip and knee replacements, cataract surgery within sixteen weeks for "at risk" patients. CIHI's conclusion: "While there have been some improvements in wait times for priority procedures over the last three years, these improvements are not being seen consistently across all procedures or across all provinces." The first results for the Wait Times Reduction Fund were therefore modest and bought at a high cost that it is hard to imagine can be indefinitely sustained, although demand will continue to be high. Nor, of course, did the fund deal with many other procedures that governments considered to be lower priorities. Wait times did not generally come down for those lower priorities, and in some cases went up, in part because what gets measured tends to draw attention and resources compared with what does not. At least the fund produced some interprovincial measurements, because provinces generally hate being compared with each other. Comparisons invite comment. Comment invites criticisms of poor relative performance. To say that the provinces conspire not to compare would be an exaggeration, but only a slight one. Let's just say they find serious, detailed comparisons not to be in their interest.

Knowing that wait times, above all else, worry Canadians about medicare, the Harper Conservatives campaigned in 2005 on something called the Patient Wait Times Guarantee. After they took office in 2006, that policy produced another $1 billion infusion in the federal 2007 budget, $612 million of which was for developing a wait-time guarantee for at least one of the five priority areas identified in the 2003–2004 accord.

To monitor the "fix" resulting from the First Ministers agreement of 2003–2004 would be the new body, the Health Council of Canada. (Quebec, of course, refused to participate, maintaining its traditional position that health is a provincial matter, so Ottawa should just cough up money and shut up. Alberta also chose not to participate.) So what happened with all those tens of billions that the Martin and Harper governments had transferred to the provinces? The Health Council's 2011 report found that provincial health-care spending had indeed galloped ahead: from $85 billion in 2004 to $125 billion in 2010, an average yearly increase of 6.7 percent. Nine of ten provinces (Quebec having refused) had indeed instituted wait-times guarantees, but few patients apparently knew about them. In addition, some of the new guaranteed wait times were up to twice as long as the guaranteed wait times announced by governments in 2005! Did governments "achieve meaningful reductions in wait times?" the Health Council asked. The answer, it said, "is not straightforward."

The council looked at Ontario's Emergency Wait Times Strategy unveiled in 2008 that promised 90 percent of patients with uncomplicated conditions would be treated and discharged within four hours. Also, 90 percent of those with complex conditions requiring admission or more treatment in emergency would be admitted or discharged within eight hours. Three years later, wait times in 80 percent of cases had declined by 5 percent for uncomplicated cases and 15 percent for complicated ones. Very modest progress had unquestionably been made. But for those who needed admitting, only 40 percent found a bed within eight hours, and on average those poor souls spent thirty hours in emergency.

The 2003–2004 federal–provincial plan was also supposed to finance a drug-information system across Canada for access by pharmacists and hospitals. By 2010, however, only 30 percent of pharmacists working in communities and 46 percent of those in hospitals were part of the system, and just 29 percent of hospitals were hooked in. As for the much-ballyhooed 2004 National Pharmaceuticals Strategy announced by the premiers, the Health Council said in 2009 that the strategy had "stalled." Two years later, in its 2011 report, the council said that the strategy "has not gained momentum." As for electronic health records, the need for which has figured in every health-care study, the council found that the infrastructure covered only half of Canadians, in part because "many physicians are not using it in the clinical decision-making and patients can't benefit fully from the technology until they do." No wonder that according to OECD figures, Canada ranks at the bottom in the use of electronic technologies.

Tommy Douglas's dream, the one that animates medicare today, was to design a health-care system for patients, regardless of income. Internationally, the Canadian system ranks poorly as a value-for-money proposition: high costs, average results. What's happened to that patient-centred dream?

Today, almost every government report talks about "putting patients first," or building a "patient-centred system." Hardly any political speech does not repeat the phrase, to the point that it has become a cliché. The Canadian Medical Association says, "The system needs to be patient-centred," as part of recommending a charter for patient-centred care. The Alberta minister of health, following a proposal from a legislative committee, recommended a patient charter for his province. The federal health minister, Leona Aglukkaq, unveiled in 2011 the Strategy for Patient-Oriented Research. Not to be outdone, the Ontario health minister, Deb Matthews, insisted in early 2012 that her government's new Action Plan (another cliché) was "obsessively patient-centred."

Repeating ad nauseam that a health-care system should be first and foremost about patients is like saying education should be for students, welfare for its recipients, roads for drivers, the courts for those seeking justice. To have to repeat the obvious — the health-care system must be "patient centred" — must mean that it is not. Or at least not as much as it should be. Something has gone awry when so many of those who administer, govern, defend and analyze the system seem to suggest by the repetition of the same phrase that patients are not actually at the heart of the system. What seems to have happened is that a system supposed to be designed for patients has become one designed for and by providers.

This criticism is not at all surprising. The health-care system features huge bureaucracies, large institutions, powerful

professional associations, formidable unions, well-paid administrators, all nominally supervised and directed by a political party
that, once in power, wishes to remain there. Each part of the
system has its own ways of doing things and interests to protect.
They are the producers and providers of a service (or product)
called health care. Patients are consumers of that service.

As is well known in public affairs generally, when the interests of producers are pitted against those of consumers, producers
win more often than not because there is no free market wherein
the decisions of thousands or millions of consumers can shape
producer behaviour. Health care should never be a free market,
given the huge gap in knowledge between patients and providers,
the high costs of some medical treatment and the need to have
all citizens covered. Market rules do not apply in the public
domain generally, so the superior organizational might, lobbying
capabilities, negotiated entitlements and focused attention of
producers overwhelm the more diffuse, non-organized interests
of consumers. Occasionally, consumers of public services can
be mobilized, and citizens can always throw a government out
of office. But in health care, consumers do not picket hospitals,
denounce physicians' practices or act collectively. Health care
tends to be a deeply personal matter not easily subject to mass
mobilization.

Once achieved, a producer entitlement is difficult to diminish,
let alone eliminate. Producers or providers become, in economic
parlance, "rent-seekers" looking to appropriate unto themselves
what they can of available resources. As the population ages,
there are fewer K–12 students but not fewer teachers, administrators or schools. As university professors' salaries go up, they often
teach less. As courts get more money, trial delays do not seem
to go down. Complex public systems, unless pushed in another
direction by politicians, the media or some external force, tend

to coalesce around the interests of providers/producers. Which is what has happened to medicare.

That medicare has moved away from its presumed goal—patient-centred health care—was underscored in a report commissioned in 2009 by the Saskatchewan government. Called (naturally) the Patient First Review, the report was done by the long-time health administrator and medicare advocate Tony Dagnone. In fairness, all reports on public policy are designed to make things better, so they do tend to focus on areas requiring improvement rather than detail what is going right. That said, Dagnone asked patients what they expected from the health-care system and what they had found. The care, they said, was good, but not good enough. He discovered too much waiting, too much landing in emergency rooms because of no other place to go, lack of basic information because people in the system are too busy, lack of electronic medical records, lack of respect because too many patients sensed they were a bother to the system. He wrote, "Patients ask that health-care workers and their respective leadership see beyond their declared interests so that the interests of patients take precedence at every care interaction, every future contract negotiation and every policy debate." This laudable series of objectives belies extensive experience that exhortation gets a government nowhere against entrenched provider groups. One might ask of a staunch defender of medicare why after four decades these obvious objectives have not been realized. To which the answer is, not bad faith or ill intention but the nature of public-sector dynamics.

Reform of a system as complex and complicated as health care will not come easily. The system is optimally adapted to existing incentives and constraints—as long as these remain much the same, it can be changed only at the margins. Provinces are trying to make changes so that the system can become more patient friendly, and in some cases they have succeeded. In too many instances, however, they cannot because they will not fundamentally change the incentives within it. Changing them is one reason why international studies continue to show that other systems work better than medicare, even if Canadians do not realize it.

EIGHT

How Much Does Medicare Cost?

Health care is straining provincial budgets across Canada. It now takes up 42 to 45 percent of provincial program spending, and the share is growing. Health-care costs have been rising faster than those of any other government program, faster than government revenues, faster than the economy. Before the end of this decade, health care will likely consume more than half the budget of every province. This pattern exists in small and large provinces, in those that have raised taxes or lowered them, in those with centre-left or centre-right governments.

Privately, many premiers have said these trends cannot continue; publicly, they are afraid of the reaction if they place facts in front of citizens. Or they fear the rows that might ensue if they took on the formidable entrenched interests such as doctors' associations, nurses' unions, local communities, seniors' groups, pharmaceutical companies, for there is an ironclad law of cost reduction: if it is done seriously and on a sustained basis, somebody has to lose money or services, or both. Which politician eagerly strides into that situation? Premiers, notably all those outside Alberta and Saskatchewan, in the post-recession era face budgetary deficits of such magnitude that whatever their reluctance to confront interest groups, they will have to seek health-care cost relief in the form of much lower negotiated agreements with doctors and nurses in the years ahead—as the McGuinty government in Ontario began doing in 2012. On the outcome of these negotiations over the next decade will rest some of the sustainability challenges of medicare.

Some provinces did put on the brakes, signing modest collective-bargaining agreements with physicians and nurses, pressing hospitals to balance their budgets and securing economies in administration. Canadians have seen this kind of pause before. Provinces had begun to rein in health-care spending before additional restraint was forced on them when the Chrétien government cut transfers in the mid-1990s. So the record shows that provinces can restrain health-care spending when forced by external pressures to do so. Once those pressures ease, catch-up spending occurs. By 1997, health-care spending had resumed its upward climb after a period of restraint starting in 1993. Since medicare arrived fully in 1972, periods of restraint have been inevitably followed by sustained bursts of increases beyond the growth in provincial revenues.

Ontario raised taxes by imposing health-care premiums ranging from $300 to $900 in 2004. Quebec introduced a health tax in 2010 and pushed up its sales tax by two points. Other provinces refused to raise taxes; Alberta and British Columbia reduced them. Whether taxes went up or down, spending on health continued to rise rapidly. Simultaneously, there were reductions in absolute or inflation-adjusted terms of spending on many other government programs. These reductions occurred by stealth, because governments do not like admitting that they are reducing spending elsewhere to make room for more health care. Talking about trade-offs is difficult because groups being traded off don't like their fate.

The squeezing of other program spending shows up in provincial budgets year after year. Within the health-care sector, predictably, all attention is focused on the health-care portion of any budget, with questions raised about how much the health-care budget will be increased. Nobody in health care pays any attention to what is happening to K–12 education, universities and community colleges, public transit, roads, justice, social welfare, the environment, recreation, assisted housing and the many other portfolios that citizens expect their provincial governments to manage. For people in the health-care sector, and for most citizens, health-care spending is *über alles*.

Governments (and taxpayers) face the challenge of the "sustainability" of the public health-care system, a word much muddied in the use. Commissioner Roy Romanow defined *sustainability* as "ensuring that sufficient resources are available over the long term to provide timely access to quality services that address Canadians' evolving health needs." There are many elastic phrases in that definition. What are "sufficient resources?" What is the "long term?" Who defines "timely access" and what is it? What will be "Canadians' evolving health needs?" No matter. All generalized definitions contain some measure of elasticity. The definition is wrong for a more fundamental reason: it misstates reality. The proper definition of *sustainability* has to include all of what Romanow mentioned, *plus* the impact of health-care spending on governments' ability to carry out other functions, and at appropriate publicly acceptable (whatever that is) levels of taxation. To isolate health care from the other responsibilities of government, and from governments' need to raise revenues to support *all* their activities, reflects health-care myopia. It therefore misstates the sustainability challenge faced by all governments.

Kevin Page, Canada's Parliamentary Budget Office director, did not misstate the sustainability challenge. In a February

2010 report, he projected that provincial–territorial health-care spending would rise to 14 percent of GDP by 2040 from today's 8.4 percent. (Remember that public spending accounts for only 70 percent of total health-care spending, so public and private health care would come close to 20 percent of the country's economy in 2040 from 11.7 percent today.) Page pointed out that to pay for the rising share of health care, governments would need to increase revenue or reduce other spending by $15.5 billion annually. The longer governments wait to start funding future liabilities, he observed, the heavier the costs for future health-care users. When discussions swirl around "equity" in medicare, they seldom deal with the intergenerational unfairness that today's costs, if not properly funded, will impose on the next generation.

Page outlined painful cost projections. It is easier politically to let silence surround the collateral damage of health-care spending rising relentlessly at rates above provincial revenues. Provincial governments do not want to raise taxes, fearing public reaction. They do not want to open the door to more private health-care spending, fearing public reaction. They do not want to explain the impact of health-care spending on the rest of their budgets, fearing public reaction. So they press on, seeking efficiencies wherever possible, rearranging regional models of health-care administration, making constant announcements about new health-care spending because that is what the public wants, while the share of health-care spending rises in their budgets each year, without any of them knowing how to contain it on a sustained basis.

The provincial pattern is, broadly speaking, similar across the country. Look at three provinces to understand better the pattern: Alberta, which lowered taxes by abolishing health-care premiums and is rich; Ontario, which raised taxes in the form of health-care premiums and is suffering economically; and Quebec, which imposed a health-care tax.

The dry bones of the Alberta budget tell a revealing story about spending in the country's wealthiest province. In 1993, Alberta spent approximately the same amount on health care and education: $4 billion. Two decades later, in 2013, Alberta will spend $16 billion on health care and $9 billion on education—health-care spending quadrupled, education more than slightly doubled.

Consider those raw numbers as a share of total government spending. In 1993, health care and education each took about 26 percent of the provincial budget, social services 11 percent and all other programs 33 percent. Twenty years later, health care will have risen to 43 percent of program spending, while education will have dropped to 23 percent, social services to 10 percent and other programs to 24 percent.

These two decades, 1993 to 2013, featured wild swings in Alberta health-care policy, from severe cutbacks to huge infusions of cash, from toying with private payment to ruling it out, from creating regional health authorities to abolishing them to create one province-wide body, from closing hospitals to opening them, from coping with diminished and then soaring federal transfers, from dealing with natural resources royalties that plummeted, skyrocketed, dived and then rose. As elsewhere, politicians promised one thing but did another. One Alberta health minister, Ron Liepert, promised a bold program of health reforms and cost control, "because the current system is not working and is not sustainable," only to be part of a government that then pledged to increase health-care spending at just under 6 percent a year for five years.

Happily for Alberta, it can absorb such increases more easily than other provinces. It enjoys the lowest personal income taxes in Canada and no sales tax. Former premier Ed Stelmach's PC government, fulfilling a 2008 election promise, scrapped health-care premiums of $44 a month for individuals and $88 a month for families. If health care seriously strained the provincial budget, any government could easily raise more revenues, except that the provincial government does not want to raise taxes. Nor do Albertans want to pay higher taxes, at least not according to a 2010 legislative committee's report on Albertans' attitude to their health-care system. Albertans, the report found, are committed to their health-care system, want it improved and expanded but do not want to pay more for it.

Professor Livio Di Matteo of Lakehead University and his research partner, Rosanna Di Matteo, did a detailed forecasting model about the fiscal sustainability of Alberta's health-care system for the University of Calgary's School of Public Policy. They looked at a variety of future possibilities for health-care spending, all of which were disquieting. Before they glanced forward, they peered into recent history. They found that between 1996 and 2007, total health-care spending grew at an average annual rate of 10.2 percent, compared with a 6.9 percent annual rate in overall government spending. True, cutbacks occurred from 1993 to 1996 in all government spending (these started in Alberta before the federal restraint budget of 1995), including health care, but the decade-long splurge from 1996 to 2007 more than made up for the cutbacks. In real per capita terms, health-care spending rose 87 percent, slightly above the national average.

Aggregate numbers can deceive. Not everything in the Alberta health-care system rose at the same rate. Hospital budgets and physicians' payments grew less rapidly than total health-care spending, although the Stelmach government later gave the doctors a very generous long-term settlement. What pushed up spending were drugs (some of which were paid for publicly), public health, capital costs (again, paid for publicly) and health services provided outside of medicare.

What of the future? The simplest, but least satisfying, method of projection is to project forward past spending patterns. Doing that, the Di Matteos took the rate of spending increases from 1976 to 2007, the year when per capita health-care spending was $3696, and concluded that by 2030, per capita spending would be $8218 in 2007 dollars; that is, after taking account of inflation. Such a continuing increase would pose serious challenges for any Alberta government. These challenges would be nothing, however, if the province's health-care spending kept rising as it did from 1996 to 2007, when it grew 10 percent yearly. If a 10 percent rate of increase continued, per capita health-care costs would be $14,215 a year, clearly so unsustainable that by 2030 health care would consume 80 percent of provincial revenues, assuming no tax hikes.

The researchers also tried to incorporate hard-to-measure factors such as aging, technology improvements and population growth into their projections. Even when factoring in these matters, the authors concluded that "health care takes up an even larger share of provincial revenues," the only question being a modest share or a very large one. They concluded that the "inescapable logical conclusion" of their projections will require "political choices of health over other expenditures, tax increases over tax cuts, and/or increasing the share of private health-care provision or maintaining the status quo." Of course, they noted another option: controlling expenditures by restructuring health-care delivery—the lure of efficiency—which is what Alberta and other provinces have been struggling to accomplish. Efficiency improvements alone, however, will not allow Albertans to avoid hard choices.

The latest boom in natural-resource royalties continues to

make Alberta's government the envy of all others in Canada. In 2010–11, revenues from bitumen oil and other fossil fuels pumped $8 billion into the Alberta budget, with a projection that in 2015 fossil-fuel revenues will be $15 billion. With that cornucopia in hand and projected, the Alberta government in 2012 announced a 7.9 percent increase for health care for the following fiscal year. From 2010–11 to 2014–15, Alberta will have spent an additional $3.4 billion on health and $600 million on all education, $700 million on social services, while cutting spending on everything else.

A twelve-person group of eminent Canadians, asked to chart a long-term path for Alberta's future (the Premier's Council for Economic Strategy), warned in its 2011 report, "Nowhere is the need to bring expenditures and revenue into alignment more obvious and critical than in health care ... The current growth in government expenditures on health care is not sustainable without tax increases or major reductions in all other govern-ment programs. If this is left unresolved, rising health-care costs clearly have the potential to undermine Alberta's future efforts to invest adequately in our future ... It is time for Albertans to face the facts on rising health-care spending." Was anybody listening?

Quebec is less fortunate than Alberta but somewhat more resolute. Quebec has the highest personal tax rates in Canada and the highest per capita debt. Whereas Alberta has plenty of fiscal room, courtesy not of superior management but of fossil-fuel resource revenues, Quebec does not, although slowly the government is raising the continent's lowest university tuition fees and increasing hydro rates. Quebec has faced the health-care spending dilemma in two ways that set the province apart from others. The government has spoken some truths to the population, and it has raised taxes specifically for health care, despite an already large tax burden.

Quebec is lucky, fiscally speaking, in two important ways. First, the French language and culture reduce the mobility of doctors, nurses and other health-care professionals. (Over 90 percent of graduates from the province's three French-language medical schools stay in Quebec.) Quebec can get away with paying health-care workers less than elsewhere, knowing that few will want to work in an English-speaking milieu. Second, Quebec receives about $8 billion a year in equalization payments from Ottawa, and $4.5 billion for health (growing faster than the provincial health budget), part of $15 billion in federal transfers that amount to 23 percent of Quebec's budget. Without these transfers, Quebec would be in very serious fiscal difficulty.

Claude Castonguay, in a controversial report to the Quebec government, recommended that citizens be told more about the costs of their health-care system. The government responded by making annual statements—*comptes de la santé*—that lay out those costs. The statement, the only one of its kind in Canada, explained that health-care rose each year from 1980 onward by 5.9 percent, whereas all other program spending increased 4.4 percent each year.

In the 2011 *compte de la santé*, the government revealed that health-care spending from 2008–2009 to 2010–11 had grown by 4.2 percent, a lower rate than previous periods. However, the government was simultaneously trying to eliminate Quebec's deficit by 2013–14 and to make a dent in the province's onerous debt. In this three-year period, while health-care spending was rising by $3.5 billion and education by $1.2 billion, overall expenses were only growing by $2.7 billion. This arithmetic meant, by definition, absolute or real (after inflation) cuts everywhere else: natural resources, justice, employment, transport,

pending increase, the government outlined a series of measures
to try to move patients away from hospitals toward community-
and home-based care and presumed no increases for doctors'
pay. Without what the government called these "transformative
changes," health-care spending would be 4.5 percent yearly,
closer to the historic average. And, of course, the provincial deficit
each year would be higher. No government anywhere had ever
kept health-care spending to 2.1 percent for a sustained period of
time. Ontario was therefore attempting something almost heroic
in health-care policy terms. History suggests, however, that even
if the province can manage this containment for a few years, the
pressure from provider groups, new technologies, rising drug
costs and an aging population will push that yearly increase
closer to 4.5 percent than 2.1 per cent in the not too distant future.

Some of the money invested in health care in Ontario over the
years before this new period of restraint (as in other provinces)
brought tangible, beneficial results. For example, in an exceptionally far-sighted move, the government committed $741 million
to diabetes prevention and treatment, anticipating the epidemic
of diabetes that accompanies the aging of the population and
the obesity of too many Canadians. Ontario fully funded insulin
pumps for children and adults with type 1 diabetes. It invested
$1 billion in home care, $1.4 billion in long-term care facilities
and it spent $1.5 billion (with help from federal funds) in the
designated surgeries, reducing wait times for cataracts, hip
and knee replacements, cancer surgeries and general surgeries.
Ontario reduced those wait times better than any province.

In his first provincial campaign, Liberal leader Dalton
McGuinty had pledged not to raise taxes while in office, dramatically wielding a pen at a photo op to sign a no-tax-increase
pledge from the Canadian Taxpayers Federation. McGuinty
was so far ahead in the polls that he did not need to make that

sustainable development and municipal affairs. The circle of
health-care increases, and smaller ones for education, could
only be squared by cutting other programs, a pattern found all
across Canada.

The circle-into-square spending choices would have been
more acute had Jean Charest's Liberal government, which
enjoyed a majority in the National Assembly in 2010, not imposed
tax increases to help pay for health care. Rather comically it
did not wish to use the word *tax* and so called the health tax a
"general contribution." The tax will rise to $200 per adult by 2012,
with low-income people exempted from any payment. At $200
per adult, the new fund will add $975 million to the health-care
budget of about $30 billion.

The government explained that the fund would "permit the
closing of a part of the growing gap between health-care spending
and revenues to finance it." The new money will go into a special
fund. It is not supposed to be used to pay higher wages for those
in the health-care system. Instead, the money is supposed to fund,
among other initiatives, more group family practices, volume
incentives for surgeries and training for more specialized nurses.
The new money will allow health-care spending to keep growing
at 5 percent, even as the government brings the deficit to zero
by keeping overall spending increases to 3.1 percent. In other
words, the government isn't really reducing the yearly increase
in health-care spending by very much. It's raising more revenue
to keep health-care spending increases going up by 5 percent, an
approach with at least the virtue of honesty. The government was
saying implicitly to Quebec citizens, if you want more health care,
pay for it.

Another change—revolutionary by Canadian standards
although used elsewhere—proved a bridge too far for the
Quebec government and citizens. To narrow further the

health-care spending/revenue gap, the government proposed a user fee, although it chose another fancy expression to avoid direct language. Low-income people would have been exempted, as well as those whose chronic conditions required frequent visits to medical professionals. The per-visit fee was fixed at $20. Rather than the patient paying the doctor, the fee would be added to the patient's income-tax statement for inclusion in annual taxes.

A political storm immediately blew up around this idea. The government backed down. Finance minister Raymond Bachand admitted that the Quebec "political culture" was not ready for such a radical departure. He could have said the Canadian political culture. Who knows what might have happened if this user fee had not been proposed in the same budget with the health tax? As it was, the combination of the fee and the health tax was considered too steep a revenue increase to pass political muster, even for a majority government.

"So the question now facing us is, how do we fund the best health care without compromising our investments in schools, helping the vulnerable or protecting the environment?" asked the Ontario Liberal finance minister, Dwight Duncan, in his 2010 budget speech. The minister did not provide an answer, but he continued, "Just twenty years ago, thirty-two cents of every dollar spent on government programs were spent on health care. Today, it is forty-six cents. In twelve years, if we don't take action, it could be seventy cents."

The next year, 2011, Duncan presented another in a long string of Ontario budgets bulging with money for health care. The budget for health care was slated to rise by 5 percent (after inflation), whereas overall expenses for the entire government would increase only 1.7 percent. Put another way, health-care

expenses were going up by $2.2 billion, but total s␂ $1.2 billion. Something had to give, and it did in th␂ way. Cuts in absolute or inflation-adjusted terms␂ portation, research and innovation, northern deve␂ promotion and sport, labour, energy, the envirc␂ resources. Duncan insisted, however, that thing␂ in health care. For the next three fiscal years,␂ budget would not rise each year beyond 3 percent␂ had never happened in Ontario.

Such a drop would represent quite a change fo␂ the health-care budget exploded by 8.5 percent i␂ 9.5 percent in 2006–2007. Now Duncan was pr␂ spending increases to an average of 3 percent, w␂ what tricks he had up his government's sleeve.␂ tricks, because to get to 3 percent each year fo␂ had to take about $1 billion from previously proje␂ growth and hard-wire those economies into the␂ these cuts would not be enough, because Onta␂ tion became so grave that it faced a $14 billion ␂ and six years of declining deficits thereafter. Ont␂ tion had become a mess, and the government be␂ something about it.

It asked the eminent public-policy␂ Drummond to review all government spending␂ the most through report ever done of a provinc␂ medicine he proposed was strong, stronger tha␂ could stomach. Except in health care, by far t␂ spending. Whereas Drummond suggested a c␂ spending of 2.5 percent (or less) until 2017–␂ percent annual increases thereafter, the gove␂ health-care spending growth of only 2.1 perc␂ 2014–15. To accomplish this unprecedented␂

foolish commitment. He did and was stuck with it. Except that in his first budget, secure with a majority of seats, he imposed health-care premiums tied to income—a tax by another name—that by 2011-12 were worth $3 billion, a sum about three times larger than the health tax imposed in Quebec. His government delisted physiotherapy, optometry and chiropractic services, in effect "privatizing" them. He also froze the budgets of twelve departments other than health. Here was the classic health-care spending trifecta: higher taxes to provide more money for health care, privatization of some services and a squeeze on other budgets.

The Ontario government's extensive gambling operations also now finance health care. Originally created to fund culture and recreational programs, Ontario's provincial lotteries, charity casinos and racetrack slot machines have become cash cows for health care, as they have in other provinces. These activities raise $1.7 billion for the Ontario government, of which culture and recreation receive only $120 million. Hospitals get the bulk of the rest: $1.5 billion. McGuinty has acknowledged, as have other premiers, that health care is now hooked on gambling. No wonder the cash-strapped government counted in its 2012 budget on even more money from gambling, including adding new casinos.

A million more Ontarians found family doctors, although since the population of the province increased by one million during those years, access did not actually improve substantially. Despite improvements in some areas, it was disappointing, even shocking, to read the 2010 report of the Ontario Health Quality Council, the most authoritative and comprehensive agency in Canada established by the provincial government in 2005 to collect and analyze data about the province's health-care system.

Among the council's conclusions are these: "Our emergency department wait times are among the worst in the world." "Only

53 per cent of urgent cancer cases are completed within the two-week target." "The proportion of family doctors who have an electronic medical record has risen from 26 per cent in 2007 to 43 per cent in 2009 ... However, we still lag behind countries such as the UK, Australia and the Netherlands where 95 to 99 per cent of family doctors have an EMR." "Compared to 10 other advanced industrial countries, Ontario and Canada have the worst record on timely access to primary care. Almost nine in 10 Ontarians are waiting too long to see their doctor, and this indicator has gotten worse in the last three years."

These damning observations came in a very long, detailed report in which the government's many initiatives to improve the health-care system were underscored, and eight impressive "success stories" were highlighted. The council had no axe to grind. It said, "Ontarians are fortunate to have a publicly funded health-care system that provides a comprehensive range of services for all." But then it painted a picture of a system that, despite all the new spending, government initiatives, some admirable "best practices" that lead the country and presumably the best efforts of those working in the system, still left distressing gaps almost everywhere. The council's dreary conclusion: "despite spending a lot more on health care, Ontario generally scores worse than many countries."

What about the future? The TD Financial Group, the best group of economists doing public-policy research in Canada when Don Drummond led it, produced a report in 2010 that outlined the province's challenge. The TD report said, "Based on a status quo projection, growth in health-care spending would absorb four-fifths of the Ontario budget by 2030, leaving only one-fifth for all other government programs. This situation is clearly not feasible nor acceptable." Even without new investments to improve the system, the TD group said population growth, aging, general inflation, health-care inflation and increased utilization of the system would mean 6.5 percent yearly increases, more than twice the government's 3 percent target. It called this anticipated increase the "Health-care Pac Man." Obviously, these TD projections were more pessimistic, but quite likely more realistic, than the long-term ones contained in the McGuinty government's 2012 budget that forecast increases of only 2.1 percent.

The same pressures appear in other provincial budgets. In Nova Scotia, where an NDP government wrestled with a large inherited deficit after taking office in 2009, the HST was raised, bringing in about $220 million in additional revenue. Cost restraint was imposed across the government because of the deficit, so expenditures overall fell slightly. The reason expenditures did not fall more sharply? The health-care budget rose $212 million. In Manitoba, from 2009–10 to 2010–11, the health-care budget under another NDP government jumped $234 million, whereas total operating spending went down $208 million. This meant smaller budgets in department after department. In Saskatchewan in 2010, the overall budget dropped $120 million, but the health-care budget went up more than $200 million. The following ministries' budgets were cut: agriculture, K–12 education, justice, First Nations and Métis relations, highways, environment and tourism.

In British Columbia, the 2010 budget offered an $820 million increase for health, $78 million for K–12 education and $55 million for transportation. The following budgets, however, were cut in absolute dollars: forests, environment, aboriginal relations, agriculture, citizens' services. The following budgets were flatlined (which meant cut after inflation): housing and social development, public safety, children and family development, advanced education. Over three years, from 2009–10 to 2012–13,

the health-care Pac Man will be at work. B.C.'s overall departmental budget spending will rise about $2 billion during these
three years, which is the same amount as the health-care budget.
As a result, there will be zero increase for all other departments combined! The 2012 Liberal budget projected more of the
same from 2012–13 to 2014–15: a health-care increase of about
$1 billion within a total spending increase of $1.2 billion for all
programs. Health care would then consume 42.2 percent of the
province's operating budget, up from 38 percent ten years earlier.
Twenty percent of gambling revenue in B.C. goes to charities, but
80 percent enters a Healthcare Account. To ease the controversy
surrounding the proposed introduction of the Harmonized Sales
Tax, the government pledged to add *all* additional HST revenue to
health care. The people rejected the HST in a plebiscite anyway.

By reducing spending on just about everything else, by
putting four-fifths of the money from gambling into health care,
by introducing a new system of funding hospitals and of course by
continuing to receive payments from Ottawa indexed at 6 percent,
B.C. could keep its health-care budget rising at 4.9 percent a year.

British Columbia has a particular challenge because the
province is such a nice place to retire. That means the share of
seniors in the population is projected to rise from 24 to 39 percent
in the next two decades. Atlantic Canada has been losing younger
people to other parts of Canada, leaving behind a disproportionately elderly population. More seniors mean more money needed
for health care.

Aging of the population definitely offers a challenge to the
sustainability of medicare, but by no means a fatal one. All sorts
of scary scenarios (the "grey tsunami") have been painted about
future costs because the population is getting older, and older

people do use and cost the health-care system more money than younger ones. Those over sixty-five years of age consumed about 44 percent of all health-care spending in 2008, despite representing only 13.7 percent of the population. Consider hospitals. Seniors accounted for about half of government hospital spending in 2008, with most being spent on seventy- to eighty-nine-year-olds. One of the health-care system's greatest challenges is to get fewer people treated in hospitals, given the huge cost per patient. With seniors accounting for half the country's hospital costs, and 44 percent of the total cost of medicare, no wonder solutions are urgently needed to get more seniors treated outside hospitals, at home wherever possible or in lower-cost institutions than hospitals.

The aging of the population is expected to add 1 percentage point to total health-care spending growth, or about $2 billion a year in today's dollars, 70 percent of which will have to come from public sources, given the seventy-thirty public–private split of health-care spending. Two billion dollars is hardly chump change, but it's almost a rounding error against total health-care budgets. Aging is therefore not a budget breaker. It is, however, an extra cost that augments somewhat the spending pressure on provincial budgets.

A few health-care economists debunk the argument about health-care spending squeezing out other government services. They agree with Roy Romanow, who said the squeezing-out argument is "overheated rhetoric." They make two assertions, often simultaneously: that a spending squeeze does not exist, but if maybe a squeeze does exist it's not related to health care—rather, it stems from governments slashing taxes. They maintain that federal and provincial governments in the past decade have cut taxes, thereby driving down the national share of revenues to GDP. The argument rests on two assumptions: that lower taxes are axiomatically bad, and that all or most of the money produced by raising them again should be spent on health care.

Some governments have indeed cut taxes, and the overall share of taxes to GDP has declined a little in the past decade. The Chrétien government cut personal and corporate taxes after eliminating the deficit; the Harper government reduced the GST by two points (at a cost of about $12 billion to the federal treasury) and lowered the corporate and personal tax rates, while raising the personal exemption level, among other changes. A few provincial governments have done likewise. Manitoba under an NDP government cut its corporate tax rate (as did other provinces). Alberta eliminated health-care premiums. British Columbia under the Liberals reduced corporate and personal income tax rates. It is also true that some governments have raised taxes, as noted: Ontario imposed health-care premiums; Quebec introduced a health tax. A few provinces raised their sales taxes (Quebec by two points) or harmonized them with the GST. So the provincial pattern is mixed. But whether a province raised or lowered taxes, whether a province's revenues rose fast or slumped, and whether a province was in a surplus or deficit position, provincial health-care spending remained on an upward track, exceeding even in the best times the increase in government revenues. The pattern of health-care spending is clear, regardless of provincial (and national) economic circumstances: health-care costs have been rising faster than the collective wealth of the population for most of the time since medicare's inception.

We do know that whatever the revenue situation of governments, the health-care bill goes up faster than their ability to pay for it at current tax rates and without any adverse impact on other government programs. The key measure for any provincial

in addition to these much higher transfers, "it would be useful for governments to consider notionally earmarked taxes for health in the future." Higher transfers followed by further earmarked taxes—a double injection of funding—was part of the commission's deemed solution to medicare's future sustainability. If indeed the public were given the facts of health-care spending, with its effects on other areas of public activity, and then clearly expressed a preference for more taxes and/or less spending on other areas, then fine, spend more on health care. But the Romanow commission did not put the question in this fashion: more health-care spending, but at what cost and with what trade-offs? No politician does either.

During the past decade, Canada began to spend more on health care than on all education combined—K–12 to postgraduate university. Put crudely, since most health-care spending occurs in the latter stages of life, health care is certainly about today, but a lot about yesterday, and only a little about tomorrow; whereas education is about today, a little about yesterday, and a lot about what lies ahead.

A country that spends more on health care than education is one that worries more about today's consumption than tomorrow's investment. In the 1999–2009 period, health-care costs rose annually by 2 percent more than education's as a share of provincial budgets, which doesn't sound like much, until we remember that this gap exists every year and gets compounded. After, say, two decades, the budget for health-care spending will have risen almost 50 percent relative to the education budget. Unless there is more investment in education and skills, there will not be enough productivity gains to power an economy with fewer people working, courtesy of aging, and supporting a rising number who are not. Also, the Canadian economy will face even fiercer competitive challenges from developing countries whose citizens understandably want a better life. The aging of the Canadian population and the competition from major developing countries are the two greatest challenges to Canada's relative economic position in the world. It is unclear, therefore, why and how spending more of our collective wealth on health care would assist Canada in meeting either challenge. Is it axiomatically true that a marginal dollar spent on health care is a wiser investment than one spent on education? What about climate change and other environmental perils? Or the country's physical infrastructure, on which we all depend? Or social services outside health care, some of which influence the health status of the population as much as, if not more than, the health-care system itself.

What about poverty reduction? Every study about health care underscores that the social determinants of health drive costs and outcomes. The healthier the population, the better for its people and the lower the cost pressures on the health-care system. Poverty is the most consequential social determinant of health. One reason among many why Sweden and other Scandinavian countries spend less of their collective wealth on health care but achieve better outcomes is that they have much lower poverty rates than Canada. They spend more of their collective wealth in taxes that, in turn, provide a better network of social services than Canada's. They then spend less of their collective wealth on the health-care system. A marginal dollar spent on reducing poverty would do more for curbing health-care cost increases than one put into today's system. In the real world of Canada, there is no such debate, because citizens want more health care now and in the future. Politically, health care is potent, urgent and tangible; poverty reduction is distant, complicated and intangible for those who are not poor.

NINE

Can Efficiencies Save Medicare?

D r. Cy Frank, a man on a mission at the Alberta Bone and Joint Health Institute in Calgary, places on the table a chart full of boxes and arrows. The chart, which depicts a patient's path through the health-care system, is too detailed to understand except after long study—which is exactly the point. Dr. Frank points out that every time a patient gets transferred within the complex health-care system, the transfer can be confusing to patients and costly to the system. What's needed, he asserts, are case managers assigned to patients who will guide them through the system. Hiring such case managers will cost money up front but will eventually save money and help patients, "because each time they get handed off in the system, they risk getting lost." Frank declares, "I am on a mission to avoid waste in the system."

The search to reduce waste and improve efficiency within Canada's health-care system drives reformers everywhere. Efficiency gains would improve patient satisfaction and reduce costs, or at least reduce the increase in costs. As the OECD said in a 2004 report about health-care systems in all its member countries, "Ultimately, increasing efficiency may be the only way of reconciling rising demands for health care with public financing constraints." In 2010, the OECD estimated that Canada could lower by 2.5 percent its spending on health care were the

Canadian health-care system to become as efficient as the best in the OECD.

Improving quality outcomes and efficiency is the standard answer, bordering on a mantra, from those who assert that medicare does not face a sustainability challenge. Efficiency gains, they insist, will blunt cost pressures, so that additional taxes will not be required, nor cuts in other government programs, nor additional borrowing, nor any private payments; nothing, in short, that would change the essence of medicare. Kenneth Fyke, who chaired the inquiry into health-care in Saskatchewan, spoke for this entire school of thought when he declared, "Quality and efficiency problems are the true enemies of sustainability."

Canadians, when asked by pollsters, believe that the financial sustainability of their system can be assured by cutting waste. This response is the reflexive one, however, to all suggestions that any public service needs more money. "Don't raise my taxes and don't cut my services, just cut waste and duplication" is the echo that weary designers of public policy hear all the time, and not just in the health-care field. Like all simple answers to complex problems, the reflex is as alluring as it is wrong.

Health-care experts provide an enormous list of efficiency gains that, if implemented, would solve all long-term financing challenges. They are invariably frustrated at the slow pace of these changes that seem so obvious in concept and easy in implementation when described in academic studies. Politicians, too, buy into the efficiency agenda but often more in rhetoric than reality. Some of the reforms might provoke confrontations with established interests in the system—and with voters. Closing rural hospitals or merging urban ones, for example, would be part of the to-do list of every "rational planner," but closures and mergers enrage local citizens who consider hospitals to be a civic entitlement. Changing the "scope of practice" so that nurses could provide some of the services of doctors might make sense, as might allowing pharmacists more latitude in prescribing, but negotiating the new rules is often contentious. Electronic health records, where Canada lags far behind other countries, have been recommended over and over again by studies, but their implementation has been painfully slow.

Commissions into the future of health care reported that efficiency gains were there for the taking, although securing them would require more money now to achieve cost relief later. Kenneth Fyke, in his report about Saskatchewan's system, said, "My advice to government is this: Invest in change." Fyke's report, a fine piece of work within the model of the "rational planner" (take the existing system and make it work better), recommended delivery and administrative changes common to almost every report on health care (fewer health districts, fewer hospitals, more family clinics, centralization of specialty care, electronic health records) to create a "just and fair modernization of Medicare." He put the Romanow commission's "buy change" argument this way: "Implementing these changes will require an initial investment, but in the long run they will help to keep costs down."

Cy Frank's work offers a microcosmic example of this search for efficiency. Chronic diseases of the bone and joint such as arthritis cost Canadians $17 billion a year, Dr. Frank estimates. More than 6 million Canadians will be afflicted with these diseases by 2024. Arthritis will afflict the largest number, perhaps 5 million. Dr. Frank, a widely admired figure in Alberta medical circles, calls what's coming the "burning platform," since many of these diseases disproportionately afflict the elderly.

Flow charts on the wall of the boardroom where we meet depict how he and his colleagues are trying to reduce waste by minimizing hand-offs within the system. Doctors, he argues, make decisions that drive 74 percent of the system's costs, but they are not evaluated for their own efficiencies, their quality of medical practice and patient outcomes. Nor are they plugged in to hospital administrators who have to manage budgets. A lack of evaluation encourages doctors to order too many tests, such as MRIs for orthopaedic work. When it is noted that Canada lags well behind other countries in per capita access to MRIs, Dr. Frank sniffs that doctors still rely too often on the machines anyway. Teams of doctors and administrators need to work on managing cost, access and quality. To make the system work more effectively for doctors, administrators and, most important, for patients, much better data are needed to improve quality and efficiency.

It is a slightly ironic complaint. The Canadian health-care system swims in data. There is more of it, from more sources, than ever, yet a common complaint is that not enough data exist. Statistics Canada collects vast amounts of data about health care. So does the Canadian Institute for Health Information, to say nothing of provincial health ministries, regional health authorities and provincial monitoring bodies. Hospitals spit out data. Anyone interested in health-care policy, let alone medical science, struggles to keep up with the volume of research, numbers and analyses. And yet, the familiar cry is that we lack much crucial information that those who operate the system, or operate in the system, need to know to make it run better.

Dr. Frank acknowledges the prevalence of data but argues that the data measure overall systems, not individual performance and outcomes. "It is true that there is a lot of data being generated in the health-care system," he says. "The issue is that it is not the right kind of data. It is not always reliable, and it is not timely enough to guide decision making." He has, therefore, devised a strategy to measure data and provide feedback on everything in orthopaedic surgery for hips and knees within the province. Everything surgeons and those who work with them on surgical teams do before, during and after operations must and can be measured—against provincial standards and against the outcomes of other teams.

For example, each surgical team's operations and outcomes should be charted. How long from referral to a specialist to assessment? How long from a decision about surgery to the actual surgery? What kind of outcomes? How long for an operation? How long for individual parts of the operation, such as incision to closure for a hip or knee replacement? What share of patients wait how long for discharge? How long before the patient resumes normal daily activities? The surgeon and the team will be shown the confidential results of a "continuous improvement report" that compares their performance with provincial norms and the results of other teams in Calgary, Edmonton and Red Deer. When teams analyze their comparative results, a plan can be devised and implemented to improve them, part of the "continuous improvement" strategy.

Dr. Frank points to a chart that shows how one surgical team saved $60,000 in less than three months. If all teams met the provincial norms—a four-day stay for hip and knee replacements—it would save $19 million a year for the Alberta health budget. Imagine what could be saved and how quality could be enhanced, he says, if such insistence on "continuous improvement" extended to all medical procedures. Efficiency gains lead to speedier release, superior quality, happier patients, doctors and their teams working more efficiently and feeling good about their improvements and, in theory, savings for the taxpayer. Dr. Frank wants the savings reinvested, however, in further improvements in quality, efficiency and access for hundreds of additional patients. He believes that with this kind of tangible evidence about efficiency, more patients can be treated with the same resources so that the "more of everything" health-care costs can be controlled. Extrapolating this strategy to all areas of health care, he believes, can maximize value for money and illustrate that the public system can be made sustainable.

Perhaps improvements will come from Cy Frank's battle for greater efficiencies. There is, however, a long way to go, in Alberta and across the country. Wait times within the province, he says, from consultation to surgery take thirty weeks in 90 percent of cases, but the period from reporting pain to consultation with a specialist can vary from fifteen to sixty weeks. This means that in 90 percent of cases, the wait time from pain to surgery ranges from forty-five to ninety weeks, or roughly eleven to twenty-two and a half months. No wonder Commonwealth Fund studies show Canadian wait times to be the longest among seven industrialized countries studied.

It would be a polite understatement with a record like Alberta's to say that something is not quite right. Across Canada, five years after the 2003–2004 First Ministers' Accord on Health Care Renewal, the Canadian Institute for Health Research found that wait times for hip replacements had declined in three provinces and remained the same in three (including Alberta), and could not say in the other four. More success was made in knee replacements, with five provinces reporting progress and one (Quebec) reporting none. But what is "progress," when measurements are as elastic as Saskatchewan's reporting that 90 percent of knee-replacement cases had been dealt with within 464 days, Nova Scotia 576 days, Manitoba 397 days, Alberta 395 days, New Brunswick 340 days and British Columbia 275 days? This is "timely access?" After all that new money provided under the accord?

Cy Frank is searching for sustainability through quality and efficiency improvements in a very microscopic, promising way inside
hospitals, the core institutions of medicare. The eye physicians
Geoff Williams, Robert Mitchell and Amin Kherani are searching
by taking procedures out of hospitals altogether.

At six-thirty on a dull, wintry morning, the three physicians sip
their coffees and talk freely about the $24 million they borrowed
to invest in the South Alberta Eye Centre off Macleod Trail in the
south-centre of Calgary. Dr. Mitchell, already wearing his cap
and gown for his first surgery of the day, at seven, is a cataract-
removal specialist. Dr. Williams and Dr. Kherani specialize in
retinal problems and other inner-eye afflictions. Their wives
considered them a bit crazy to borrow that much money. Now
they declare themselves happier in their new clinic handling
about twice as many patients daily, they estimate, as when they
practised only in the hospitals.

The Eye Centre gleams with bright lights, shining fixtures,
colourfully painted walls, comfortable waiting rooms and
state-of-the-art equipment. It is the kind of place that drives
unreconstructed defenders of medicare wild with loathing: a
privately financed building, services in a setting that looks and
smells like private medicine, even if patients are fully covered
by Alberta Health Services (AHS) and do not pay a nickel from
their own pockets. No matter. To those dedicated to the purity
of medicare (all public, all the time), the Eye Centre presages
the proverbial slippery slope toward private medical services,
privately paid for, and the parallel public–private system of the
kind many countries have, and have had, for years. So controversial has the idea been of providing publicly paid eye treatments
inside privately financed clinics that other clinics in Calgary and
Edmonton have opened and closed, caught in fierce, shifting
political winds.

Those winds, Drs. Williams, Mitchell and Kherani admit, are their biggest fear and that of their bankers. They had to bid for an Alberta Health Services contract in 2010 and meet all AHS specifications and quality standards. The Eye Centre and another clinic were winners in the bidding; three other clinics lost. The AHS would give them only a one-year contract. In 2012, however, the Eye Centre signed a new five-year agreement with the AHS.

Dr. Kherani calls the centre "ultra-public" because he and his colleagues—there are about six other surgeons who practise there but are not owners—get paid on a fee-for-service basis like all other surgeons. Patients' charges are covered by the AHS. Patients come from all over southern Alberta, from Calgary south to the U.S. border. Some of them have to be treated fast, as in cases of retina detachments, and speed is more likely found in this clinic than in the emergency rooms of Calgary hospitals. Dr. Kherani and his colleagues also operate in those hospitals for complicated cases when patients have more than one problem and need the full range of services that only a hospital can provide—in trauma cases, for example. "The difference," Dr. Kherani says, "is that in the public system you get a quota allocation of operating rooms during regular hours, whereas here 50 percent of retinal surgeries are done in off-hours." When you control patient flow in a smaller clinic, he explains, you can better organize operating times for patients and staff.

The result, the trio asserts, produces more efficient use of their time and more patients being treated. Their centre is integrated into the hospital system, because straightforward cases come from the hospital to the centre, very complicated ones from the centre to the hospital. For the eye surgeons and, they say, for patients, it's a win-win result. Quality is maintained and efficiency is enhanced by more patients being treated at lower per-patient costs. Nurses are not unionized—which is why nurses' unions hate private clinics, regardless of the public payment for patients—although the centre's nurses are paid union rates. If nurses did not receive union rates, the doctors say they could not attract qualified staff. Clerical and secretarial staff receive lower salaries than in hospitals, a saving for the clinic. The Alberta government did compare costs of delivering eye procedures in private clinics and public hospitals but refused to make the results public. Leaks to the *Calgary Herald* suggested that the report found costs in private clinics on average to be 28 percent lower per procedure.

Processing more patients, especially for repetitive kinds of surgeries, enhances any doctor's income when he or she is being paid on a fee-for-service basis. More patients means more money. Without the ability to set rates individually, doctors can enhance their incomes under the fixed-fee schedule only by seeing more patients. Obviously, therefore, the gross incomes of Drs. Williams, Mitchell and Kherani are higher than if they worked only in the hospitals because they can see more patients and bill accordingly. Ophthalmologists are among the best paid of all specialists across Canada, with those in Alberta being the highest earners overall. (The Canadian Institute for Health Information reported that doctors who specialize in cataract surgery earned an average of $551,666 a year in 2010.) There's a very good case to be made that certain procedures such as cataract removals have become much simpler and faster owing to new technologies, so fees should be reduced.

Seeing more patients, of course, does not axiomatically reduce costs for the AHS. More patients being treated requires more per-patient payments to physicians. The centre obviously takes some patients out of the hospital, thereby freeing up operating-room time for acute-care cases, which is what hospitals are uniquely equipped to handle. The centre's doctors will make more money, but the doctors also have to defray the $24 million cost of the investment. When they retire, they expect to have at least their share of the equity in the business to sell or pass on.

Today, the Eye Centre flies below the political radar, but it was not always so for clinics that operated outside the hospital system in Alberta. Throughout the 1990s, private clinics became a political football, dragging Alberta and Ottawa into fights, pitting the Friends of Medicare and unions against the provincial government, and causing the PC government of Premier Ralph Klein to wobble back and forth from enthusiasm for extending private delivery to retreat. One flashpoint was the use of so-called facility fees, direct charges to patients to meet overhead and other costs placed atop the medical charges absorbed by the province. Chrétien's federal government claimed that these fees constituted a kind of extra-billing and thus violated the Canada Health Act. It reduced federal transfers to the province by $3.6 million in 1995. Later, the Alberta government retreated in the face of these penalties and public opposition, so clinics such as the Eye Centre now have their facility fee paid by the government as part of the contract to deliver services. The centre's costs, even including the facility-fee payment, will be lower per patient than at a hospital because it does not have to sustain the large overhead expenses of any hospital.

The squabble over facility fees was part of a much larger storm around private health care that erupted after the Klein government cut the health budget from $4.2 billion in 1992–93 to $3.4 billion in 1996–97 as part of an assault on the provincial deficit and a reduction in the increase of federal transfers. Whereas the previous PC government of premier Don Getty had been building full-scale hospitals in rural areas, Klein cut acute-care beds and closed hospitals, including three of eight in Calgary. Acute-care beds fell from 4.5 to 2.4 per thousand population. With public facilities contracting, wait times expanded. The debate began inside cabinet, and in the public, about substituting private facilities for the disappearing provincial ones.

This sort of debate breaks out every time restraint of whatever severity is imposed on the public system. Wait times rise, citizens get unhappy and some elected officials begin to think about private clinics to deliver certain services. The Klein cutbacks produced that kind of debate. The later recession of 2008–2009 that damaged every government's fiscal position produced the same effect. Whereas 10,500 cataract surgeries a year were being done before the recession in Alberta, 75 percent within sixteen weeks, restraint caused by the recession's dire impact on public finances pushed total surgeries down to 8500 and extended wait times to up to forty-six weeks. The contract given to the Eye Centre and another clinic was supposed to increase cataract surgeries to 12,000, thereby significantly reducing wait times again. Such a reduction could not be accomplished within hospitals alone, given the constraints on availability of operating time.

The logic is obvious and compelling. Almost every reformer of health care agrees that patients should be kept away from expensive hospitals wherever possible, without impairing their health. There are some medical procedures that might be called "repetitive," and basic eye surgeries would be among them. An expensive operating room might have been needed for such surgeries years ago; today, technology makes these surgeries just as safe in operating rooms within clinics. So, too, diagnostic tests for eye problems do not have to be done in hospitals; clinics such as the Eye Centre are well equipped to do them. Technology, cost control and shorter wait times for these repetitive surgeries make eminent sense, provided that quality is high and per-procedure costs are lower than in public facilities, but they still create political waves for those who dislike anything other than services delivered within public facilities, no matter how crowded, how long the wait times and how inconvenienced the patient.

The emergency department of the local hospital in Bridgewater, Nova Scotia, is not very busy in mid-afternoon. There are no genuine life-and-death emergencies from heart attacks or injuries sustained in car accidents. The paramedics are idle. The hospital has available beds, if necessary, so patients in the waiting room are not there because of bed blockers occupying beds upstairs. Patients tell a visitor that they are frustrated by the one to four and a half hours they have spent there. No official person briefs them regularly on what is happening, why they are waiting, how long it will be before they receive medical attention.

Behind the doors separating them from medical personnel, a doctor busies herself with paperwork, presumably not because she wishes to avoid seeing the patients beyond the doors but because the demands of routine have to be respected. She checks two patients in forty minutes. An elderly woman who had fallen and hurt her wrist is admitted. Presumably, a life-threatening case from a car accident or a heart attack would have galvanized everyone into action. On this quiet day, however, the serenity of routine permeates the ward.

Some of those waiting patients at the emergency department should not have been there—a situation that prevails across Canada. They should have gone to a local clinic or been steered to the hospital not far away in Lunenburg, assuming that the Bridgewater hospital knew the waiting time at the Lunenburg hospital was much shorter. But the two hospitals were not connected by a communications system, the administrative equivalent of the left and right hand not knowing what the other is doing.

They are sometimes there because they could not get an appointment with a family doctor. Emergency doctors are paid on a fee-for-service basis, so getting through as many patients as possible augments income; anything out of the routine and ordinary takes more time. In small communities, family doctors sometimes work in emergency, which pays more per patient, so it is in their interest to see patients there—an example, among many, of the wrong incentives.

"No one is riding herd on the emergency departments. You and I were at the emergency department at Bridgewater today. We both noticed there wasn't a sense of urgency," says John Ross, an emergency-room physician who guided me that day. Dr. Ross did a thorough study of the province's emergency system at the behest of the government. So when he speaks, he is in a position to analyze the province-wide system.

"Partially because it's been like that for so long that mediocre service is okay, no one is really complaining. Patients come into a visually not pleasant environment. There are a bunch of signs. The whole thing is about not serving and not making you feel welcome or comfortable. So we're all complacent and complicit in mediocre service."

Why are there no complaints?

"The culture has been present for so long that it is just the way it is. You have to wait. We are busy, and we like to remind you that we are busy," he replies. "I think patients are just afraid to ask questions. They don't feel like they have a right to. Our *disease-care non-system*, as I like to call it, is so overburdened that [people say] we are just lucky to have what we have, and we'll just accept it ...

"People who wind up there are often people who are

disenfranchised, or less empowered than some of us are. They tend to be elderly, so they don't complain as often."

John Ross is far from an ideological critic of medicare. He has worked intermittently in Africa on humanitarian medical projects. He's a case study of the concerned, politically progressive and medically skilled physician, clinician and professor. He believes strongly in public medicine, which is one of the reasons why the Nova Scotia government asked him to study the emergency health system. His study, with its many commonsensical recommendations, offered a menu of better practices that would produce efficiency gains that, in turn, would assist patient care, improve quality and might bend the rising cost curve of health care. He travelled all over Nova Scotia, talked to medical practitioners, patients and members of the general public. He presented "symptoms and diagnosis of a system not working ... The emergency department is simply the canary in the coal mine, alerting people to troubles that are putting the entire health-care system at risk."

Among the problems that Dr. Ross discovered almost four decades after the full introduction of medicare: people wait too long for care and to see their doctor; they are confused about where to go; they fear losing any health services; they trust doctors and nurses and want more of them. People in rural Nova Scotia were particularly concerned about losing their emergency department, or perhaps their entire hospital, if they had one. (Some citizens feared that if rural doctors lost the extra money they could earn from working in emergency departments, they might leave the area altogether and head for more remunerative posts elsewhere.)

Ninety percent of patients who present themselves at small emergency departments could be treated in a clinic. Dr. Ross found that 85 to 90 percent of people who go to emergency are not admitted to hospital, but too many do not receive a timely assessment. "Tens of thousands of hours of people's valuable time is spent waiting." It seems logical that people should be diverted away from emergency departments, but there are too few clinics, and Dr. Ross found that "many communities reported a six-week wait for a doctor's appointment."

The problems of the emergency departments could not be divorced from those of the entire Nova Scotia health-care system. Dr. Ross described the evolution of the problems. Detailed accounting imposed by governments on hospitals were replaced by global budgets in the 1970s (the same system remains in place today). At first, these global budgets worked well, "but over time, the costs of equipment, new treatments and staff skyrocketed. So has patient demand for more services." Physicians have a "very limited understanding of the cost of the tests, treatments and procedures they order." His sober conclusion: "The result is that increasing consumer demand—caused by an aging population, more expensive technology and treatments, and the perception that health care can cure almost everything—has created immense pressures inside provincial health-care budgets. But the lack of accountability for how tests and treatments are ordered is equally problematic. We continue to try to pay for everything within a budget that is unrelated and unresponsive to the pressures from within. This leads to unacceptable wait times and one crisis after another."

Reading Dr. Ross's recommendations, and talking to him about them, raised a simple question: why have these things not been done years ago? It's the same question that the proponents of major efficiency gains in Canadian health care need to answer. If efficiency gains are so obvious and achieving them so easy, why haven't they been harvested? And if they haven't been harvested thus far, why does anyone think it will be easy to harvest them in the future? Change is difficult for all sorts of reasons, and the difficulties are not entirely because of greedy doctors, fat-cat bureaucrats and lazy health-care administrators. One reason, among many, is how hard it often is to change established patterns of behaviour.

The complexity of the system is compounded by the local leadership and responsibility for the system as a whole. Yes, ministers are collectively responsible, and the health minister of any government in particular, but that minister has no idea what is happening on the ground throughout such a complicated system. He or she tends to respond to headlines, opposition-party taunts and periodic crises. In an unfortunate but understand-able way, the people who run and work in the system respond rationally to the constraints and incentives before them. Serious efforts to change those constraints and incentives usually smash against the system's complexity and lack of overall leadership, which dilutes or frustrates change and produces a return to a self-sustaining status quo.

There is also a sense of helplessness when working in a huge, complicated system. As Dr. Ross discovered, "The impres-sion from travelling around Nova Scotia is that staff in most urban emergency departments are so accustomed to the norm—over-crowding, patients staying in the emergency department for days, hospital flow problems, a lack of support for innovation—that they have given up trying."

Dr. Ross's proposed changes were quite straightforward, even elementary: streaming patients within emergency waiting areas into urgent and non-urgent; having a senior decision maker see the patient as quickly as possible; informing those who are waiting what is happening and why; using the Ontario and British Columbia benchmark of eight hours from first assessment to leaving the emergency department. Dr. Ross offered dozens of other changes—all of which the Nova Scotia government, to its credit, accepted as part of a three-year reform plan for emergency services. Other efficiency gains are in progress, such as one province-wide purchasing agency for all the regional health authorities, combining the back offices of hospitals, reviewing drugs used in nursing homes, giving doctors access to data about health outcomes of patients so that doctors' performances can be measured, keeping remuneration increases for physicians to 1 percent.

In an attempt to drive efficiency and reduce costs, senior Nova Scotia officials are reviewing many existing practices within the health-care system, but some efficiencies are easier described than achieved. The NDP government, on taking office in 2009, pledged to keep open all emergency departments twenty-four hours a day at all hospitals, even little rural ones, an eye-rolling expense. Senior Nova Scotia officials know that some rural hospitals should close and their emergency wards with them. They also understand that a province with 975,000 people has no need of nine regional health authorities. But just try closing a hospital or combining regional health authorities, however, and wait for the howl. As one official said, "Health care is very political, and is therefore difficult to change."

Change it must, and radically too, believes John Ross. The sustainability challenge is real and pressing. The woes of the emergency system, he concluded, cannot be remedied without wholesale changes to the entire system, starting with putting the patient at the centre. In Nova Scotia, John Ross found that "patient care ... has become more of a slogan than a practice of a foundation for a strategy ... Much of today's disease-care system is provider centred—designed for the convenience of the practitioners. By that measure, it is a rousing success. Patients, however, have a different perspective."

Dr. Ross dismisses the argument that health care needs more money. "Our disease-care system is driven by people like me, a disease-care specialist," he says. "Once you hire someone like me, I'm going to wind up ordering more tests and costing more money. We've made this health-care system so opaque and so magical that wonderful things can happen, and all that is required is to put more money into it so I can get this impossible-to-treat thing fixed." Nova Scotia is spending about $3.5 billion for health care for 975,000 people. "A Grade 4 kid would say that's a lot of money," he says. "Surely we could spend the money more creatively."

Months after our first conversation, Dr. Ross's outlook had brightened. The government pushed ahead with his recommendations. Targets for wait times were being met. Communications improved with patients waiting at emergency departments; waiting rooms have been given a facelift, including at Bridgewater. Good people throughout the system are working to make it better.

Dr. Ross has pointed emergency care in correct directions. It was reassuring to hear that things had improved, with more improvements to come, but it still remains doubtful that efficiency gains alone can make medicare sustainable, although that is what Canadians want to believe and health-care experts keep telling them can happen. There is no shortage of suggestions about how to make the system more efficient, from the micro changes for surgical improvements developed by Dr. Cy Frank to the systemic ones envisaged by Dr. John Ross for emergency medicine. Every day, hospital and health-care administrators, civil servants, doctors and researchers are trying in good faith to wring greater efficiencies from the system, sometimes with success.

The health-care system, however, is immensely complicated, containing within it large institutions such as hospitals that are themselves extremely complicated; powerful vested interests such as doctors associations and nurses' (and other) unions, all working under negotiated agreements on employment conditions and pay; vast health-care ministries; federal–provincial agreements; demands from patients with every conceivable ailment and illness; media reports highlighting problems and presided over by provincial governments operating in a charged, partisan environment. Changing any one element of the system—the way a hospital or home-care delivery is run, the pay scales for doctors or nurses, how medicine is practised, how to encourage patients to use the system more responsibly—would be a major challenge for the sturdiest administrator or toughest politician.

Public institutions and policies, and not just in health care, develop what social scientists call "path dependency," meaning that the way things were previously done carves patterns of behaviour and creates entrenched assumptions that are strongly resistant to change. What looks so simple to a health-care expert writing an article, or a commissioner producing a report or an author penning a book—outsiders, in other words—invariably confronts the "path dependency" of any long-established policy, the iconic nature of medicare, the entrenched ways of health-care providers, the insistent demands of patients, the fears of citizens, the re-election prospects of a government and the sheer complexity of the system.

Think of the health-care system as a jigsaw puzzle of contoured pieces. Each piece touches three or four other ones. If one piece were to change, it would push others, causing them to move, and so on across the board. So it is with efficiency: a change to achieve better results necessarily means a series of shifts, which makes the entire process of change more difficult. In the private sector—not that it is without faults—the imperative of the bottom line can drive change, since a private enterprise's ultimate survival can depend on change, often disruptive and radical. The disappearance of companies that were household names several decades ago testifies to that cruel reality.

No such pressures attend public enterprises. As long as the health-care system is publicly organized and financed, especially the way that Canada has chosen to structure medicare, it will be governed by public-sector norms, which means ultimate political control, a high degree of unionization, very strong "path dependence," large and not very nimble bureaucracies, a high value on process over outcomes and an inherent tendency to expand. Economists have long noted that productivity improvements— that is, efficiency gains—in the service sector, writ large, are harder to achieve than in the goods-producing sector, and they are especially hard in the public sector. The health-care system, being largely public, suffers from something called Baumol's cost disease, named after the economist who demonstrated that wage growth eclipses productivity improvements in the public sector.

In the private sector, wage growth is determined by productivity and competition for skills. Neither of these factors applies to the same extent in the public sector. As a result, labour-intensive sectors such as health care tend to have lower productivity growth than capital-intensive sectors. As long as the demand for the labour-intensive outputs such as health care is sustained or grows, the number of hours worked in that sector will grow relative to the hours in the capital-intensive sector. To keep workers in the labour-intensive sectors means wage growth that is roughly parallel, which in turn means the total wage cost for the labour-intensive sectors such as health will capture a steadily growing portion of the economy. This shift is what has been happening in health care, efficiency gains notwithstanding.

The "buy change" assumption that underpinned the Romanow commission implicitly presumes that more money, properly directed, produces efficiency gains over the medium term. Alas, the new money doesn't all buy change, because in large, complicated systems those who are best organized and mobilized will grab a disproportionate share of the new money for themselves. This is precisely what happened once governments began pouring money back into the system following the federal–provincial accord of 2003–2004. Providers—doctors and unionized employees—saw their fees and wages rise sharply, without any commensurate productivity gains, thereby wrecking the hopes of the "buy change" theorists. Romanow, a former politician, was aware of the risk when he wrote, "Additional funds should not become a target for increasing salary pressure from health-care providers. There is a serious political risk to all parties—governments, health-care providers and their organizations, and regional health authorities—if the bulk of the additional funds simply goes to pay more for the same level of service, the same access, the same quality. This simply will not be acceptable to Canada." Maybe not, but that is what happened.

It could be argued that no more new money "buys change" more dramatically, if painfully, than more money. The less-is-more school of management argues that only this kind of pressure forces new thinking about ways to achieve greater efficiencies, because as long as providers and administrators know that they cannot count on more, they will have to make do with less, which in turn forces at least some kind of creativity. These short-term bursts of restraint, however, usually crumble under the pressure of labour unrest, media headlines about heartless governments and opposition party attacks. They also crumble because health-care demand always exceeds available supply. Any squeeze on supply faced with constant demand—without productivity gains— produces more triaging of care, longer wait times and generalized patient unhappiness.

The reports in the 1990s about health care produced a surprisingly common list of changes designed to improve efficiency. Many of these sensible recommendations have been, or are being, implemented, although the "rational planners" who proposed them say they have not happened fast enough. They blame a variety of villains, starting with governments and doctors, rather than accept that the sheer complexity of the system is more to blame. Almost every province has established varieties of family clinics bringing doctors, nurse practitioners, nurses and even physiotherapists, nutritionists and pharmacists together. Many are trying to move doctors away from fee-for-service to some form of salary. Electronic health records are being introduced, albeit slowly and with much controversy. A few provinces are toying with new methods of financing hospitals. A great deal of money is being spent on home care to keep people out of hospitals. The number of new doctors in or emerging from medical schools has almost doubled. Six provinces have created their own health-quality councils to monitor outcomes and performance measures, although of course there should be a national body to end this unnecessary duplication, but provinces, being provinces, prefer to do their own thing. So the system is changing slowly. Changes do not come fast enough to suit proponents. Or changes do not work out as planned. Or even if they do, the efficiency gains fall short of what had been hoped.

For example, over the past two decades, provinces have created new structures to administer their systems as recommended by various commissions. Health care presents a specific governance challenge because it is so costly, employs so many people, is everywhere present (or ought to be), must cater to so many different challenges, contains powerful vested interest groups and is, at heart, a political creation in theory run for the people, by the people. Good governance of such a complicated system is difficult to manage with the best will in the world and smart people in charge. But it does have to be managed, since large sums of public money are involved, and the stark alternative—free-market medicine—lacks centralized control and tends to be much more expensive to administer. Getting governance right has therefore been on the agenda of every "rational planner," and rightly so. Predictably, getting governance right has not been easy, judging from the massive changes that governments have imposed.

The only province that created a governance structure and left it in place is Manitoba, which set up twelve regional health authorities in 1997. In New Brunswick, nine regional health corporations, established in 1992, were shrunk to two in 2008. Nova Scotia set up four boards in 1994, then created nine District Health Authorities in 2001. Newfoundland had thirteen boards in 1994, then cut them to four in 2005. Quebec created local authorities in 1972 and merged them with other health organizations in the early 1990s to form Health and Social Service Regional Councils. The province still has eighteen regional boards that theoretically manage the system but constantly spar with the health ministry in Quebec City.

British Columbia had twenty regional boards and eighty-two Community Health Councils in 1993, reduced their number in 1996 and then amalgamated administration into five regional health authorities and one provincial health service authority in 2002. Saskatchewan created thirty-two health districts in 1992, then merged them into twelve in 2002. Alberta's changes can fairly be described as dizzying. Seventeen regional health authorities were created in 1994. These were reduced to nine in 2003. In 2008, one big provincial board was created, ostensibly to bring the greatest possible efficiency to the system (and to cut down on the rivalry between Calgary and Edmonton). When predictable local griping began about the new, province-wide authority's insensitivity to local concerns, new local zones were created within the province-wide authority. Ontario established its Local Health Integration Networks (LHINs) in 2006 but gave them little effective power, then announced in 2012 that LHINs would become responsible for family practitioners.

Regional structures make good sense in theory and, in contrast to the alternatives, in practice. Imagine a huge health-care ministry trying to micromanage the system; or a non-system in which hospitals did their own thing (as they do in a private health-care system) with patients as profit-drivers and no coordination among the hospitals. That regional institutions have been changed so often suggests that, as with so many putative efficiency gains, their promise exceeded the reality. Governments hoped new governance would produce better outcomes for patients and some bending downward of the cost curve. When the reductions did not materialize, governments' instinct was to reorganize the regionalization, hoping for better results the next time. If the past be any guide, given the cost pressures on the health-care system, more reorganizations lie ahead in the search for savings and efficiencies. "Change fatigue," already a complaint in Alberta and Ontario, is likely to grow. So will the search for efficiencies everywhere in the health-care system. If past results presage the future, efficiency gains will be harder to achieve than they appear to proponents. Although necessary and useful, they will not be enough to remove the challenge of making medicare sustainable.

Efficiency gains are desirable to improve patient outcomes and the quality of medicine and to lower the increase in health-care costs. There is no shortage of suggestions about how to accomplish these objectives, everything from substituting nurses or nurse practitioners for doctors, to improving data collection, to focusing on the 1 percent of patients (in Ontario) who account for 49 percent of total hospital costs and 34 percent of total health costs, to diverting people away from hospitals and getting them out of hospitals faster, to focusing on micro-efficiencies in medical procedures, to clamping down on excessive drug prescriptions ... The list goes on and on. One important improvement would be the creation of a national council on clinical evaluations and outcomes, rather than the potpourri of provincial ones, to guide physicians. Each proposed efficiency gain is easier to describe than to put into practice, but collectively they could make a difference in helping the health-care system get better. Beware, however, of believing that efficiency alone answers the challenges of medicare.

Professor Harvey Lazar, formerly of Queen's University in Kingston, pulled together thirty researchers to examine some of the results of health-care reforms from 1990 to 2003, everything from creating regional health authorities to new ways of delivering medicine. The reforms, the researchers found, "were aimed at improving the existing health-care model rather than replacing it. In this sense, the love affair between Canadians and their health-care system remained intact." The reforms' results, however, were "slight to at best moderate." Saskatchewan seemed to have embarked on the most ambitious reforms, Newfoundland the fewest.

The strongest force for reform came not from within the system but from without, especially the period of government restraint in the mid-1990s. "The crisis," writes Lazar, "helped place reform proposals that promised cost containment, efficiency and effectiveness on to the decision agenda of governments." Less is more, according to these studies, apparently produced results that the "buy change" theory did not. The biggest reforms, for better or worse, came from new governments. Political "values" (public attachment to medicare's egalitarian principles) and "insider interest groups" (doctors and unions) acted "mainly as protectors of the status quo or an improved status quo rather than as forces for radical reform or transformative change." The picture presented from these thirty studies helps to explain why efficiency gains from within are so hard, as change comes more from external than internal forces. The strongest opponents of change were organized groups within the system who were motivated to protect what they had.

TEN

Is Private Health Care
the Answer?

"Everything has changed over the last forty or fifty years. We organized a system in the '60s, and it has not evolved, really, since then. The system continues to be managed pretty much the same way it was forty years ago. The system no longer meets the needs of the population," Claude Castonguay told me one afternoon in his office at a Montreal think tank.

Creators of the Canadian health-care system are elderly now, but age has not dimmed a passionate commitment to their brainchild, except for the questions that have crept into the analysis of the father of Quebec's health-care system, Claude Castonguay. Emmett Hall, summoned in 1980 to review medicare sixteen years after his Royal Commission recommended it, pronounced the system fundamentally sound and suggested ways of reinforcing it by, among other things, banning extra-billing by doctors. Castonguay was asked by Quebec in 2008 to review the health-care system he designed. Unlike Hall, he looked back on his creation with a mixture of pride and dismay.

After the commission that Castonguay chaired recommended a public system similar to the one Hall proposed for all of Canada, he entered politics and became provincial minister of health to oversee the implementation of his ideas. Four decades later, Castonguay considers his system resistant to change, excessively centralized, clogged by bureaucracy and interest groups, costly to maintain, burdened with sagging productivity. Still committed to the idea of a public health-care system, he would allow private delivery and payment for some health-care services—heresy for true believers in single-payer, government-run health care and quite a departure for someone who designed Quebec's medicare.

"I still think we should have a good public system, as efficient as possible," he says. "But I feel—and this is not unique to Quebec because pretty well everywhere public systems cannot cope as a result of the rapidly increasing cost of these systems—you have to do a certain number of things." That "certain number of things" would include private health care alongside the public system.

Payments to hospitals should definitely follow the patients, rather than global budgets, he argues, because such an incentive would make hospitals more efficient. "It might rearrange services toward those hospitals that are more efficient. But then if the public system is not able to cope with the demand, and you have alongside a private hospital at the same price that will help relieve pressure on the system, that is one way private services could be developed," he continues. "It could be a hospital owned by private interests who will manage it under the public system.

"You can also have a system where people will pay for some or all of the services. You can also have private rooms in hospitals where for a limited number of hours each day and a limited number of hours each week, if there is demand and doctors are ready to use them and are ready to charge patients, it seems to me that everybody would win. It would be an additional source of income for the hospitals. It would take pressure from the public system. Doctors would make more revenues, and people who are ready to pay would get service sooner."

What about equity? Would people with less income receive

fewer services and in a less timely manner than those with more money? "Look at the situation here in Quebec with radiology exams," he replies. "If you go to a hospital, it will be free of charge. But if you are not ready for the long waiting periods to get that X-ray or some other exam, you go to the private clinics and you get the service immediately. The clinics are busier than hell. They make a lot of money and people pay for the services, and not only the wealthy people."

Quebec has more private clinics than anywhere in Canada. Even in Quebec, where health care is not as iconic as elsewhere in Canada, public opposition caused the government to decide not to license more. So whereas Castonguay would encourage more private delivery and payment of health-care services, the Quebec government treads quietly and the public does not rise up to demand more.

"The only explanation," Castonguay suggests, "is that in the public system jobs are unionized and in the private sector they are not. Labour unions in Quebec have been among the most active fighters against anything private.

"Patients don't have much to say. It's a very strange thing, and I wish I knew what the answer is. We will have to have some kind of a crisis even to have people be ready to discuss this issue. People are very passive. They accept what they would never accept from any other type of service. Some of our hospitals in Montreal, if you go there in the morning, what you see is long lines of people sitting in corridors, dirty floors, very grey atmosphere, depressing.

"And yet people accept all this. Why? I don't know. They feel if they can get into the system, they are not paying anything, so they seem to be happy. They know that medical services cost quite a lot. When they get into the system, they are well treated. So you don't hear too many complaints. People are very patient. I am always surprised by their willingness to accept what to me are pretty unacceptable situations."

The Charest government imposed a health-care tax on everyone who pays income tax that will bring in almost $1 billion a year for the health-care system. Castonguay is a skeptic. "In the last five years, the health budget has increased by about 35 percent, yet we haven't seen any improvement in the productivity of the system. So why add a few more billions?" he says.

Private health care makes Canadians angry, nervous and confused. In dogma and according to the Canada Health Act, patients should not be allowed to pay for medically necessary services; in practice, private health care is slowly growing. The Canada Health Act is supposed to stop extra-billing and user fees and halt all forms of private payment for essential health care. How can it be, then, that anyone standing on Parliament Hill who looks across the Ottawa River into Quebec will see the site of an old garage now converted into a clinic where for $1000 a patient can get an MRI within forty-eight hours, a test for which the wait time would be many weeks in the public system, except for emergency situations? How can it be that advertisements at the Calgary airport inform passengers that fast surgical service is just a flight away in Vancouver at the Cambie Surgery Centre? Or how can it be that those wanting much faster orthaopedic surgeries than in the public sector can pay for them at Dr. Nicholas Duval's private clinic in Laval, Quebec?

The majority of Canadians, according to polls, do not support private health care, because it offends the principle of equity, or care based on need, not income. On this principle Tommy Douglas introduced medicare in 1962 in Saskatchewan. That health care should be available to all, regardless of ability to pay, remains a foundational icon of contemporary Canada. Canadians are nervous about any private health care because they do not know how far down the proverbial slippery slope private health care might lead. And they are often confused about private health care because different meanings and realities are attached to the use of the word *private*.

Private health care has been part of medicare from its creation. The greatest of all the compromises at the heart of medicare was between the state and doctors, as previously noted. The state would take over the organization of the health-care system. It would pay the bills for "medically necessary" services, thereby guaranteeing the principle of equitable access. But doctors would remain entrepreneurs, earning their money from a fee schedule negotiated with the state, deciding what hours to work, how to practise. They would not become employees of the state—their deepest fear—but remain individual practitioners, part of a self-governing body of professionals who happened to be paid by the state. They negotiated the right to practise outside the medicare system, but very few of them did. Doctors would practise medicine using the state's facilities such as hospitals where required, then bill the state for their services. As long as the state paid, patients/taxpayers/citizens didn't seem to mind how doctors organized their affairs with the state. If doctors insisted on being self-governing professionals and business entrepreneurs, fine, as long as their services were available, medical quality was high and patients paid only premiums and user fees of the kind originally implemented by the Douglas government in Saskatchewan but subsequently eliminated by the NDP government of Premier Allan Blakeney. This was very different from the National Health Service in Britain, where doctors were employed by the state and received salaries from the state, although some worked exclusively in private, fee-paying health care.

Private practitioners working within a state-organized system defined Canadian health care. It is curious, therefore, that private delivery of publicly paid for services should be so controversial in certain settings. If a single practitioner/professional works on a fee-for-service basis, as most physicians still do, Canadians do not get upset, perhaps because it's been that way since the beginning of medicare. But if a group of private practitioners form a clinic to provide services for which they charge the state on a per-procedure basis, rows break out. In both cases—single doctor in an office, group of doctors in a clinic—the patient does not pay because the state does. Even in Quebec, this private delivery of publicly paid for services can be controversial. Just such an arrangement between a clinic of surgeons in Rockland in northeastern Montreal and Sacré-Coeur hospital—an arrangement that gave patients quicker access to surgeries—was abruptly cancelled by the minister of health who listened to union objections.

The same fate befell Canadian Radiation Oncology Services (CROS), established in 2001 in Toronto to deal with desperately long wait times for radiation oncology. So long were the waits that the Ontario government had to send 2018 patients to the United States at a cost of about $30 million. In an attempt to stop the drain, Cancer Care Ontario signed a contract with CROS to run a private clinic with public money. CROS lasted slightly less than three years and achieved 60 percent efficiency gains compared with hospitals, measured by patients treated versus costs. But it was closed down by attacks that it offended the spirit of medicare—another example of putting ideology before patients' well-being. In a patient-satisfaction survey conducted by Cancer Care Ontario a year after CROS began, 100 percent of patients said care was excellent, and 94 percent said they would recommend the clinic to friends. No matter.

The critical distinction is therefore between privately organized health care financed through tax dollars, and privately organized health care financed by private cash or insurance payments. This distinction, however, causes fear and confusion, again because the word *private* has become so emotional in Canadian medicare. Private has come to mean profit. The whole ethos of medicare is that profit is bad, un-Canadian and a threat to Canadian values. If somebody is making a "profit" from health care, this profit has to come from somewhere, and that somewhere is the patient either through direct payment or tax dollars. Canada pays doctors handsomely by international standards, but if they wish to make more than their fee-for-service payments or salaries by extra-billing, the Canadian Health Act prohibits the payments. Doctors can work exclusively outside medicare, but they receive no services from the public system such as hospital privileges, so few of them do. But what if a group of doctors, usually specialists, form themselves into a private enterprise and take procedures out of a hospital into a clinic? What if they finance the clinic themselves, do more procedures than can be done in a hospital where space and time are more restrained, operate under quality-control supervision of the state and then bill the state, thereby charging patients nothing?

Here is where, strangely, all hell can break loose. In theory and in practice, such health-care delivery and payment is consistent with the Canadian Health Act, which says nothing about delivery methods but which is emphatic about public payment. It is consistent, too, with the logic that if one doctor can be his or her own entrepreneur, billing the state for services rendered, then six or eight or ten or twelve doctors practising together and billing the state for services rendered should be considered to be functioning within the same boundaries of medicare. Except that theory and practice can clash with dogma, abetted by confusion.

The word *private* connotes for defenders of the medicare status quo a decisive move away from the values of medicare. Maybe private delivery of publicly paid for services would be the starting point, but just you wait, they warn. Before long, these institutions will be charging some of their patients directly, and down the slippery slope they will go until they become profit-maximizing, patient-pay clinics. Those who insist that all procedures must be done in a "public" hospital or other public setting, albeit by private entrepreneurs called doctors, believe that anything outside a hospital setting risks compromising medical quality. They also think anything done outside hospitals risks "creaming off" the easy procedures, leaving all the complicated cases with their attendant costs for hospitals. Nurses and other unions deplore the idea of taking anything out of hospitals because jobs anywhere else might not be unionized. If doctors work in a clinic that they have financed, they have to somehow make a "profit" to pay for the equipment, staff and other overhead, so something fishy must be going on. Corners must be cut, standards compromised.

The notion that certain procedures could be done more efficiently outside a hospital, wherein clinical time is restricted owing to shortages of space and staff (and union rules), thereby allowing doctors to make their "profit" (and more money perhaps), suggests to the critics a perversion of medicare's values. So although these privately organized clinics—or outpatient institutions, as they are sometimes called—are growing in number, their growth is sometimes attended by fiery debate. The Romanow commission wanted a reformed and more efficient public system, so disliked any move toward "private" delivery or payment. The Senate committee led by Michael Kirby—whose report was longer, more comprehensive and more challenging of the status quo than Romanow's—also favoured a public system but one based on an "indifference principle" about how services were delivered, privately or publicly, as long as the public purse paid.

The report that Claude Castonguay produced following his 2008 review of Quebec's health-care system stood out among the heap of government-commissioned studies of health care, because it asked an essential question: how much health care can we afford? Castonguay was interested in improving health-care access and quality, but his report had a specific mandate: to recommend "additional sources of health-care funding," to study the role of the private sector and to investigate how to better inform citizens about the costs of health care. The government asked for answers from a man with long experience in public policy and the reputation for being the father of public health care in Quebec. No doubt the government figured that these qualities would deflect furious opposition of the kind that greets any proposals for fundamental reform.

Castonguay did not disappoint. He offered a gloomy assessment of the province's public health-care system about four decades after he had created it: "Our health-care system is a monopoly installed at every level with the culture inherent to monopolies, whether public or private. The culture is based on regulation and budgetary controls, closed to the outside world, impermeable to real change, adaptation and innovation. It is a culture that favours inefficiency."

He outlined some unpalatable truths: "On the political level, any reconsideration of the system and its funding modes risked denunciation as an attempt to introduce a two-tier system. To control the growth of public health spending, successive governments have thus resorted to rationing methods and authoritarian governance. Wait times have lengthened. The system's productivity has declined. Employee motivation has plummeted. Public dissatisfaction with the health-care system has been accentuated. We must face facts: today, the public system does not seem to be able to satisfy public demand."

Then Castonguay reached the nub of his mandate: "The growth of public health spending is the number-one challenge of our public finances. Above all, it is encroaching ever increasingly on the State's other missions. The growth rate of public health spending is unsustainable, because of all the implications arising from it. This is an inevitable certainty."

An "inevitable certainty." Whereas Romanow, writing at a time of large budgetary surpluses, invited Canadians to ignore the threat of unsustainable health-care increases, Castonguay forced readers to confront it. Castonguay also offered a more sophisticated understanding of "values." He agreed, as one would have expected from the father of medicare in Quebec, that the health-care system had to be founded on the principles of universal access and social solidarity so "every person must have access to the medical and hospital care required by their state of health, regardless of their socioeconomic status or income." But, he argued, solidarity must be shown between generations, because today's generation "does not have the right to bequeath an undue financial burden for the future." Another profound difference emerged: whereas Romanow had spoken only of rights and obligations of the state toward citizens, Castonguay spoke of responsibilities of citizens toward the health-care system, which meant, in part, contributing "to the health-care system's funding according to his means and, complementary to this, in relation to his consumption of care."

In the decade before the Castonguay report, the Quebec economy had grown at 4.8 percent yearly, whereas health-care costs had risen by 6.4 percent. In 1980–81, the report said, health care took 30.6 percent of all program spending; by 2007–2008, that share had risen to 44.3 percent. Health care as a share of government spending was rising by 5 percentage points a decade.

Castonguay outlined the challenge—specific to Quebec but apparent everywhere in Canada: the government was predicting yearly health-care increases of 5.8 percent from 2008 to 2018, but the economy and government revenues would grow by 3.9 percent. This 2 percentage point gap didn't seem like much each year, but over a decade the gap would amount to $7 billion. More revenue would be needed, and spending increases had to be reduced to what Castonguay called the "growth of collective wealth."

"Collective wealth." Here is one of the most controversial ideas in health care. There is no right amount that a society should spend on health care, especially a rich country such as Canada. Rich countries always spend more on health care than less affluent ones. Advanced industrial countries are all wrestling with health-care spending rising faster than their economies, or their collective wealth. Germany and the Netherlands succeeded in restricting health-care increases to only slightly above the level of economic growth, but in Canada the idea that health-care spending should be allowed to rise only at the level of the increase in collective wealth remains heretical. The navel-gazing of those who work in and those who comment about the health-care system, the immense power of interest groups within the system, the unwillingness of Canadians to confront hard truths about health care and the political fear of talking sensibly about health care means that it is easier for governments to borrow money to cover the gap between spending and revenues, or to squeeze other spending, which is what governments have been doing for a long time.

In the early days of medicare, following Emmett Hall's Royal Commission, it had been assumed that health care and collective wealth would move in lockstep, each growing at about the same rate. Very soon after medicare's introduction, that hopeful analysis was blasted by the reality of slower economic growth and faster health-care spending. Ever since, governments have fed money into that gap. So have individual citizens for the many areas not covered by medicare. Castonguay faced this reality: "If public health spending is allowed to continue increasing at the current pace, this could only be achieved to the detriment of the State's other missions—or by increasing the tax burden. Both of these options are dead ends."

Like all who study health care, Castonguay saw inefficiencies and rigidities, the curtailing of which could reduce cost increases. These inefficient practices, of course, were easier to analyze than change. For example, the government could curtail certain services through establishing a group of experts to constantly review the scope of public coverage, but as he acknowledged, "reviewing the basket of insured services is taboo in Quebec. It is perceived as a Pandora's box which must not be opened." Better health promotion and prevention might help. The Quebec government (like those of other provinces) had taken many health-promotion measures in recent years, but the population was not getting healthier. Even if more emphasis was placed on health promotion, the impact would not be felt for many years, even decades.

From the beginning of medicare in Quebec, doctors were supposed to work together in family clinics with other kinds of practitioners. Quebec was often lionized elsewhere in Canada as the model province for this kind of care. Yet unbeknownst apparently to people elsewhere, Quebec had the lowest per capita access to family doctors in Canada—75 percent access compared with the Canadian average of 86 percent. Medical students preferred specializing rather than training for family practice. Clearly, family clinics were a more efficient method of delivering front-line health care, and Castonguay said Quebec needed more of them. They would establish better links with the local community if each patient registered and paid a yearly fee of $100 (eligible as an income-tax expense). Doctors who worked in the clinic would be paid by a combination of salary and the number of patients on the clinic's roster, the so-called capitation system of payment.

Better governance, the dream of reformers everywhere, inspired Castonguay. None of these dreams were especially new, as in the creation of regional health authorities that would then purchase services from hospitals and clinics. This attempt to split buyer and provider was quite common in Britain, Sweden and Australia. But Canada was far behind the reform curve in using this model, as in so many other areas. Castonguay recommended electronic health records, a staple of reform agendas everywhere. He called for better clinical measurement of outcomes so the best treatment at the lowest cost would be assured as often as possible. He recommended a new institute to evaluate quality and measure outcomes, another priority of health-care reformers everywhere. Except that Castonguay had been around long enough, and had acquired enough world-weary experience, to know that "Quebec physicians and other clinicians to date have shown little interest, if not resistance, to measurement of the quality of care and clinical performance."

He offered another the dream of a "new unionism," although he seemed to understand the unlikelihood of the dream's realization. In Quebec, he wrote in words that could apply elsewhere: "In the health and social services sector, unionism has mainly empha-sized monetary questions and job descriptions." He continued to say that "in our health-care system, labour relations, to all intents and purposes, still bear the stamp of a climate of confrontation throughout the pyramid from top to bottom ..." where "labour relations continue to be based on bargaining power." Unions exist, above all, to negotiate "monetary questions and job descriptions." They are especially powerful in Quebec, but they are well organized elsewhere too. Unions, like medical associations, can always find some situation somewhere in Canada or the United States to justify why they should be paid more or have their work conditions improved.

Into this description of Quebec's health-care system, Castonguay wove his ideas for private health care becoming more evidently part of the system. One of three commissioners dissented from these ideas, so the three-person report was not unanimous. And the Quebec government, having specifically asked for a study about more private money in the health-care system, rejected Castonguay's ideas. They were too politically hot.

The debate over privately delivered medicine—paid for privately or publicly—has intensified, because medicare did not evolve as rapidly as medicine and the society it served, which is not surprising given how difficult changes are to achieve in any complex system. Hospitals are extremely costly institutions. Cost pressures on hospital budgets caused patients to be moved through the institutions as rapidly as possible. More rapid discharges might well have been good for patients, but it cast them immediately outside the purview of public payment for their health-care needs as soon as they exited the hospital.

All sorts of new or improved procedures—from cataracts to angioplasty to joint replacements—took up time, space and money in hospitals. Lives were significantly improved by these medical advances. Some of these procedures saved the state money in the long run because medical conditions were not allowed to deteriorate to the point that later treatments would be more expensive.

Angioplasty is cheaper than critical care following a heart attack. But these improved procedures did put pressure on operating-room time in hospitals and on hospital budgets, adding to the cost pressure on overall government health-care budgets. The new procedures made triaging more difficult for hospital administrators and made wait times longer without sizable infusions of additional cash. Some governments responded by no longer paying for some publicly financed services. Ontario, for example, delisted physiotherapy, optometry and chiropractic services as a cost-saving measure. Patients then either had to buy private insurance or, most likely, pay from their pockets.

Some treatments that once required hospital procedures and recuperation time in hospitals can now be done, in whole or in part, by pharmaceuticals, such as the treatment of ulcers by drugs instead of stomach surgery. As the population profile gets slowly older, more people need care in institutions other than acute-care hospitals or at home. The trouble was, and is, that state budgets are so stretched at existing levels of taxation to pay for doctors' bills and hospital costs that the rest of the health-care system has been left outside the public system.

This example will vary from province to province, but suppose en route to work tomorrow, you have the misfortune to be struck by a car. You break, let's say, your pelvis or suffer an injury that requires hospitalization followed by recovery. From the moment of injury to full recovery is what might be called the continuum of care. Again, depending on the province, you might be billed for the ambulance that takes you to the hospital. While hospitalized, your financial cares are covered by the state: beds, food, nursing, surgery, drugs. Once you are discharged, depending on your age and province, your drugs may no longer be completely covered by the state. Physiotheraphy will cost you money. You might have to buy crutches or rent a wheelchair. In other words,

the Canadian system fulfills its secularly sacred mission of equity
through public payment when you are in the hands of a doctor
and/or in a hospital, but on either side of those parts along the
continuum of care, the mission falls apart. Similarly, if the definition of health care is broadened to include dental and eye care
and pharmaceuticals, the Canadian public system offers nothing
or a patchwork, far short of what public systems supply in Europe.

That is why—to the surprise of most Canadians who do not
know the facts—Canada uses tax money for a smaller share of
its total health budget than almost every other country with a
public health system. As noted previously, 70 percent of health-
care spending in Canada is public, but 30 percent comes
from private sources. Only Switzerland, the Netherlands and
Australia, countries with essentially public systems, spend
more health-care money privately. The Scandinavian countries
(minus Finland), Japan, New Zealand, France and Germany,
among others, spend less private money. This seventy–thirty
distribution makes Canada an outlier in the world of public-
health systems: almost complete public coverage for what we
have come to define as "essential" medical needs—doctors and
hospitals—but a patchwork or non-existent public coverage for
other health-care needs, even though as medicine has evolved
these have become "essential." Deep, narrow and expensive, as
opposed to the systems elsewhere that are somewhat shallower,
wider and cheaper. This unique shape of the Canadian system
is what history has handed down, even though it no longer fits
the health-care needs of a somewhat older population and taking
into consideration the changes to medicine.

Where do we spend private money in health care? In 2008,
Canadians spent about $50 billion of private funds on health care,
with spending rising 5 to 6 percent a year. Of this, $12 billion went
to prescribed drugs, roughly two-thirds paid for by insurance,

one-third out-of-pocket. Another $11.2 billion went to dental care, with a little over half covered by insurance; $3.6 billion for eye care, with only about a quarter of the payments insured; $4 billion for in-hospital services, such as single rooms, to patients; $4 billion for institutions other than hospitals (long-term care facilities, for example); $2.2 billion for professionals other than doctors. With so much left out, per capita incomes rising and the costs of some services outside the public system growing fast, private insurance spread to cover many of these costs. It grew from 24 to 41 percent of all private health-care spending from 1988 to 2008. Governments understand that the shape of health care has somehow got to change so more care is provided across the entire continuum of care, but they are so stretched financially that expanding public care is proving difficult. One big trade-off of expanding public coverage along the continuum of care, with the new costs defrayed by asking for people to pay for some portion that is now "free"—a trade-off that is common in some other countries—is deemed far too politically risky. So, too, is another possible trade-off: asking people to pay higher taxes to expand medicare. And so, too, would be an explicit endorsement (as opposed to an eye-averting one) of more private, profit-making medicine of the kind Nicholas Duval practices.

ELEVEN

Dr. Duval's Option

D r. Nicholas Duval is a medicare outcast, a private, for-profit doctor. Duval does not advertise; his website is mundane; his private orthaopedic clinic sits along a busy boulevard strip in suburban Laval, north of Montreal. Thousands of weekly commuters could easily miss the sign in front of the Duval Orthopaedic Clinic.

Inside, a patient can get a hip replacement for $18,000, a knee replacement for $16,000, a hip resurfacing for $18,000, an Achilles-tendon reconstruction for $7500, an arthroscopic knee procedure for $3000, roughly the cost of similar procedures within the public system, although patients do not know how much anything costs in a hospital because they do not pay directly. The charges for these interventions are posted on the wall in the waiting room of the Duval Clinic like room rates on a hotel door.

Standard procedure would see a patient book an appointment, visit Duval's wife, a family practitioner who works in the clinic, and undergo standard physical and blood tests to ensure the patient is ready for surgery. A week or so later (late November and early December are especially busy because patients want surgery before they head south after Christmas), the patient returns, makes a down payment of $1000 and gets the surgery. The financial package also includes a week in a private room at the clinic (flat-screen television, squeaky clean, lots of space), two daily physiotherapy sessions (for which the patient must pay), a checkup at the clinic after six weeks and another after six months.

Is the Duval Clinic a canary in the mine shaft for Canadian health care? In countries with largely single-payer public systems, such as Sweden, Australia, Britain and New Zealand, a Duval-type clinic, or private hospitals or wings in hospitals, would be more common. They would be at the margin of the countries' overall health-care system, accounting for perhaps 1 percent of patients in Sweden, 10 to 15 percent in Britain and a somewhat larger share in Australia and New Zealand. In Canada, however, private paid-for medicine remains an outcast, even though the Supreme Court authorized it in the Chaoulli decision that centred on Charter of Rights and Freedoms protection of private provision of health-care services. Provinces such as Ontario will not allow private medical practice for services covered by the Canada Health Act. Other provinces such as Quebec and British Columbia turn a blind eye, as with Dr. Brian Day's orthopaedic clinic in Vancouver that does private surgeries for private payment but also takes patients from the public lists such as Workers' Compensation Board cases paid for by the government. The Duval Clinic accepts patients willing to pay from their own pockets, with no patients referred from the public system. "We're the only one," Duval says.

Timeliness of access and fear of hospitals drive patients to Dr. Duval.

"About 10 percent of the patients are not from Quebec, and most of those are from Ottawa. It's only a two-hour drive, and wait lists in Ottawa are very long," he says, adding that he has operated on a smattering of patients from Atlantic Canada, Alberta and even Yukon. "There are two major reasons why they come. One is the wait times. The other is that they are scared of infections in their hospitals. They know that if they go into a public hospital, they are going to share a room with someone else. They have been there. They see it's dirty and they are a bit scared. In the public system, you could wait for a year for an operation from the time you see an orthopaedic surgeon."

Duval is expanding slowly to make sure his business and medical models are sound. In 2010, his clinic did 464 surgeries, of which 197 were joint replacements. When he started in 2002, there were 230 surgeries, including 90 joint replacements. He and his wife are the only owners. They began with a $3 million bank loan, then secured another for $6 million to build a new wing. Another orthopaedic surgeon who opted out of Quebec's public system performs surgeries at the clinic; two other doctors alternate between the public and private systems. "You are allowed to alternate if you send a letter to the government thirty days before you opt out and you send a new letter eight days before you go back into medicare," Duval explains.

The clinic employs thirty people, not all full-time. The fifteen nurses are not unionized. They receive about 90 percent of the money that their equivalents would earn in a hospital but presumably without the benefits. "We have no trouble recruiting," Dr. Duval insists. Joint-replacement surgeries are done on Mondays and Wednesdays, minor surgeries on Tuesdays, clinical visits on Thursdays and Fridays. Duval comes to the clinic on Saturdays to check on patients operated on the previous week.

"There is a lot of profit. I make the same income as any orthopaedic surgeon. It's not a problem," he says. "The reason it works well is because it's specialized. The fact that you always do hips and knees means your nurses are very efficient; the orderlies become very efficient at taking the patients up, giving them a shower, making them walk. It's always the same thing. By being efficient, there is a lot of money you don't waste."

What of the cost to the patient? Patients go to the United States for similar procedures and pay between $40,000 and $90,000 for surgery and three days in a hospital. His clinic offers the same service for much less. Still, $16,000 to $18,000 is a lot of money, although money buys a patient an operation within one or two weeks instead of many months. "I'm not sure I would pay that," Duval says. "Maybe I would wait in line to get my surgery done. I would hesitate before making a decision. What I hope will happen is that government will say, 'Look, our wait times are ridiculous and our surgeons are not able to do some of their surgeries.'

"Why don't they put the money on the patient instead of putting the money either on public or private? Let's say a hip or knee replacement is $16,000. You go where you want and we give the public hospital or the clinic $16,000. It seems that private is the bad guy in health care …

"It's not fair in a hospital. Orthopaedic surgeons get three days, with the hip-and-knee guy one day, the sports-medicine guy gets one day, the general surgeon gets one day. In a hospital, it doesn't work. It's war."

That kind of "war" drove Dr. Duval out of the public system, "I had almost two years of wait time for some of my surgeries," he recalls.

Even a for-profit, private practitioner needs the public system. Duval deals with standard cases, not complicated ones that only a full-blown hospital can handle. An arrangement with a local hospital means that should an unexpected emergency occur during surgery—a heart attack, say—the patient is dispatched as soon as possible to the hospital.

Critics of private clinics deplore this "creaming" of patients— that is, accepting only the routine cases. To them, "creaming" means the for-profit doctor makes easy money on routine cases, while the public system absorbs the costs for complex ones. Defenders such as Dr. Duval reply that such a division of labour is better for at least some patients, who use their own money to attend to their own health needs. If they do so outside the medicare system, their needs are met more swiftly without harming anyone in the public system. Health care is a right, and an intensely private matter, for which an individual should be able to decide how and if to spend his or her own money, especially if the public system suffers from bottlenecks and delays. To which critics would reply that draining routine cases from the public system makes the overall per-patient costs of that system greater, leeches experienced health-care professionals away from the public system, thereby weakening it, and sends the country down the slippery slope toward two-tier health care.

But as the population ages, placing more demands on the system for the kind of orthopaedic procedures that Duval offers, the public system's wait times are likely to lengthen. If so, a clash beckons between the timelines set by governments and those set by some seniors for their health care.

The biggest threat to equity principles of medicare from the aging of the population does not come from the observable fact that older people use and cost the health-care system more. That they do is incontestable. In 2007, for example, the average yearly cost was $3809 per capita for youths aged one to adults aged sixty-four. For those aged sixty-five to sixty-nine, the cost was $5589; for those seventy to seventy-four, $7732; for those seventy-five to seventy-nine, $10,470; and for those eighty years and older, $17,469. In the coming decades, there will be many more Canadians as a share of the total population over sixty-five years of age, and more above eighty, or even ninety.

Aging poses a range of challenges for the health-care

system—notably, how to treat as many ailments as possible outside a hospital—but, surprisingly, a huge upsurge in costs will not be among them. The aging of the population will definitely add costs, but these are estimated in a range of studies to be only about 1 percent a year, or several billion dollars in today's money. Several billion extra dollars, year after year, is not chump change. Governments, paying 70 percent of all health-care costs, are struggling with how to pay today's health-care bills without raising taxes or cutting other programs. But given what the country is spending on health care (public and private), roughly $200 billion a year—the public share of the new money for seniors stands between a rounding error and something to be modestly concerned about finding.

A bigger threat from aging comes from timeliness. Will the public health-care system be there for us when we need it? Will it be there within a timeline that is convenient to me or a time frame established by a government? What if my timeline, given the shortening of the years left to me, is a good deal shorter than the government's? Obviously, no public system can respond immediately, or even very quickly, to each and every ailment. The system has to triage, mobilizing resources to deal with those who are most in need of treatment. Some waiting is therefore inevitable in a system in which money cannot buy speedier access (although waiting time for some patients needing certain procedures, and with the ability to pay, would diminish if Duval-type clinics sprouted). At what point, however, does waiting become aggravating, even intolerable? The public system, triaging as best it can, establishes one timeline; the patient, especially an older one, might have another. He or she might say: These are my remaining years. I want to feel better as quickly as possible so I can enjoy a higher quality of life in the time I have left. If the public system can relieve my pain or make my life more comfortable within a reasonable time frame—one that I define as reasonable—that is a good solution. If not, why should I not be able to use my money as I see fit to improve my own health as quickly as possible to maximize the enjoyment of the years I have left? It's my money, my ailments, my life, and why should the state, if it cannot provide timely access, deny me the right to relieve my pain as quickly as I can? The older the population becomes, the greater the number of people who will ask that question. No one likes to wait unnecessarily for health care. The shorter a person's timeline, the more the urgency to reduce the wait.

This clash—a senior's timeline versus the system's time frame—will intensify political pressure to bypass the public system by creating private outlets for health care that will deliver faster care for certain types of ailments. The pressure for private-delivery, privately paid-for medicine will come more from an aging population than from free-marketers in medicine, of whom there are few in Canada. Obviously, seniors who are not economically comfortable will be unable to pay for their health care. But there will be some seniors for whom improved health will be the most important consideration for their shortening lives. This attitude is the nightmare of defenders of the public system: "middle-class flight," as more and more people no longer believe they can get what they, not the state, consider timely treatment and demand an alternative outside the system.

Some seniors with resources, as part of the middle-class flight, will pay what it takes for faster improvement of their health, either because they have the money already or will change other aspects of their lives to find the money—using savings, forgoing vacations, moving into smaller accommodation, whatever. If such sentiments grow, political parties will begin to sense that a political market exists for private-payment health care.

Health care would seem the classic political issue in the broadest sense of the term, since it is largely publicly organized and financed. And yet, as often happens in the Age of the Charter of Rights and Freedoms, courts have barged into this political field, including the Supreme Court of Canada. In particular, courts have pronounced on the role of private medicine in Canada, which one would have thought to be inherently and exclusively a political concern. But there are few subjects that judges cannot choose to see through a legal prism, health care apparently being among them, although they have no expertise in the field.

Quebec was one of four provinces (Alberta, British Columbia and Prince Edward Island being the others) that prohibited private health insurance for medically necessary services provided by the public system. The province did so under two statutes, because it feared that private insurance would lead to privately paid for services that would draw doctors and patients from the public system, thereby weakening it. George Zeliotis, a patient, and Jacques Chaoulli, a doctor, joined forces to ask the courts to find the statutes unconstitutional because of the prohibition against private medicine. They argued that without the option of private delivery of medically necessary services, they would find themselves on the public waiting lists, whose lengths were so long that persons on them risked prolonged pain and suffering in contravention of their rights under the Quebec Charter of Human Rights and Freedoms and the Canadian Charter, especially section 7 that protects the "security of the person."

What came to be known in legal shorthand as the Chaoulli case began with a Quebec trial judge. She heard many weeks of testimony, including expert witnesses from Canada and abroad, before concluding that, yes, the Quebec government had justifiable reasons for the prohibition on private insurance. Such insurance would weaken the public system and create a "two-tier" health-care system. The preservation of the public system in the interests of all citizens overrode the individual rights of patients to pay for faster access outside the system. A Court of Appeal judgment upheld her ruling. And that was that.

Except that Zeliotis and Chaoulli were especially determined. Their case had caught the attention of provincial governments, medical associations, private clinics, social action groups and labour unions who saw the case raising such crucial issues that only the Supreme Court of Canada could settle them. Onward therefore went the case to the Supreme Court in 2004, which revealed itself in a 2005 ruling to be as divided as the country. There were three decisions from seven judges (on a court where sharply split decisions were rather rare). Two of the decisions, supported by four judges, reached the same conclusion, albeit by slightly different analytical means: the prohibition on private insurance did contravene basic human rights protected by the charters. By a four-to-three decision, the Supreme Court struck down the provincial ban and opened the door to private insurance, which, in turn, was thought would lead to a flood of private medicine. Except that what followed was a trickle, not a flood, because whatever the state of the law, the state of public opinion remained angry, nervous and confused about private medicine; and politicians were more worried about the state of public opinion than the state of the law.

The Chaoulli decision articulated passionately the pros and cons of private medicine. None of the Supreme Court judges were health-care experts, but they plunged into reviewing the "facts" previously examined by the trial judge, an exercise that Supreme Court judgments had lectured appeal courts against doing. No matter. The judges cherry-picked studies that suited their judicial preferences. The international evidence about the impact of private insurance on public systems does not reach a consensus. That countries differ widely about using, encouraging or prohibiting private insurance speaks to the uncertainties about it.

Our learned judges were divided but not uncertain. Madame Marie Deschamps, arguing against the ban on private insurance, agreed that "no one questions the need to preserve a sound public health-care system." Private insurance, as shown in other countries, does not threaten the public system, she argued. The judge had little time for dissenters. The judges who disagreed with her, she said in her judgment, illustrated an "emotional reaction," and some of those groups who intervened were using a "socio-political discourse that is disconnected from reality." Governments, she argued, had promised numerous times to find solutions to long waiting lists. They had consistently failed. "The governments have lost sight of the urgency of taking concrete action. The courts are therefore the last line of defence for citizens."

Beverley McLachlin, the chief justice, argued that the state had developed a health-care system but then failed to deliver "a reasonable standard within a reasonable time." The state's "virtual monopoly ... results in delays in treatment that adversely affect the citizen's security of the person." She ranged over evidence from abroad and concluded that "many western democracies that do not impose a monopoly on the delivery of health care have successfully delivered to their citizens medical services that are superior to and more affordable than the services that are presently available in Canada. This demonstrates that a monopoly is not necessary or even related to the provision of quality health care."

Ian Binnie, writing for the minority, pleaded for judicial humility. Chief Justice McLachlin had written about a "reasonable standard within a reasonable time." Who among the judges, Binnie asked rhetorically, could and should define constitutionally a "reasonable standard?" He argued, "The public cannot know, nor can judges or governments know, how much health care is 'reasonable'... It is to be hoped that we will know it when we see it."

Health care was properly a matter for legislative democracy and not courts. Nevertheless, he thought that private insurance would lead to a two-tier system used not, as McLachlin suggested, by "ordinary" Canadians but by those who can afford it, namely, the better-off. "Those who seek private health insurance are those who can afford it and can qualify for it. They will be the more advantaged members of society," he wrote. "The concern is that once the health needs of the wealthiest members of society are looked after in the 'upper tier,' they will have less incentive to continue to pressure the government for improvements to the public system as a whole." The Quebec government, and by extension others, was constitutionally entitled to prohibit private insurance.

The gifted health-policy amateurs of the country's highest court had wrestled a central complexity of any health-care system almost to a draw. Nonetheless, a thin majority decision emerged that produced a legal precedent that went nowhere in the real world of politics. No government grabbed the Chaoulli decision and used it to justify opening up health care to private insurance for matters covered by the public system. No further cases built on the Chaoulli precedent to force governments into action.

The Supreme Court could not have predicted when it heard the case in 2004 that the federal and provincial governments were negotiating a $41 billion health accord, a portion of which was specifically targeted at reducing wait times. Governments were in fact trying to tackle (again) the wait-time problem that a majority on the court said so imperilled the well-being of citizens as to justify private insurance. There the matter has stood: a legal decision largely ignored, although by definition capable of being revived; a federal–provincial deal that has brought down some, but not all, wait times.

There is no consensus about the impact of private health care on a public system, although to advocates and detractors the virtues and evils of private health-care insurance (PHI) are clear. The evidence very much depends on what is being studied, by whom, in what context and, critically, the kind of private health care and its financing and relationship with the public system. Sweeping generalizations nonetheless abound in all discussions of private health care that often reflect the ideological convictions of the analyst. Most Western industrialized countries have, and will continue to have, some kind of private health-insurance market, often for basic health care and not just ancillary matters such as cosmetic surgery and upgraded hospital accommodation. Canada is an outlier. Private health-care insurance for basic services is theoretically allowed in parts of Canada, but so many restrictions apply that it either does not exist or exists at the margin of the system.

Apart from the Castonguay report, private payments for health care have only been suggested once in recent years. In 2001, the Alberta Premier's Advisory Council on Health, chaired by former Progressive Conservative deputy prime minister Don Mazankowski, recommended a parallel private health-care system. It called for an "opening-up" of health-care delivery and financing to reduce reliance on public revenue sources that the council suggested had become too onerous. "People who can afford to pay more would be able to use the private system and open up more space for services in the public system. This option would provide the most choice to consumers," it suggested.

It appeared that perhaps something might happen in Alberta to contest the principles of the Canada Health Act that forbade private payment for essential services. Premier Ralph Klein at the apogee of his political popularity mused about a health-care "Third Way." Iris Evans, Alberta's health minister, talked about a parallel private system that would compete with the public one. A caucus committee began studying the Mazankowski report. That is where the "Third Way" became the No Way. When the private health-care issue came before caucus, as it did several times, PC MPs, especially those from rural areas, rejected the idea. Their constituents were nervous about such a fundamental change. That nervousness twitched the premier's political nose. The Mazankowski proposal disappeared.

Finding reliable, objective, international and comprehensive results for private insurance is hard to locate amid the plethora of studies. The OECD in Paris has done voluminous work on the subject, because controversies about the role and existence of private insurance exist in many of the OECD's member countries. In a careful, comparative study, the OECD said PHI presents "both opportunities and risks." PHI injects new resources into health systems, adds to consumer choice and helps make the systems more responsive. But it poses "considerable equity challenges" and adds to total health-care expenditures, including for the public sector.

The OECD survey concluded (as per Judge Binnie's ruling) that "high-income groups are more likely to purchase private health coverage." The very issues argued about in the Chaoulli case—wait times and what they reveal about the problems of the public system—are those that led to more private insurance in Australia, Ireland, Denmark and Britain. Reported the OECD, "there is a strong link between demand for private health insurance and waiting times for elective surgery," precisely the driving force behind the plaintiffs' complaints in the Chaoulli case. Operating either outside or within public institutions, privately insured medicine can be used to improve access to timely care (for some), and give individuals with PHI "enhanced peace of mind, less anxiety and less pain—and better health outcomes when waiting times are very long." Moreover, PHI has created a market for new hospitals or clinics, and so has shortened wait times caused by rationing of services in public hospitals. Australia, which spends much less of its GDP on health care than Canada but gets comparable outcomes, has encouraged PHI as the principal means of shifting demand from overburdened public hospitals. In France, 90 percent of the population has private health insurance paid by individuals and employers that tops up coverage from the public system for essential services. The OECD, in an important conclusion, found that "only a few OECD countries have both long waiting times and high levels of population covered by PHI."

PHI is some respects, however, can aggravate problems in public systems. There's some evidence that PHI increases overall health-care demand, so that wait times do not necessarily fall and overall health-care costs rise. The OECD, being careful, unlike advocates on both side of the emotional divide over private insurance, said the relationship between PHI and the length of wait times "has proven difficult to ascertain." PHI does seem to increase health-care utilization (and therefore costs), but is that because of latent demand caused by aging of the population and/ or increased availability of care?

PHI will get the private-insurance policyholder to see doctors faster. If PHI pays doctors more per visit than the public system, the financial incentive is obviously to shortchange patients from the public system by doctors who work in both the private and public systems. Governments have introduced a variety of means to try to reduce the inequalities of access and treatment between private and public systems, with mixed and sometimes financially costly results. Across the OECD, private insurance is becoming more expensive relative to inflation, putting it out of reach for more individuals, especially low-income ones. And there is always the challenge that PHI providers obviously prefer healthy persons to those with pre-existing problems or an age or lifestyle that suggest illness is not far away. If PHI patients can opt out of the public system, their departure changes the risk pool for those who remain, since the PHI holders will tend to be younger and healthier. Similarly, it is an open question whether the PHI holder will care much about the public system.

Boosters of private care claim that it creates competition, stimulates innovation and improves quality. As with the Scottish jury verdict, the case is "not proven." The OECD discovered that private insurers did not find it in their interest to invest in quality improvements. Nor should anyone assume that PHI automatically reduces the overall cost of health care; if anything, overall costs rise. The removal of some patients from the public system in theory reduces the number of those on the wait lists, thereby shortening them, but if physicians work outside the public system, thereby reducing supply, the wait times might not shrink and in some cases might lengthen. If PHI is subsidized by the state, as happens in a few countries, public costs rise. And PHI, by definition, features a number of health-care producers, none of which can match the purchasing power and single-payer simplicity of the state, so administrative costs are higher. With PHI comes more complexity, too, as governments try to establish regulations to protect consumers and, where possible, to promote access to PHI.

In its major survey of Canada's economy in 2010, the OECD noted that "Canada is almost unique in the OECD in offering consumers so little choice in the area of health insurance." It suggested that "if even a small portion of the population chooses to opt out of public insurance and purchase private insurance for core services, the presence of competition from private plans would give politicians and managers of the public plan a strong incentive to operate more effectively and reduce costs, since otherwise they would lose market share." This conjecture is based on a classic market principle: one firm gains at another's expense. The declining firm pulls up its socks or loses market share and profit and, at worst, goes out of business. But the public health-care system can't go out of business. It has no internal incentives to lower costs, and demand will still be enormous even if some patients leave the system. The OECD plan can work if, within the public system, there are privately organized and public providers, as in Sweden, with money following the patient within the system. At the very least, the public–private issues are a great deal more complex than the selective certainties expressed by the gifted health-care amateurs on the Supreme Court and many of the passionate advocates for and against private insurance. But the OECD evidence does suggest that if wait times are a serious problem, as they are in Canadian medicare and as they might increasingly be if they conflict with seniors' own timelines, the pressure for private care will grow.

TWELVE

Can We Make
Ourselves Healthier?

Making the public healthier, thereby preventing illness and improving individual happiness, is a health-care mantra. What has been called the "wellness agenda" runs through every health-care discussion. It seems axiomatic that if we could just make everyone fitter, we would need the expensive health-care system less. This assertion is correct, but only up to a point. The wellness agenda is politically unassailable. It has also been politically oversold.

For example, in the summer of 2010, federal, provincial and territorial ministers of health issued a ringing Declaration on Prevention and Promotion, titled "Creating a Healthier Canada: Making Prevention a Priority." Wading through statements of the obvious—"Canadians value their health"; "Disease, disability and injury remain a serious concern in Canada today and must be addressed"—the unsuspecting reader might have been tempted to believe that this portentous declaration would produce action. It said all the right things about the importance of preventing disease by making the population healthier, encouraging people to eat more nutritious foods, get more exercise and make better "lifestyle choices." It said, "To create healthier populations, and to sustain our publicly funded health system, a better balance between prevention and treatment must be achieved." Canada, ' the ministers asserted, "is showing leadership in making prevention and promotion a priority."

If Canada were indeed "showing leadership," it does not show up in international comparisons. Canada ranks in the middle of the pack for health outcomes in studies by the Organisation for Economic Co-operation and Development. According to a Conference Board of Canada report, Canada came fourteenth of twenty-four countries in overall health outcomes.

If Canada were "showing leadership," why are Canadians fatter than ever and why do they exercise less? Obesity rates have climbed such that obesity is now considered an "epidemic." In 2009, 24.1 percent of Canadians were deemed to be obese, compared with 14 percent in 1979. Among two- to seventeen-year-olds, 18 percent were overweight and 8 percent obese. According to a Sport Canada report in 2008, the share of adults aged fifteen and older who reported actively participating in sport had dropped from 45 percent in 1992 to 34 percent in 1998 to 28 percent in 2005. As all health researchers know, health outcomes are more related to low income than to any other factor. Since income inequalities have risen in Canada, that swelling group of low-income Canadians remains unfit, at considerable cost to themselves and the health-care system. On the positive side, smoking rates have declined to 17 percent nationally from 32 percent in 1984 and 46 percent in 1964. The decline in tobacco use constitutes the greatest public-health success of the past generation. It will pay dividends for those who quit smoking or never start—and for the long-term costs of the health-care system. Canada can still do better, since the country's smoking rate remains higher than that of seven other OECD countries.

Just eight months after their 2010 declaration, Canadian health ministers were at it again. They announced in 2011 a "national dialogue" in the battle against obesity. The ministers had apparently forgotten about the 2005 federal/provincial/territorial plan called "Integrated Pan-Canadian Healthy Living Strategy," which had the same wellness agenda and could be piled atop a stack of government reports, plans, policies and declarations of intent to promote healthy living and thereby prevent health problems dating back to the earliest days of medicare.

Canadians therefore have not lacked for studies or policies or programs from their governments to make them healthier. Those policies and institutions and good intentions, alas, have largely failed.

A healthier population and relief from cost pressures. Who could oppose these objectives? They command overwhelming support among health-care experts. They were goals outlined by commissions into health-care policy by Roy Romanow and Michael Kirby. They were recommended as urgent priorities in a 2009 Senate committee report under Dr. Wilbert Keon, a distinguished cardiac surgeon. Canadians buy into these object-ives, too, according to public-opinion polls, except when it might mean taking more personal responsibility for health and life-style choices. When confronted with uncomfortable trade-offs for sustaining medicare's financing, making the population healthier provides an escape from hard choices.

Properly and vigorously pursued, the wellness agenda might make progress over time in improving overall health and shave small costs from the system. Control of blood pressure has helped reduce the incidence of heart and stroke problems, for example. Better nutrition, it has been reported, can help reduce the inci-dence of cancer and heart disease. But anyone who seriously believes that the wellness agenda will reduce the costs for medicare has been reading and believing too many of those plati-tudinous government reports. The gap, sadly, between the fine intentions and the distressing realities should make everyone cautious in placing too much hope in the wellness agenda. In this sense, the wellness agenda is a mirage, because thus far it has not made the population appreciably healthier or relieved pressure on health-care costs. The wellness agenda's short-term returns will be modest and certainly will not allow avoidance of hard choices about medicare.

Emmett Hall insisted in his Royal Commission report that gave rise to medicare that individual responsibility was crucial in health care, although the system he designed imposed no penalties on those who failed to shoulder such responsibility. He wrote, "Positive and enlightened attitudes towards his health and habits to promote it are part of the individual's responsibility which cannot be replaced by compulsion or by public health measures."

Hall was right in one sense: the state cannot compel people to live healthy lives, and even the healthiest of persons can be struck by illness. Nor has the state found a way to penalize or reward citizens for taking (or not) "positive and enlightened attitudes" toward health. Instead, the state has relied on "public health measures" that are long on information, regulations, exhortation and examples to coax changed behaviour from the populace. In some instances, the state has taken action against harmful products to make them less affordable and desirable (cigarettes), implemented laws to promote safety (seat belts, bicycle helmets) or stiffened penalties for dangerous behaviour (drunk driving). Taxes and regulations, therefore, have been used with considerable success to prevent bad health outcomes for individuals and lower costs for the state. Some of the debate today swirls around whether to extend those same tools of taxation and regulation to make less desirable health choices more costly, as in taxing sugary drinks or requiring the use of less salt. Flu shots for all, immunization programs for children, more nutritious menus and anti-smoking campaigns in schools, more awareness of sexually communicated diseases such as HIV/AIDs—the list of initiatives taken by governments to improve public health is long and impressive.

Still, the share of health-care budgets for public health remains a small fraction of the total. For example, the budget of the Ontario Health and Long-Term Care Ministry in 2011–12 was $47 billion; the budget for the Ministry of Health Promotion and Sport, created in 2005, was $400 million, or less than 1 percent of the health-care budget. When Canadians demand more spending on health care, they generally focus on the needs of today and tomorrow rather than on the longer-term benefits of better overall societal health. A marginal dollar put into hospitals, doctors and drugs will trump a dollar spent on promoting health around every cabinet table in the country. The general public and cabinet ministers would never dream of taking a dollar from the existing health-care delivery system and putting it into prevention. Zero-sum does not work in health care.

Medicare, remember, was created to cover costs for physicians and hospitals, even though its founders hoped that eventually it would be extended to other health services. It was designed as a medical system to treat medical problems, not a social-service system to promote certain lifestyle choices, reduce income inequalities or limit traffic and workplace accidents.

The wellness agenda, much in vogue these days, has been around for a long time. Monique Bégin had wanted to add health promotion as a sixth principle in the Canada Health Act. Instead, she could only persuade her cabinet colleagues to include a reference to it in the preamble. As long ago as 1974, a decade before the Canada Health Act, the federal health minister Marc Lalonde had issued a document, "A New Perspective on the Health of Canadians," that was hailed by health-policy experts internationally as the best of its kind. It framed almost forty years ago many of the issues around today's wellness agenda before anyone used that term. The report's analysis and recommendations were considered radical at the time, but today they are commonplace in almost every discussion about promotion and prevention. The report had very little impact in Canada, however, outside the small world of public-health-policy experts.

The Lalonde report of 1974 drew attention to a problem still acutely relevant today: "The annual rate of cost escalation ... is far in excess of the economic growth of the country. If unchecked, health-care costs will soon be beyond the capacity of society to finance them." It wondered about how to "control costs while removing all incentives to patients, physicians and hospitals to do so. The existence of a generous supply of hospital beds and of increasing numbers of physicians makes it easy for patients to seek care even for minor conditions and for physicians to hospitalize more patients, particularly when there are no financial barriers. Thus the goal of ready access to health-care services, both physical and financial, conflicts with the goal of controlling costs."

What the report called the "traditional" approach to health care—doctors and hospitals—defined medicare, but health care extended well beyond doctors and hospitals into the entire society, or what was called a "health field" concept. It encompassed biology, environment and lifestyles. Health had to be looked at not just as the treatment of disease and illness but also as a government- and society-wide set of challenges to make people healthier. Governments urgently needed to tackle that broader challenge for the sake of individual health outcomes and for the reason that "if the incidence of sickness can be reduced by prevention then the cost of present services will go down, or at least the rate of increase will diminish."

The Lalonde report laid out everything relevant for a serious public-health agenda. Since then, governments have been reinventing the wheel. Not to be outdone, the Mulroney government in 1986 produced its own health-promotion report, "Achieving Health for All." It ploughed much of the same ground, with two notable exceptions. More than a decade after Lalonde's bold analysis and prescription, this new report acknowledged a difficult truth that "prevention is a far more complex understanding than we may at one time have imagined." And the report put much more stress on the hidden truth of health care: that "people's health remains directly related to their economic status." (The reverse is also true.) The report continued, "We have not done enough to deal with ... disparities. As we search for health policies which can take this country confidently into the future, it is obvious that the reduction of health inequalities between high- and low-income groups is one of our leading challenges."

The international evidence that links socio-economic status to health is overwhelming. The World Health Organization Commission on the Social Determinants of Health, published in 2008, amassed a huge amount of data to underscore the links. The WHO concluded starkly but irrefutably that "social injustice is killing on a grand scale." In a report to the British government, Sir Michael Marmot analyzed health inequalities in England and concluded, "Inequalities in health arise because of inequalities in society." Whereas much government activity in Canada and elsewhere revolves around changing behaviour, the Marmot report said that such efforts would never be enough. "Serious health inequalities do not arise by chance, and they cannot be attributed simply to genetic makeup, 'bad' unhealthy behaviour, or difficulties in access to medical care, important as those factors may be. Social and economic differences in health status reflect, and are caused by, social and economic inequalities in society."

If governments and their citizens were truly serious about health promotion, they would confront the social determinants of health, which would include employment and working conditions, housing, standards of living, early child development.

It is little wonder, thinking about this analysis, that government efforts to promote healthier living and prevent illness have met with such limited success, for governments are loath to make the link, except rhetorically, between the social determinants of health and health outcomes. It is easier, and less costly, to develop health-promotion programs and to pursue a wellness agenda than to tackle entrenched income inequalities. Almost completely gone from Canadian political and public discourse is a sustained debate about such inequalities, so the debate about public health seems as worthy as it is removed somewhat from reality. Just as the health-care system is criticized as being too removed from the urgency of preventing illness, so the wellness agenda seems too removed from the urgency of thinking about ways of reducing socio-economic inequalities, or the so-called social determinants of health.

In the self-absorbed world of health care, it is just assumed by those employed in the field and by the experts that marginal government dollars, if they are available, should go into health care. People can debate how those dollars should be spent within the health-care system, but they assume that health care trumps every public priority. Canadians, too, seem to think governments should spend more on health care, which means pushing more dollars into the system. But it could be argued that if people really do worry about sustaining the system's rising costs over the long term at existing levels of taxation, then dollars should not be spent on the health-care system but on preventing people from entering the system as patients, and that the best way to accomplish that objective would be by reducing socio-economic inequalities. A dollar spent on poverty instead of the existing health-care system, or even some public-health programs, would be the best long-term investment not only in health but also in lessening cost increases.

The trouble with such an argument is that it flies in the face of political realities that people want health care now, and woe betide a politician who denies it to them by arguing that dollars will not be spent on reducing wait times or training more doctors or buying new technologies but on reducing income inequalities. And woe betide, too, the politician who says money will be spent on poverty in the face of doctors, nurses and other unionized employees who demand, and often receive, considerable wage increases whenever new dollars appear. In other words, the political reality of where dollars for health care have gone and will continue to go trumps the logic of where they should go. The political reality centres on the demands of today; the logic points to a longer-term horizon. The political reality can be quantified—how many doctors, technologies, prescriptions, hospital beds—whereas the logic of spending dollars elsewhere does not lend itself to such easy measurements. The political reality is about me, now; the logic is about others, later.

So commissions, reports and intergovernmental declarations pile atop each other. New institutions are created, programs developed and funds spent on what is an important objective: to make the population healthier. And yet, Statistics Canada's massive 2009 Canadian Health Measures Survey (CHMS)—the first comprehensive national survey to determine fitness levels—was enough to make the most ardent proponents of public health wonder what had been happening.

Many studies of fitness had relied on a measurement of body mass index (BMI) because it can easily calibrate an ideal ratio of height to weight. It is true that some health experts question the BMI method, noting that it cannot differentiate between muscles and fat, does not account for genetic variations and cannot easily be applied to different ethnic groups. But since no consensus has emerged about what should replace the BMI, it remains the measure most frequently used by doctors and health researchers.

The Statistics Canada survey, using BMI data, showed that Canadian adults had become heavier over the previous twenty-five years. (The populations of most OECD countries had also become heavier.) The CHMS survey went beyond the traditional BMI measurements to include fitness tests and other body composition measures. It found that "fitness levels of children and youth have declined significantly since 1981, regardless of age or sex. Fitness levels of adults have also declined, particularly among younger adults." Among youth fifteen to nineteen years of age, the share of those whose waist circumference put them at an increased or high risk of health problems had tripled. Decreases in fitness levels since 1981 were particularly pronounced for young adults aged twenty to thirty-nine. In the 2007 to 2009 period, just under 38 percent of adults were at a healthy weight, with many more men than women being overweight. In raw numbers, 4.4 million Canadians aged eighteen and older were classified as obese. The share of the population in that category is rising every year. Health Canada recommends a daily 1500 mg limit of sodium, but the current daily average is 3400 mg. The government is counting on voluntary action by food companies and public information campaigns, approaches almost certainly bound to fail, to bring daily consumption to 2300 mg, still well above the recommended daily intake.

Beyond income inequalities, the wellness agenda, so extensively studied and urgently preached, crashes up against various intractable realities of Canadian life that largely defy the best intentions of government policies. Among the main enemies of wellness is television. Watching television is, for the most part, as vacuous for the mind as it is unhelpful for the body. It is, after all, mostly a medium of escapism and entertainment and, as such, is the preferred way to spend leisure time for the largest number of Canadians. To television have now been added the computer and the smart phone. Together, they provide physically inert activities that defy the wellness agenda's prescriptions for a more active lifestyle. Depending on which study is consulted, the television is on in the average Canadian home twenty to twenty-four hours a week, or roughly three hours per day. Although a few people watch television while pedalling a stationary bicycle or following exercise programs, most people are anchored to their chairs or couches. The CHMS study referenced above asked twelve- to seventeen-year-olds how many hours a week they watched television. The weekly average was nine hours, to which was then added time playing video games and using a computer or smart phone to bring the total of screen-time viewing to twenty hours a week. How does any government policy combat this widespread societal preference for television and other electronic devices over more active pursuits?

Canada is also increasingly a suburban society. There has

been, and continues to be, a migration from rural areas to urban/ suburban ones; and the majority of immigrants to Canada land and remain in cities. Although urban planners struggle to intensify downtowns, with some success it must be said, the largest growth areas still lie in suburbs, which are built around the needs of the car. It is difficult for many suburban dwellers to walk to any store, movie theatre or other commercial establishment, even if they wanted to, because of the nature of suburbia with its shopping malls, sprawling neighbourhoods and wide thoroughfares. Rural residents have an even more difficult time walking anywhere, except for strolls in the country. The observable fact remains that cars are the principal method of transporting people. The entire North American continent's land transportation networks have been built around cars and trucks, for which no easy substitution exists. Even if massive investments were made in public transit, for which a strong case can be made on environmental grounds, the shift from cars would take time and not pull more than a small minority of drivers from their vehicles.

The number of jobs that require physical labour is dropping, and the number of desk-bound jobs is rising as the service sector of the economy eclipses the others. Even some blue-collar jobs have been converted into ones that require computer skills to operate mechanized assembly procedures. The Canadian climate in most of the country makes bicycling difficult, if not impossible, for months of the year and renders walking sometimes unpleasant too. The Canadian diet is heavily dependent on dairy products and red meats, with many items containing dollops of sugar and salt. Canada is also fast-food heaven, from Tim Hortons to McDonald's. Canadians have a very sweet tooth and are the world's largest per capita eaters of doughnuts. For many years, the federal government has produced the widely acclaimed *Canada's Food Guide*, an excellent source of information about nutritious eating and an outgrowth of the policy emphasis on health promotion. How many television advertisements are there promoting the guide compared with those for Tim Hortons or McDonald's?

A large gap also exists between the apparent urgency of health promotion and prevention and understanding with some precision what works across a whole society. We do know that a healthier society is obviously better for individuals, and that it can relieve a little cost pressure over the long term on the health-care system. We also know, courtesy of OECD research, that a strong correlation exists between levels of education and obesity. The higher an individual's education, the lower the probability of being obese. Higher levels of education, according to OECD research, allow greater access to health-related information, a clearer understanding of lifestyle choices and improved self-control. If this research is correct, Canada doesn't have all that much to gain in fighting obesity by making the population better educated, since the university and high school education rates here are already among the highest in the world. Of course, they could be higher still, but pushing up overall levels of education would only contribute marginally to reducing obesity.

What about all the other methods being tried by governments? The OECD tackled that question in a comprehensive 2009 report. It examined 150 studies of health prevention and promotion policies, a majority in the United States but some from Britain, Australia, Canada, New Zealand, ten other OECD countries and six developing countries. It made for sobering reading for all who believed that health prevention and promotion efforts would axiomatically be effective, reduce costs and be easily implemented.

Many prevention policies, it concluded, would bring better health returns but not for a long time.

The report found that "overweight and obesity rates have been increasing relentlessly over recent decades in all industrialized countries," another salutary reminder that many of Canada's health-policy challenges are not unique. Governments, the study said, have implemented many policies nationally and locally but "without a strong body of evidence on the effectiveness of interventions, and virtually no evidence of their efficiency and distributional impact." Specific policies do a little or some good, but since so many factors contribute to the obesity problem, one or two policies "will not reduce significantly the scale of the obesity problem."

Many health-prevention and -promotion policies, of course, cost money in the short term, and "they do not always generate reductions in health expenditure even over the longer term." Why? "Individuals may live longer with chronic diseases, as a result of prevention, and may survive long enough to experience unrelated diseases which they would not have experienced otherwise," the OECD found. As always in health research, the biggest variable tied to health was socio-economic status, rather than society-wide or targeted health promotion or prevention strategies.

Nonetheless, governments in Canada and elsewhere are pushing a variety of wellness plans, when they are not busy drafting declarations and gathering more information. So which ones work best? The sad answer from the OECD: "Most interventions were shown to have only a limited impact on the overall scale of the obesity problem." The least effective results in changing behaviour came from mass media campaigns and tax changes on foods, the best from targeted work with at-risk individuals, doctors and, critically, dietitians.

Imposing higher taxes on fatty foods such as sugary drinks is now a popular option in certain health-policy debates. Indeed, machines that sell such drinks are being withdrawn from schools in North America, either under government regulations or because companies wished to make a gesture that would deflect a tax. The objective of a higher tax would obviously be to lower consumption, and the OECD study estimates that a 10 percent tax would reduce consumption by 2 percent. The trouble is that low-income people, who spend a larger share of their income on food than others, would be disproportionately affected by such a tax, because consumption patterns would be only slightly affected. Administratively, such a tax would be difficult, since how would a distinction be made between, say, sugary drinks and so many other products with sugar? What about sodium, or other additives consumed in large quantities that are deemed injurious to health? How would a government tax such products? The more compli-cated the tax regimen, the higher the administrative costs. Looked at from only the cost-to-government perspective, tax increases on unhealthy foods are best, since they put money in governments' pockets. These taxes, however, do not appear to influence behav-iour very much. The OECD's study suggests soberly that "common beliefs about the potential impact of preventive interventions are often based on simplistic assumptions, which may lead to exceed-ingly optimistic expectations."

These international results are not what proponents of the wellness agenda want to hear. This agenda has its merits over the long haul, and it sounds appealing to politicians and citizens who want to avoid hard choices. Its logic on a personal level is impec-cable: the more an individual takes care of his or her own health, the better for him or her, and perhaps for the health-care system. The agenda, however, is also a diversion away from the much harder questions of socio-economic inequalities that are among the most evident drivers of health-care costs (to say nothing of human unhappiness) and of how to finance a health-care system without raising taxes or cutting other government programs. It is an agenda that is alluring and important but also not likely to produce anytime soon the results sought by its most ardent proponents. It is a necessary consideration but by no means a sufficient answer to the dilemmas of Canadian health care.

THIRTEEN

What Does the Public Think?

People in every country have symbols that define their national identity, but only Canadians believe the health-care system to be their most important national symbol. According to a Focus Canada survey done by the Environics Institute in 2010, 85 percent of Canadians ranked health care as the country's most important national symbol. When Environics first asked this question in 1997, 89 percent of Canadians had ranked health care at the top. Over that thirteen-year period, health care eclipsed in importance (in descending order) the Charter of Rights and Freedoms, the flag, national parks, "O Canada," the Royal Canadian Mounted Police, multiculturalism, Canadian literature and music, hockey, bilingualism, the Canadian Broadcasting Corporation, the national capital and the Queen. A 2008 survey by a leading Canadian pollster, David Herle, asked respondents how important were certain institutions and values to "the Canadian identity." Medicare came first (91 percent), ahead of freedom of speech, democracy, educational opportunity, compassion, freedom of religion and everything else on the list.

A 2007 Pollara poll of 1223 Canadians found that during the previous decade, health care far eclipsed all other issues in importance, except for a brief spike of interest in climate change in 2007. A 2010 Ipsos Reid survey for the Canadian Medical Association showed health care as the most important issue by an almost three-to-one margin over the economy and recession. During the 2011 federal election, Nanos Research found that health care topped the list of issues of concern. In November 2011, an Ipsos Reid survey showed health care at the top of the list of national concerns, above jobs, taxes, poverty and all other issues. Year in and year out, then, with a few exceptions, health care eclipses all other public concerns. No wonder politicians consider health care the third rail: touch it and you die.

Pollsters have repeatedly tried to figure out what Canadians think about the actual health-care system. What emerges is a confusing mélange of passions, convictions, fears and mythologies. For example, Canadians are constantly being told medicare is the best in the world and, according to a 2006 Pollara poll, 51 percent of Canadians believed it. In a Deloitte 2011 survey, by margins ranging from five to one and twelve to one, with younger Canadians the most positive, respondents agreed that "our system works better than most systems in the world," which of course has no basis in fact.

A 2011 Deloitte survey of consumer satisfaction found half of Canadians willing to give their health system an A or B grade, a higher share than in Germany and Britain but a lower share than in Belgium, Switzerland, France and Luxembourg. Most of the positive respondents must have given a B grade, since only 32 percent of Canadians said they were "satisfied with the performance of the health-care system." Predictably, 57 percent of Canadians gave a D or F grade to their system for "wait times." A majority of Canadians were pleased with the medical innovations, up-to-date technology and buildings in their system.

A survey done for the Romanow commission in 2002 found

very strong attachment to the public system, but only 37 percent of respondents believed the system was fine the way it was. The federal-government-sponsored Health Care in Canada survey of 2006 found that although 57 percent of respondents thought they were receiving "quality health care," 59 percent thought wait times were lengthening, and 55 percent favoured a "complete rebuilding or some major repairs" to the system. The Ipsos Reid survey for the CMA found generally higher satisfaction rates for people who had used the health-care system, but a large majority worried about the impact of the baby-boom generation on future quality, access and financing of the system. If the system needed more money, most respondents did not think they should themselves pay more in taxes or fees. When forced, however, to choose between a reduced level of health services and two alternative forms of increased funding, only two in ten preferred fewer services. Forty percent opted for more taxes on all citizens, and 40 percent said let the wealthiest pay directly from their own pockets.

A large and crucial difference appears in attitudes about people paying privately for health care and people receiving care in private facilities within a public-payer model. When people were asked, as Environics did in its Focus Canada reports of 2007 and 2009, 72 percent said they would support a system wherein health-care services provided by the private sector were covered by tax dollars. Contracting out "delivery of public covered services to private clinics," an option tested in 2005 and 2006 Health Care in Canada surveys, was approved by majorities of 55 and 51 percent, suggesting that Canadians had moved past the ideology of medicare as an all-public-all-the-time delivery system.

Environics asked about support for specific financing changes. The approval rate for pay out-of-pocket for faster service was 51 percent; pay extra for use beyond routine services, 46 percent;

a small user fee, 41 percent; higher taxes, 46 percent; delisting services, 26 percent. Environics concluded that "when it comes to privatization, Canadians prefer having one public system of health care over a two-tier system (even when being presented with arguments for and against private health insurance). However, paradoxically, there is clear and increasing support for private-sector delivery of publicly funded health care and for paying out-of-pocket for faster access ... Canadians also continue to show openness to various ways of financing the current health-care system, including user fees, paying for use beyond routine services, and even raising taxes, but are less open to the delisting of health-care service."

What seems clear from a wealth of polling is Canadians' apparently abiding belief that they can demand and should receive more from the public system, without being prepared to pay for it. For example, Environics gave respondents sixteen areas for "high priority spending"—everything from more physicians to home care to end-of-life care to aboriginal health. Of the sixteen high-priority areas, Canadians agreed that more should be done in fifteen of them by majorities ranging from 52 to 80 percent. Asked about drugs, approximately two-thirds of respondents said governments should pay for all prescription drugs.

A Strategic Counsel survey of 2009 asked for suggestions about improving the system: five of the six top suggestions involved spending more public money (more doctors, shorter wait times, more nurses, more emergency rooms, generalized increase in funding). A Deloitte 2008 survey gave respondents twenty-five changes to health care to consider, many of which involved more government spending on health care. Twenty-four received a positive response. The only one that was rejected would require all Canadians to purchase supplemental insurance. Any politician therefore faces the clash between demands for more services, better access and higher-quality care—demands that would normally require additional revenues that taxpayers do not wish to provide.

David Herle's Gandalf Group conducted one of the most recent (2011) and comprehensive surveys about health care, although only of Ontarians. Not surprisingly, 71 percent of respondents said health care was the provincial government's most important responsibility. By somewhat less than a three-to-one majority, Ontarians did not think the health-care budget needed to be curtailed, perhaps in part because they were so ill informed about the system costs. Health care in 2011 took up 42 percent of the provincial budget, but two-thirds of respondents thought it took up 40 percent or less, with 39 percent believing it took up less than 30 percent. Asked where, if necessary, the government might cut $100 million in spending, health care was the area to be most spared the knife. For such a precious matter as health care, however, people did not want to pay more in taxes. Thirty-nine percent refused to pay higher taxes for health care, although 51 percent said they would pay "slightly" higher taxes. Reported Herle, "All ideas for raising additional revenue are unpopular," an observation that explains, in part, why politicians are so frightened of even raising that option. Asked if the government were to increase spending, where that spending should go—surprise!—89 percent said health care.

Herle then discovered what pollsters had long noted: people think that if indeed the health-care system faces a financing problem, the answer lies in reducing waste and inefficiency. That is the answer people give to almost every question about finding new resources for any government program or reducing fiscal deficits.

Ontarians did not know how much money in their province was being spent on health care. They had no sense whatsoever that it might be crowding out other areas of spending, no sense that the province's deficit was large, or that health care was becoming more expensive. Herle reported, "All that is assumed by the policy elites is unknown to most of the public."

Herle's findings dovetailed with those from the 2011 Deloitte survey. It asked Canadians if "it is possible to improve quality and reduce costs simultaneously in our current system of care." By a five-to-one margin people said yes—the dream answer of those who want to avoid hard choices.

Another pattern clearly emerges from polling data and patient surveys: patients in the system, or those who have recently had dealings with the system, have a somewhat more positive attitude toward it than those who have not. Just as "bad news sells" is a media maxim, so the heath-care system is victim of the tyranny of the anecdote, whereby people relate to others their experiences. Human nature being what it is, the exceptional and the negative get more attention in the retelling than the normal and the positive. There is evidence that wait times, long as they often are, do not stretch as long as the public often believes; that the perception that the system is deteriorating clashes with positive accounts of experiences within the system; that Canadians believe they have the best health-care system in the world but also seem to think it is getting worse or will start deteriorating. An Angus Reid survey of 2010 found that 50 percent of the residents of one province, Saskatchewan, rated the delivery of health care as "good," the highest positive rating in Canada. And yet, people who had used the system for seeing a family doctor or specialist, having an advanced diagnostic test or having stayed in the hospital, offered much higher levels of satisfaction. Given a choice between a public system with new resources and a commitment to ensure access within a reasonable time frame, and parallel public and private systems, Canadians choose the public option.

The trouble lies in asking where will the new resources come from, and what is a reasonable time frame? Who would not choose the option of a public system delivering more timely access with high-quality service and excellent outcomes, at no additional cost to the taxpayer? This mirage beguiles Canadians who seem to be saying to pollsters, politicians and themselves, *Do not burden me with further taxes or fees, do not cut services on other government programs, give me more services (drugs, home care, long-term care, shorter wait times, more diagnostic tests) and make this possible by improving efficiencies and population health.* Only the bravest of politicians will force Canadians to waken from this dream.

Many governments have sent legislative committees to consult the public about health care. The latest exercise occurred in Alberta in 2009 and 2010 when a committee travelled to twenty-three communities, conducted twenty-nine workshops with over 1300 participants. The committee further received eighty-five written submissions from organized groups and fifteen hundred responses to an internet survey. The report tried to capture the passions, fears and ambivalences of Albertans.

Albertans, the report found, "overwhelmingly agreed that the Alberta government should continue to provide a universal, publicly funded health system that is accessible to all Albertans regardless of their ability to pay." Moreover, the population apparently wanted amendments to the Alberta Health Act with principles that would go beyond those of the Canada Health Act. These would include such principles-cum-banalities as "foster a culture of trust and respect," "quality and safety," "put people and their families at the centre of their health care," "enable decision-making using the best evidence available." They even wanted an Alberta patient charter (remember the clichés around a "patient-centred" system), setting out what citizens should expect from the health-care system and correspondingly what responsibilities citizens should shoulder—a discourse almost entirely missing from Canadian discussions of health care. These "responsibilities" should include "using services appropriately and wisely," "learning how to better access health services and use them appropriately," and "making healthy choices where possible."

Asked about "what's working" in the system, respondents underlined the care and compassion of Alberta's health-care professionals, the high quality of the province's health facilities, the expanded role of pharmacists and nurse practitioners, Telehealth for people in rural communities, family-health clinics where they had been established and universal access. But, noted the committee, "timely access to the system is still a major challenge—whether for a doctor's appointment, a diagnostic test, or an elective surgery. As more than one participant said, 'once you get in, the care is great.'"

What Albertans most complained about, as elsewhere in Canada, was timely access. "People spoke about delays they had experienced at each care point in the system," the committee reported, "from visiting a physician to receiving a hospital bed, and how these delays added up to a significant impact on their health and wellness." They worried about the lack of long-term care and assisted-living spaces, hospital emergency departments, the problems of accessing health care in rural areas and the need to promote wellness for the sake of individuals and removing cost pressures from the health-care system.

The belief that improved efficiencies could help patients get better care and deal with cost pressures ran through the hearings.

If the system were more transparent, patients would know how to use it better; if team-based medicine became the rule (as in family-health clinics), patients would receive improved and more timely care; if doctors were paid by salary rather than fee-for-service, costs would be reduced (although wait times might increase); if standards, guidelines and principles were clearly articulated in a charter, everyone would know what to expect, and the system would operate more effectively.

This belief that a better-organized system can solve cost problems helped Albertans avoid working through the hard choices about how to sustain their medicare. They told the legislative committee that they wanted health care to cover a wider range of services, and to offer more timely access too, but they were unwilling to pay higher taxes and user fees. They were deeply conflicted about whether the private sector should play any additional role in medicare.

The committee captured the passions and ambivalences about private health care: "Issues around publicly funded versus privately provided services are difficult ones to discuss, and they generate passionate responses. Some people expressed a desire for greater choice to improve their access to services, including the right to purchase private health insurance or pay directly for certain health services now only available through the publicly funded system. Others were open to private sector involvement in health if there were clear benefits from such involvement in terms of access or affordability. Their voices were countered by many Albertans who were very strongly opposed to the presence of for-profit elements in health care, and who argued that such elements introduce additional costs in the health-care system and undermine access, standards and quality."

Being only concerned with health care, the committee asked Albertans about health care in isolation, without inquiring whether citizens wanted more health-care coverage at the expense of other public expenditures, part of the generalized inwardness that plagues almost all discussions about health care. Accordingly, the committee reflected the rather widespread insouciance among Canadians that they can keep their existing system, expand it where possible and demand more of it, while recoiling from paying anything to use it directly, shouldering higher taxes or knowingly reducing government spending on other programs. Since the committee did not ask questions about health care in this context, which is the one that politicians must confront, it was not surprising that most of their respondents did not tackle any of these trade-offs.

Commissioner Roy Romanow listened to Canadians at public meetings. There, he encountered the challenge of all such cross-country hearings: the open microphone. Such a public process invites anyone to speak. Those who avail themselves of the opportunity tend to be eager to vent passion and grievances. Open microphones encourage interest groups that have money, organizational muscle and commitment to a cause. Public hearings, therefore, are seldom representative of overall public opinion, which is why the Alberta report, diligent though its members undoubtedly were, should be given some latitude as a full portrait of public opinion. It is also why the Romanow commission sought deeper probes of Canadian attitudes toward health care than open microphones could provide.

The first probe was conventional: a poll with many questions and a large sample size; the second was an innovative "deliberative poll," or dialogue, in which groups of citizens were selected and made to spend a day together debating issues. The process forced them to arrive at trade-offs and conclusions. Deliberative polling's virtue is that it forces participants to take into account many factors, struggle for compromises and try to see issues in the round. Deliberative polling's fault lies in being just that—deliberative—because the public's reaction to issues in the world of ten-second television clips, government spin, Facebook and Twitter is anything but deliberative.

In any event, the Romanow commission asked Canadian Policy Research Networks (CPRN) to organize twelve deliberative sessions across the country, each attended by about forty people who spent a day listening to presentations about health care, debating the subject and arriving at conclusions. They were given four scenarios: more public money for health care; user fees; increased private choice through a parallel private health-care system; reorganization of health-care delivery by making citizens sign up with a team of professionals working together. These alternatives were by no means the only ones available along the spectrum of health-care options, nor were they mutually exclusive. The scenarios, however, offered options about health care in isolation, not in the context of higher or lower taxes, and other government services. But forcing people to spend five hours wrestling with health-care issues at least produced more mature responses than conventional pollsters usually find.

The generalized pattern of analysis from the twelve groups went like this, according to CPRN. At first, people hoped the health-care system could be "fixed" by eliminating "waste" and improving efficiencies. Their response mirrored Focus Canada's surveys from 2003 onward: when asked for the "main cause of problems in our health system, more than half of the respondents said 'inefficient management of the system.'" As CPRN reported, participants discovered rather quickly about the lure of massive efficiency gains "that hope begins to fade as they work through the issues and the current and projected costs of health care."

Next along the train of thought came changing the system "consistent with the values of access based on need, fairness and efficiency."

Participants liked the idea of professionals (doctors, nurses and pharmacists, among others) working in teams. They believed this coordination would bring more "cost-effective care" and help to focus on prevention and patient education. Participants thought it reasonable to sign up with such a team and use an electronic health card. Unfortunately, in talking through and supporting this option, participants soon realized what proponents of these changes seldom acknowledge: changes might be better for patients, and even make parts of the health-care system more efficient, but they do not necessarily save money. As CPRN reported, "Even with these changes, participants come to realize that more funding will be required to sustain the health-care system they value. They struggle with where the money should come from."

At least CPRN participants were forced to "struggle," unlike the bulk of Canadians, whose leaders and commissions such as Romanow's did not ask them to think where new money for more health care might come from. As participants struggled, they rejected a parallel private system (by 47 to 39 percent), concluding that it would "drain valuable resources" away from the public system. What about user fees? "Participants were very uncomfortable with charging user fees for basic services, believing it would discourage those who are less well off from seeking needed care. This concern remains even when a subsidy for low-income citizens is proposed." So then what? "In the end, participants turn to public funding and, reluctantly, to tax increases rather than cuts in current programming." Initially, participants hoped that "transfers of funds from other programs can be used, but as citizens work through the possibilities, and one by one eliminate the candidates (such as education and social programs), they are left with tax increases as the only viable choice."

"Reluctantly," therefore, participants came to accept tax increases. They were not asked which taxes—sales taxes, personal income taxes, health taxes, corporate taxes—to increase or by how much, but they assented to the nominal idea of higher taxes with conditions. Principal among these was that the new revenues be earmarked only for health care (again, the inwardness of health care), with more transparency about where the money was being spent, a desire that led to the idea that perhaps health care needs a national ombudsman and a special auditor general. That more stringent oversight is required reflected "a distrust of the way in which the health-care system is being managed." Distrust permeates attitudes toward many governments and their programs, so there is nothing unique about such distrust toward the health-care system. Said CPRN, "The elites have spent ten years reforming the system to make it more efficient. But what citizens seem to be saying is that this restructuring has not improved the day-to-day care which they experience on a regular basis. They are paying more and getting less. Nor has it raised their confidence that the system is now more sustainable."

The conclusions of those who participated in this deliberative polling exercise were quite representative of what pollsters have found in more superficial soundings. All the earlier options— eliminating waste and duplication, efficiency gains—preferred by the participants were the easy ones and the ones that come to mind as answers to conventional polling questions. The easy options did not require any sacrifices or the loss of other government programs. It was only after working through the easy choices and recognizing that the sustainability of health care could not be assured by them that participants began "struggling" with the hard ones. In the real world of government, politics and the contemporary media, citizens make fast decisions—in the case of health care usually on the basis of their own experience with the system and almost never because they are confronted with serious options by their political leaders in order to replicate anything remotely like CPRN's deliberative polling exercise.

In 2011, PricewaterhouseCoopers tried a variation of CPRN's method. The firm chose twenty-eight people, who had volunteered from across Ontario and reflected the province's population and geography, to spend three weekends together working through options for the health-care system. This Citizens' Reference Panel listened to presentations from health-policy experts, some of whom had advised the Romanow commission. They represented the analytical school that argues that massive efficiency health-care gains are available and would, if implemented, erase any concern about the system's sustainability. With such advice being given to them, it was perhaps not surprising that the twenty-eight people leaned heavily on the efficiency analysis as the path to a better and more sustainable medicare.

They rejected the argument that the system needed more public money or private financing. Instead, they sought greater "innovation" and, of course, efficiencies—the default answer of the general public to concerns about the cost of any public service. Again, perhaps because of whom they had listened to, the panel bought recommendations from the efficiency school that had been around in some cases for decades. Some of these reforms had never been acted on. Others had produced action that, alas, did not bring the hoped-for results of proponents. Still others had failed. A few had worked. Typically, while the panel apparently expected that the efficiencies they suggested would save money and improve quality, the members also wanted more public health care, which would inevitably cost more money, not less—as in more social housing, counselling and psychotherapy, more doctors for the North (and financial incentives to attract and keep them there), more money for mental health and expanded "government assistance" to help people with increasing pharmaceutical costs.

The panel's recommendations, in and of themselves, were old but useful: family-health teams instead of physicians practising alone (already spreading across Ontario), models for physician payment other than fee-for-service (again, already spreading), moving people out of hospitals to in-home treatments (being tried), better information for patients and those entering the health-care maze (being tried), more emphasis on health promotion (being tried), "best practices" emergency departments (being tried), electronic health records (being tried), a hesitant nod to "government to study the cost-savings potential of a provincial pharmacare plan and to act on the evidence" (done and rejected for reasons of cost).

These twenty-eight citizens did a very good job and produced a report with worthwhile suggestions. The report could have been written by the provincial minister of health, so closely did the recommendations hew to what the ministry was already doing or intending to do. Like the Ontario government itself (and provincial governments everywhere), the citizens' panel rejected all the hard options of cutting spending elsewhere, raising taxes, allowing more private money, or some combination of these changes, preferring to believe that by efficiency gains alone the hard options could be avoided, the system made better for patients, quality outcomes improved and cost pressures eased.

The Canadian Medical Association held hearings about health care across the country in 2011 and produced a summary document of public attitudes. The CMA found that a majority of Canadians did believe that the system needed more money and that Canadians needed to take more responsibility for their own health. But did "responsibility" and the belief that the system required more money mean higher taxes or some kind of levy for using the system? Apparently not. "There was little agreement on whether taking responsibility for health also means contributing directly to the cost of health services," the CMA found. The search for anything but hard alternatives extended to the "general agreement that people should use the health system responsibly and not draw on health care resources unnecessarily," a terrific idea that flies in the face of the reality of moral hazard endemic in a "free" system. Some people who attended CMA meetings did think that perhaps an annual statement of how much an individual consumed of health-care resources would modify behaviour. Alas, that dreamy idea had been studied extensively in Britain, where it was found to have had no influence on use of the health-care system. But then dreams permeate Canadians' thinking about medicare, and no politician wants to shatter them.

FOURTEEN

What about Other Countries?

Health-care systems reflect a country's political culture. History frames systems, which is why it is important to understand how Canada got the system its citizens love so much. To change a health-care system is to challenge history's framing.

What works in one country might not work in another, because of differences in size, population, political systems, economies. It would be wrong, therefore, to drop holus-bolus something from one health-care system into another. To compare, however, is to learn and to wonder if comparable countries are doing things better. Comparisons with countries other than the United States are the most instructive, since these countries have largely public health-care systems, whereas the U.S. does not.

Like Canada, Sweden, Australia and Britain have comprehensive, largely single-payer (government) public health-care systems. They do not use the social-insurance component prevalent in some continental European systems that provide very good health-care outcomes but operate quite differently. Their single-payer systems are the most like Canada's.

Their systems have changed much faster than Canada's. Broadly speaking, these countries encourage more competition in health-care delivery within the public system or, in Australia's case, parallel to it. They have all moved away from Britain's initial National Health Service model (the one that inspired Canada's), which provided universal, taxpayer-supported medical care from salaried doctors and nurses, in hospitals and other institutions, according to centralized dictates. They offer wider public coverage for basic health-care needs than Canada, and they spend less of their countries' national income doing it. They also achieve comparable or better health-care outcomes. They are less transfixed by the ideology of health care than results.

SWEDEN

Stefan Ackerby, director of budget control for the Swedish Association of Local Authorities and Regions, reads a sentence from his own agency's latest report: "Inflation-adjusted costs rose by 2.9 percent nationwide from 2006 to 2009." Can that level of increase be sustained, he is asked? "Absolutely not," he replies. It's too high, he says, and has to be reduced, even though Sweden's 2.9 percent increase during that period was only about half the yearly increase in Canada.

At the Karolinska Institute, Sweden's most famous medical research institution, Professor Johan Thor refers to another study that shows the rate of increase in health-care costs higher than the rate in the growth of the economy. "Obviously, that gap cannot keep widening, because it's not going to be possible to support that," he says. "I understand the challenge. I don't know how to solve it ... I see a number of attempts, one of which is to increase efficiency in the system. There's definitely room for this. But I have seen studies that suggest that even if we are able to increase efficiency by 1 or 2 percent per year, there will still be a widening gap."

His colleague, Mats Brommels, professor of medical management, adds that "2 or 3 percent is quite moderate in an international perspective. It would not, however, be possible to fund this solely by tax income. So the prospect is that maybe we are moving away from a single-payer system."

Sweden, like Canada, has a single-payer for most health care: the state. The Swedish system, however, covers more health needs than Canadian medicare, yet Sweden spends about one-quarter less of its collective wealth on health—9.5 percent of GNP compared with slightly less than 11.7 percent for Canada. Swedish health costs are relatively lower, not only because Sweden is a more socially equal society but also because Swedish medical practitioners (doctors and nurses) are paid far less than in Canada. Were Swedish salaries imposed in Canada, every medical practitioner would go on strike immediately.

The Swedish system covers with public money services by doctors and those in hospitals, as in Canada, but it also offers more coverage for pharmaceuticals, hearing aids and some dental costs. Whereas public money covers 70 percent of Canada's total health-care bill, in Sweden it is 83 percent. Along the entire health-care continuum of needs, and not just what is provided by doctors and in hospitals, Sweden covers its citizens much better.

Sweden's challenge is, among others, that the room for increased taxes is quite limited. Swedes already pay among the highest personal income and consumption taxes in the world to support its social welfare system. Sweden needs to find efficiency gains in its health-care system to avoid further tax increases. Accordingly, pursuit of those gains has been relentless, the methods radical and the outcomes thus far quite satisfactory. The speed and scope of Sweden's changes leave Canada's reform efforts looking feeble.

Like all single-payer systems, including Canada's and Britain's, Sweden's system was and, to some extent, still is plagued by wait times. Wait times remain the biggest complaint that Swedish citizens offer about their system. No matter what previous Swedish governments tried, wait times remained stubbornly high, until recently.

"I'm surprised by the progress we have made in reducing waiting times in the last two or three years, because it has been a chronic problem in Swedish health care," said Goran Stiernstedt of the Swedish Association of Local Authorities and Regions. "If you compare health-care systems in the Western world, Sweden has always done well in life expectancy and quality and outcomes, but we had not been doing well in waiting times. That's been the major problem. We have worked on it for decades. The government put billions into the system trying to reduce waiting times, with no result at all. The county councils used the money to produce a small dip, and then the waiting times returned."

Repeated, expensive failure produced a counterintuitive solution, one hard to imagine ever being contemplated in Canada. Rather than doing what governments always do—give new money to poor performers to boost their showing—the Swedish government gave additional money to the best performers. In Sweden, health care is organized by twenty-one county councils and by municipalities for elderly care. Under the new approach, the national government set targets for wait times, then allocated a yearly sum of 1 billion kroner, or about $130 million, to the counties exceeding the targets. The best were rewarded; the worst got nothing.

"I was involved when the voluntary model was used—a billion kroner at that time also," recalled Fredrik Lennartson, director-general of the Swedish agency for Health and Care Service Analysis. "Everybody received it up front. The effects were very difficult to measure. It didn't really work. There was no significant change.

"What has happened now is that they don't get the money if they don't do anything. There's been a big change. It has actually triggered a lot of action." The government makes the targets tougher each year, as an inducement to further improvements. The result, Lennartson said, is that "county councils can just keep getting money if they keep improving. The carrot is that good councils get money, the stick is that if other councils do not improve, they will be punished politically."

Stiernstedt of the Association of Local Authorities and Regions describes the councils' reaction as "running for the money." Poor performers were shamed by the media and prodded by their own medical institutions to get better. The association's yearly book has become the reference point for comparing county-to-county performance. Provinces in Canada hate inter-provincial comparisons and do what they can to avoid them; Swedish councils might hate detailed comparisons but cannot avoid them.

Comparative county measurements show that wait times are down across the board for access to specialists, the main target of the 1-billion-kroner investment. Turning conventional wisdom on its head—rewarding winners and encouraging others to catch up—has worked, although it's too soon to measure quality outcomes. Some councils manipulated their data to make their wait-time lists look better on paper than in reality, but these tricks were found out and eliminated. Public-opinion surveys show that patients are satisfied, although many still grumble about wait times being too long.

"The other way was the old Soviet style: the longer waiting times you have, the more money you could get," remarked Lars-Erik Holm, director-general of the National Board of Health and Welfare. "You'd want to have those long waiting times. This billion, however, has helped to reduce waiting times.

It has helped the top leaders in the counties to focus on that problem. We are now approaching the European average for wait times ... We have looked at waiting times for all counties, and they are going down."

Canadians think of Sweden as the prototypical social democratic country, with high taxes, an extensive welfare system, a high degree of egalitarianism, governed forever by the Social Democrats. That image is out of date, at least politically. A non-socialist coalition of four centrist and moderate conservative parties has been in office in 2007. Some of the biggest county councils, including Stockholm, have been governed by non–social democrats for even longer. Swedes were shocked when their country suffered a banking crash in the early 1990s. They were shocked again when the country scored only modestly well in international education tests. In a world of fierce economic competition, and after joining the European Union, Swedes began to look at their cherished social welfare model and, while still preferring it to others, realized the model needed a shakeup.

Astonishing changes occurred in health care and many other social policy areas. These changes—centred on more choice for taxpayers—have been driven by non–social democratic parties. Almost no one believes, however, that if the Social Democrats returned to office they would undo the changes. Said Hanne Kjoller, editorialist for the newspaper *Dagens Nyheter*, "The Social Democrats have been against everything that the liberals have been in favour of, until it's settled, and then they are in favour of it."

In health care, and other social policy areas, the state retains the role of payer but is blind to private or public providers. The new Swedish model is about competition within a public-payer model to drive innovation, improve services, offer choice and lower costs.

For example, all pharmacies in Sweden used to be state owned and operated, as liquor distribution still is. Today, private pharmacies are everywhere, competing with public ones, although the state retains a monopoly over ordering pharmaceuticals. In education, anyone can open a private school, provided that it follows the public curriculum, with the costs defrayed by the state depending on the number of students that the school attracts. Similarly, daycare centres can be organized privately with fees paid for by the state. Ten years ago, changes to such essential services would have been hard to imagine; today, they are considered the norm.

The private-provider/public-payer model now permeates Swedish health care, unlike in Canada where the word *private* sends defenders of the status quo to the barricades. The new private–public model began hesitantly under the Social Democrats but became the preferred policy of the non–social democrats. The model builds on a previous effort to goad councils to provide shorter wait times in the form of a national decree. It stipulated that patients who could not see a general practitioner within seven days, or a specialist within three months, had the right to travel to another county at the cost of his or her own county. Few patients availed themselves of this option, and it did not spur counties to improve their health-care delivery. The guarantee remains in law but has been overtaken by the drive for greater competition within the public system.

How does the private–public model work? First, every county council is required by national law to provide freedom of choice in primary care to patients. No longer does a patient have to be attached to his or her local clinic. By Canadian standards, this is hardly revolutionary since Canadians are free to select their family doctor or clinic—providing they can find one. Second, any group of doctors can organize themselves privately, meet council requirements for care, opening hours and range of services and start practising. The more patients they attract, the higher their income. This arrangement scarcely exists in Canada, as yet.

Third, family doctors receive a mixed payment system of a fixed amount for all the patients on their clinic's list, plus a sum for each treatment. Fourth, more and more hospitals are being given money for how many patients they treat rather than global budgets fixed every year. Fifth, one private company in Stockholm operates an entire hospital on a contract with the county council, while another in effect rents its facilities to private doctors or health-care companies, with payments coming from the state.

For years, Canadian health-care experts have urged primary-care doctors to stop working as solo practitioners on a fee-for-service basis and join local clinics with a capitation payment system (a fixed salary blended with payment for the number of patients). Governments have offered financial incentives to doctors to switch to this system. Many younger family practitioners have done so, but the shift has been too slow. In Sweden, by contrast, almost all family doctors work in clinics of four to ten general practitioners, nurses, physiotherapists, psychologists and other professionals. The opening-up of health care has resulted in many general practitioners organizing privately and having their clinics compete against others for improved outcomes and patient satisfaction, because if a patient walks to another clinic, money follows wherever he or she goes.

Results vary across the country. Patient choice means little in remote communities, which are lucky to have one clinic. Counties with Social Democratic governments have been less keen to change than those run by other parties. In the city of Stockholm, governed by a coalition of conservative non-social-democratic parties since 2006, 50 to 60 percent of primary-care doctors are now privately organized. The comparison with Canada is mixed: Canadian doctors are all private entrepreneurs, or at least are not employees of the state. But most of them still operate on a fee-for-service basis, and the existence of family clinics varies widely among provinces.

"Access to care has improved. The population is happier with how they are treated. But we don't know anything yet about changes in quality," said Anders Annell, a professor at the University of Lund, who has written extensively about the changes to primary care. "There are more providers, more liberal office hours and doctors are more accessible over the phone. They are paid on a capitation basis, so if they lose one individual, they will lose money. That goes for public clinics as well. Here in Stockholm, there is no difference in productivity between private and public. In 2008, a study showed an increase in productivity for both public and private."

A small proportion of payments by councils to clinics are tied to actual performance, with incentives for targets such as access over the phone, good results in patient satisfaction surveys and compliance with councils' drug formulary recommendations. Penalties are imposed for not complying with council's requirements or poor results on satisfaction surveys.

The rapid shift of general practitioners into private clinics has taken two forms: stand-alone operations or clinics that form part of a national chain, the largest of which is Praktikertjänst, whose chief executive officer, Carola Lemne, explained why the number of private clinics has exploded.

"The money is not the primary lure. Yes, they [doctors] can earn more in the private sector, but not enormously more. You don't get to be a millionaire, but they get to decide what hours do

I work, which people do I work with ... A lot of this was politically driven. On the conservative side, there was a wish to have more actors, not just the public sector, in the belief that competition is good, that if you have others competing on quality it is good for the patient. The private sector has always managed to have much higher accessibility, even when publicly funded. It has always been enormously appreciated by the patients. When there have been big national surveys of patient satisfaction, in dentistry and primary care, the private is always better appreciated."

Her company started with three doctors in the late 1950s. It has become one of the biggest in Sweden, employing nine thousand people. It signs up doctors who want to work privately, helps them establish their clinics, centralizes all their administrative costs (for a fee) and makes them shareholders in the company. If the company makes money, as it usually does, the doctors-as-share-holders earn a dividend, which is taxed less heavily than income earned as salary. Specialists can sign up, too, and Praktikerjänst helps them group their practices together.

There are other, smaller companies run by risk capital companies or large European private health-care companies. Some controversy attends their operations from critics who claim it is wrong for the private sector, especially from outside Sweden, to make money from public payments. The debate, however, revolves more around how much money the companies are making, not whether private delivery per se is a bad development. Not every new private clinic is going to be successful. The expansion of them has been so rapid that some will not find enough patients and will close. "There are new general practitioners all over the country," Lemne said. "Some of them have overreached. We feel sorry for some of our competitors. We feel some places will be shutting down."

In Canada, fiery debate often attends any attempt to expand

private delivery of publicly paid services. Critics warn that big U.S. health-care companies will creep into the Canadian market, sign up Canadian doctors and eventually press for a full private health-care system. The spectre of "for-profit" medicine haunts Canadian health-care debates, and the problems inherent in the U.S. system are decried.

A for-profit, private-payer health-care system does exist in Sweden, apparently without much controversy. It accounts for less than 1 percent of total health-care spending. It is limited to some family clinics in big cities and a few specialists, serving wealthy Swedes and companies that buy private insurance packages for their senior employees. Private medicine might expand a little as companies use it as part of recruitment packages for employees, but it is not expected to expand greatly, especially since competition within the public system has improved access and patient satisfaction.

"We have a health policy group at my centre, and they have scrutinized Stockholm County," said Professor Brommels of the Karolinska Institute. "What they show is that, by and large, there has been an increase in cost, but that is related to an increase in volumes, which means that the political goal of increasing access to care has been fulfilled. The additional costs have not been overwhelming.

"The second important element of the reform was the possibility for everybody to establish a new enterprise or practice. The county has an authorization system. You need to comply with a number of requirements. The fear was that these new practices would be established in affluent areas, and that they would drive consumption among those citizens who needed it the least, but that has not taken place. We have seen the establishment of new practices in areas where we have immigrants, and relatively speaking, those poorer areas have increased their volumes more than in the affluent areas."

This private–public approach revolutionizing Swedish health care can barely get off the ground in Canada, where fierce ideological adherence to the status quo and fear of change paralyzes conversation, let alone action. The same applies for the non-debate around the hobgoblin of Canadian medicare: user fees. If there is one aspect of Canadian medicare that cannot ever be debated, it is the idea of a citizen paying for what the Canada Health Act defines as "medically necessary services"—that is, anything provided by a doctor or in a hospital.

In Sweden, by contrast, paying for any visit to a doctor or a hospital is almost universally accepted as normal and necessary. Every political party except the Communist Party accepts the logic of paying. The widely accepted Canadian argument that such payments discriminate against poor patients, and are therefore inequitable, has little resonance in Sweden, in part because the law exempts all those on welfare from paying fees.

Patient fees have been part of Swedish health care for a very long time. In 1970, the government lowered the fees to 7 kroner for a visit to a doctor, but the fee rose to 25 kroner in 1972, and to 100 kroner in 1991 (all under Social Democratic governments). Today, fees vary from council to council but are in the 120 to 150 kroner ($18 to $22) range per visit to a doctor and 300 kroner ($28) to see a specialist without a referral. A ceiling of 1800 kroner (about $360) exists for each patient per year. A patient pays the money at the point of contact with the health-care system, except if he or she has already hit the 1800 kroner yearly ceiling. If Sweden wanted to finance more of its health-care system through user fees, they would be set at a higher level. Why bother with user fees when they raise only about 2.5 percent of the total public spending on health care?

It's apparently an article of faith in Sweden that user fees deter frivolous use of the health-care system and signal to taxpayers the need to use the system responsibly. "There is no debate about it. No one is questioning it," said Lars-Erik Holm of the National Board. "It's there to assign a value for the service ... It's there to stop people from overusing the system, so people who are in the most need will get the attention they deserve." His colleague Mona Heurgen added, "We don't have a debate because everybody recognizes that this is a good idea. We want to have services given to the right people, not to people who are not in need of the service." Commented Lovisa Stromberg, senior adviser to the minister of health and social affairs, "There's no discussion here. I think that's because it's always been this way."

Swedes also argue that fees tend to steer people to the proper part of the health-care system. Since fees are lower for a patient to see a general practitioner at a family clinic than to present at a hospital emergency ward, the differential funnels at least some people to clinics rather than hospitals, thereby saving the health-care system money.

Proponents of the reforms believe they will bend the health-care cost curve downward. These reforms are not the principal reason, however, why Sweden's per capita health-care spending is much lower than Canada's.

Research demonstrates conclusively that inequality of income is among the biggest cost-drivers of health care, if not the biggest. As noted, poor people experience worse health than more affluent people and therefore use any health-care system more, and Sweden, with its long social welfare tradition and societal commitment to equality, does not have as many poor people as Canada as a share of total population. The Swedish social welfare system is more generous than the Canadian. Rule one of health-care cost sustainability is therefore this: produce a more equal society. Sweden follows that rule more than Canada does.

Sweden also pays its doctors and nurses much less than Canada, and since 1971 has put them all on salary, although capitation methods are being used for family doctors. Payment by salary allows government agencies to control costs better than the fee-for-service system widely used in Canada. The average Swedish doctor might earn $80,000 to $100,000, a quarter to a half of the earnings of most Canadian doctors. Swedish doctors do have avenues to increase income, such as piling up overtime, then using the extra time off to practise for a month or so in Norway where fees are higher; or receiving dividends from a private health company if their practice is associated with such a company.

Little sympathy extends to the argument that doctors are underpaid. Their association, unlike the powerful Canadian medical associations, seldom squawks about insufficient income for its members. Said Lisa Blohm, managing editor of a weekly medical newspaper read by doctors, "In Sweden, they are well paid compared to other groups, compared to nurses, for example. There is more discussion about that—the differences between nurses and doctors. Some doctors do think they are paid too little in contrast to other countries, but I don't think that people in general believe that they earn too little money … In Sweden, it's not so nice to speak about what you earn." Some Swedish doctors have gone to other European countries in search of higher incomes, but the numbers are small. Canadian doctors, by contrast, have periodically headed for the much higher incomes available in the United States, as happened in the latter part of the 1990s.

With its emphasis on the importance of keeping costs down, Sweden built its entire system over the past three decades to steer people away from hospitals. Some critics think Sweden has gone a trifle overboard, with Europe's lowest per-patient hospital bed ratio. As a result, Sweden has a much more extensive home-care program, financed by municipalities that impose taxes to discharge their responsibility for elderly care. This home-care system, and the acute-long-term-care system, eases the bed blocker problem that plagues large hospitals in Canada. Lower user fees for presenting at a clinic as opposed to a hospital are intended to keep people away from hospitals. A large system of outpatient care offers services equivalent to those provided in Canada more expensively within hospitals.

One of the ambitions of the expanding private-public model will be to move even more non-acute treatments, repetitive operations and standard procedures out of hospitals and into privately organized clinics. In Swedish hospitals, as in Canadian, patients are being whisked in and out as quickly as possible. It is all the rage in health-policy circles in Canada to hear about de-emphasizing hospitals. For patient expectations to change, for public institutions to adjust and for government policy to put the right incentives in place takes a very long time. What Sweden did decades ago, Canada is now scrambling to accomplish.

AUSTRALIA

Australians are Canadians' distant cousins. Basic characteristics of the two countries are different but their essential structures are remarkably similar. Both are vast territorial land masses, with most of the population bunched in cities. Both are former British colonies, with parliamentary systems and federations. Both are wealthy, with huge natural resource endowments, indigenous populations and private-enterprise systems mixed with extensive public services, including health care.

The distant cousins' health-care systems, as you would expect, have some close resemblances. Both countries provide universal health insurance for all medically necessary services provided by doctors and in hospitals. Both systems have the bedrock principle that health care is a right and that income should not influence the exercise of that right. Public payment covers about 70 percent of all health-care expenses in Australia and Canada, and physicians are largely paid by fee-for-service. Both countries cover with public money a share of pharmaceutical costs. Both have populations with similar health profiles: growing life expectancy but an aging population, with looming upsurges in cardiac diseases and diabetes. Both health-care systems' costs have been rising by about 5 to 6 percent yearly. Each country's aboriginals have health-care outcomes significantly worse than those of the general population.

The distant cousins' health-care systems diverge, however, at critical points. Australia spends less of its GDP on health care than Canada—8.8 percent for Australia versus 11.7 percent for Canada. On a per capita basis in 2009 (in U.S. dollars), Canada spent $4363, Australia $3445. Australia's health-care bill grew at 2.8 percent per year after inflation from 2000 to 2008, compared with 3.7 percent in Canada. So Australia's rate of spending has been lower to achieve roughly the same aggregate health outcomes. Australia has better results for life expectancy, heart disease, cancer, infant mortality, diabetes. It has a higher ratio of doctors and nurses per one thousand population. It leads Canada in consultations with doctors, CT scanners (it trails for MRI machines), hospital beds, hospital discharges, angioplasties, hip and knee replacements, flu vaccinations. Australia's wait times to see a specialist and for patients to have elective surgeries are both lower than Canada's.

In fairness, there are a handful of categories from OECD data where Canada beats Australia, and some categories where the differences between the two countries are too small to be significant. Nonetheless, in overall terms of value for money—health outcomes versus dollars spent—Australia's system compares favourably to Canadian medicare, although one could fairly argue that factors other than the health-care systems influence the slightly better overall Australian health-care outcomes.

Australia lets private insurance play a larger role in some areas, such as hospitals, but the state covers a bigger share of pharmaceutical costs. The Australian system is also much more centralized. The national government pays a greater proportion of the national health-care tab, and therefore directs overall health-care policy far more than in Canada.

Now comes the big divide between the distant cousins: the Australian national government allows, indeed encourages, a parallel, private system for delivery of essential health services in hospitals. What would strike Canadians as the fundamental inequity of the Australian system—that people can buy private insurance and be treated differently and faster in hospitals than those without such insurance—is considered by Australians to be quite normal. Australian political parties occasionally squabble about the degree of private insurance and its cost. But even the leftish Labour Party has never favoured abolishing the private option. Labour's answer to complaints about the public system, especially wait times, has generally been to spend more money on the public system, not to shut off the private option. By contrast, no federal or provincial party in Canada today would dream of proposing what in Australia is a *fait accompli*.

Australians accept that a private system means a trade-off between faster access for some citizens and a dilution of equity. They reckon that as in education where private schools co-exist with public ones, all health care should not be entirely public—provided that the state offers a high-quality health-care system available to all. As an experienced Australian health-care analyst, Andrew Podger, remarked, "You can liken the Australian approach to airline classes. People accept that people can choose to sit at the front and pay a lot more, but they will not accept being put in a different plane with lower safety standards." The metaphor is intriguing, because in addition to private hospitals in Australia, there are some public ones where doctors treat both private and public patients. Two kinds of patients in the same hospital; two (or more) categories of fare-paying passengers in the same plane. The advantage for the private patients is twofold: they get to choose their own doctor, and they tend to get faster access.

Australia spent a decade, 1974 to 1984, going back and forth between launching and rescinding a public health-care system. Medicare finally arrived in 1984, more than a decade after medicare in Canada, paid for by a levy on personal income tax with the money going into general government revenues. By the 1990s, frustration with wait times, inefficiencies and cost increases in the public system drove the national government to provide subsidies for private insurance companies, the theory (and ideology) being that private insurance would ease the burden on the public system. By the end of the 1990s, the government was providing a 30 percent tax rebate (not geared to income) for the cost of private insurance as an inducement for people to buy it. The subsidy rose to 35 percent for those aged sixty-five to sixty-nine, and 40 percent for those over seventy. Later, inducement became almost a requirement for some citizens when the Liberal (actually conservative) government of Prime Minister John Howard imposed a 1 percent personal income tax surcharge on all higher-income families that did not buy private insurance. The cost of government subsidies for private insurance exceeds AU$3 billion. A defender of the Canadian system would argue that if governments are going to shovel out $3 billion, the money should be spent in the public system. Australians apparently believe public money is well spent to provide some degree of choice within their health-care system by supporting parallel private payment.

Those with private insurance still get 75 percent of a physician's costs while in hospital reimbursed by the public system. Their private insurance covers the remaining 25 percent, and also pays for whatever accommodation costs hospitals charge plus a wide range of ancillary services. The privately insured can also get coverage for the "gap" between what family doctors charge and the 85 percent that Medicare Australia is willing to reimburse patients. Since most doctors charge Medicare rates, private insurance is not often used for that purpose. Through choice and strong inducement, then, 45 percent of Australia's population at the end of 2009 had private insurance for covering the gap, using private hospital facilities, being able to choose their own doctor in hospital, covering ancillary fees and drug costs not paid for by the state.

Here is another big difference between Australia and Canada. Australia's national government, unlike Canada's, runs a drug plan, the Pharmaceuticals Benefits Scheme (PBS). Given the importance of pharmaceuticals in medical treatment, PBS puts the national government squarely into the health-care system, not just as a cheque writer for the Australian states but as a buyer and provider of drugs. The result is one national scheme with similar benefits across Australia, unlike in Canada, where provincial drug plans offer a hodgepodge of different coverage.

The Australian national government determines whether a proposed new drug is clinically effective, safe and cost-effective compared with other treatments. Then it negotiates the price with pharmaceutical companies on behalf of 22 million Australians, instead of the inefficient Canadian system whereby every province negotiates for itself. In Canada, the federal government determines if a drug is fit for use; provinces then negotiate with the manufacturers. A more fractured and cost-ineffective system could scarcely be imagined.

Once purchased, drugs are then subsided for citizens by the Australian government. Citizens paid AU$34.60 (CA$1 = AU$0.95) for each prescription in 2011 (the cost is indexed each year to inflation), no matter what the cost of the drug, up to a limit of AU$1317 per person per year, after which the cost per prescription drops to $5.60. The $5.60 price is what those on "concession"—the elderly and those with chronic conditions—pay for all drugs. The average subsidy is about 55 percent of all prescription costs across Australia, higher than in Canada.

Australia also moved some time ago on reforms that Canadian provinces are only now contemplating. Australia gave up the system still in place in Canada of financing hospitals on a global budget basis. A funding formula now more than a decade old in Australia sends money to institutions for treating each patient, the "follow the patient" formula. It's another example of the Australian system being more open to change than the Canadian.

BRITAIN

When Britain's National Health Service celebrated its fiftieth anniversary in 1998, a service was held in Westminster Abbey and a commemorative stamp was issued. Declared the British health minister of the day, "The NHS remains the envy of the world." Whether the world envied the NHS or not, it spawned imitators, including Canadian medicare.

As was the case in the early years of Canadian medicare,

early estimates of the NHS's costs were wildly wrong. Within five years of its arrival, NHS costs had risen much faster than the Labour Party founders had anticipated. But such was the NHS's profound popularity that even Conservative governments left it alone, dripping whatever additional money into its veins that the treasury would allow.

The minister's words in 1998 about the NHS being the "envy of the world" were ironic. Shortly thereafter, the minister's own Labour government would embark on reforms more radical than those previously tried by the Conservative government of Margaret Thatcher. The reforms started by Thatcher, then pursued even more vigorously by the Labour government of Tony Blair, were directed at introducing more competition into the public system, widening patient choice, lowering wait times and improving outcomes. They are still being pushed by the coalition Conservative–Liberal Democrat government of Prime Minister David Cameron.

For roughly the past quarter of a century, the NHS has been changed in ways that would astonish its founders. The changes have gone far beyond anything done in Canada. The NHS's original conception of how to organize a health-care system lives on more robustly in Canada than in Britain or Australia, which is another way of saying that the Canadian system has been the most resistant to change.

When the minister spoke about the world's envy of the NHS, British health care was underfinanced by international standards. The country spent much less of its national income (about 6 percent) on health care than European countries, Australia, New Zealand and Canada. For the previous quarter-century, the NHS had vacillated between being fed and starved. An increase after inflation of 10 percent one year would be followed by six years of zero to 3 percent real growth. Prime Minister Blair was determined that the NHS would be his government's top domestic priority, and it showed. Money started coursing into the NHS at 6 to 9 percent yearly. Unlike the money that poured into Canadian medicare after the 2003–2004 federal–provincial accord that was supposed to "buy change," in Roy Romanow's famous phrase, the Blair money did indeed "buy change."

Two waves of reform washed over the NHS. Observers called the first "terror and targets." Policies descended from the prime minister's office and the health ministry, not always compatible, introducing private-sector involvement in delivery, quality controls, peer review, performance reporting, account-ability, patient choice and new ways of remunerating physicians. This direction had been signalled by the previous Conservative government and had been predictably denounced by Labour in opposition. In power, Labour moved faster in the very direc-tion it had decried. The "targets" for improved delivery, better outcomes and reduced wait times came from the top; the "terror" came from new audits, new managers required to meet targets, new national watchdogs to report on performance. Sir Richard Branson of Virgin Airways was hired to advise how to make hospi-tals more patient-friendly.

Frustrated by slow progress, despite the new spending, Blair unleashed another wave of reforms. The direction was the same; the methods to "buy change" were different. Targets were still used; indeed, wait-time targets were reduced. For example, the Blair government set a target that all persons who showed up in emergency rooms should be treated within a maximum of four hours, and 98 percent of people got that treatment—in contrast to Canada, where emergency wait-time targets range from four to eight hours. The government set another target of eighteen weeks from a consultation with a family doctor to the end of surgery, again a target far tougher than Canada's. In recent years, the average wait has been nine weeks. Canadians can only dream of that sort of timely service.

The NHS was to be decentralized, with regional health authorities buying services for patients from either public or private providers. This split between purchasers and providers that began under Thatcher exploded under Blair. The private sector would be given 15 percent of the operations within the NHS. Private health care went from being only a safety valve for the public system to being among the options for delivering publicly financed care.

Budgets were shifted from hospitals to community care. Patients could electronically book visits to family doctors. They could shop among hospitals, because global budgets for hospitals were replaced for a variety of procedures by how many cases they handled and what outcomes they achieved. Patients became potentially a source of income rather than cost. Physicians were enjoined to improve clinical outcomes, in part by adhering to research and guidelines developed by an agency, the National Institute for Health and Clinical Excellence (NICE), whose work has inspired many reformers in Canada who hunger for something similar. Physicians' pay was tied to the number of patients they saw and the quality of care they provided. Local authorities were fined if patients were ready to be discharged but could not find facilities such as nursing homes or long-term care.

Labour's many changes can be condensed into four thrusts: regional authorities (called Primary Care Trusts) to organize, deliver and provide service from any provider, greater overall use of the private sector within the NHS, patient choice and payment by results. Whether Labour's changes produced the clinical improvements, reduced wait times and reaped the greater efficiencies that proponents promised remains a subject of debate. Wait times did come down dramatically, patient satisfaction did rise and outcomes improved. How much was due to all the new money and how much to the changes is likely impossible to tell. What can be said is that the Labour Party examined what its forebears had created, reaffirmed its belief in the principles of the NHS, but decided they could not be met without broad changes in how to achieve them. Such an intellectual revolution has not occurred anywhere in Canada, and certainly not on the political left whose progenitors created medicare.

What can also be said is that the changes first launched by the Thatcher Conservatives, then accelerated by the Labour Party, are being driven still further by the Conservative–Liberal Democrat coalition. No party wants to return to the monolithic bureaucracy that ran the NHS for the first decades of its existence. The Conservative–Liberal Democrat government proposes to shrink that bureaucracy drastically and abolish regional health authorities by giving general practitioners new powers to group themselves into "clinical commissioning groups," which will, in turn, buy services for patients from hospitals, specialists and clinics, public or private. Primary-care physicians in these groups will control 60 percent of the NHS budget. The principles of splitting purchasing and providing service remain intact; the group doing the purchasing would change, and centralized bureaucracies would be reduced and local control enhanced. It is too soon to tell whether these innovations will work, but they do represent a continuation of efforts to change the NHS that began a quarter of a century ago.

Provincial governments in Canada are toying with elements of the new British model: moving some doctors away from fee-for-service, paying more attention to standardized clinical results, basing hospital funding on patient numbers and outcomes rather than global budgets. The moves are tentative at best. The wait-time targets established by provincial governments in Canada would be scorned in Britain as much too lax. Clinical outcomes are comparable or better, yet Britain still spends approximately 2 percentage points less of its national income on health care than Canada (9.8 percent versus 11.7 percent). The parent country of public health care has shaken up what it created to achieve better results. Canada remains wedded to a British model that no longer exists, like a child transfixed by a picture of parents taken decades ago.

The Swedish, Australian and British systems are not without flaws. Citizens in those countries still complain about wait times, although they are lower than in Canada. According to the OECD, single-payer systems generally have the longest wait times. Governments in these countries wrestle with higher costs. Populations are aging. The systems are highly politicized. When something goes wrong, political hell can break loose. As one wise observer of British reforms noted, when politics and markets collide in health care, politics usually wins. Systems often look better from afar than up close, because foreign observers miss details; they aren't using the systems, as local citizens are.

Still, these systems perform at the very least no worse than Canada's and, by most standards and outcomes, better. They provide a vital public service that is taken very seriously by their citizens. Yet these countries have been able to bring about far greater changes to health care than Canada has. They have been willing to stick to their principles while changing their methods, whereas Canadians are stuck with their principles, while being too fearful of new methods.

PART FOUR
REMEDIES

FIFTEEN

Doctors and Nurses

Doctors and nurses, hospitals and drugs are the heart of the health-care system. They are its three costliest parts. Any hope of easing future cost pressures and getting better patient outcomes depends on changing each. Of course, many other changes would also help, such as electronic records, better clinical evidence, changing the scope of practice for professionals by letting lower-cost personnel in the health-care system do routine work. On changes involving doctors and nurses, hospitals and drugs, however, rest the most promising opportunities to improve quality and access and reduce the increase in costs. These are the three urgent health-care priorities to improve a system that does not provide Canada adequate value for money in health. In the search for remedies, begin with medical personnel, then turn to hospitals and drugs.

Canada has a very expensive health-care workforce. Canada's 69,000 doctors are among the highest paid in the world. Their pay cost taxpayers more than $27 billion in 2010, or about $390,000 on average per doctor in the public system, or about $800 per Canadian. Their pay represented about 14 percent of all health-care spending, compared with about 29 percent for hospitals and

16 percent for pharmaceuticals. According to the OECD in 2010, Canadian specialists had the third-highest ratio of remuneration to the average wage of thirty-three countries; family practitioners had the fifth highest.

Doctors and nurses are not culprits in Canada's health-care problems, but the system cannot change without more flexibility on their part and that of their associations and unions. Doctors, nurses and hospital administrators have seen considerably increased incomes in recent years, and this trend cannot continue.

Only governments can check these increases, since they are the paymasters, although it would help if physicians' associations and nurses' (and other) unions understood the impact of their salary settlements on the sustainability of medicare. Governments can, and should, continue to change the method of doctors' pay, and look for ways of delivering care more cheaply. Governments' objective—no, their imperative—must be to restrict increases to provider incomes to the rate of inflation for the next decade. British Columbia and Ontario led the way in 2012 with tough negotiations that held doctors' incomes to increases less than the rate of inflation.

The financial sustainability of the system is not the providers' associations and unions' principal objective. When the issue of sustainability is raised, union leaders too often answer, raise taxes, especially on corporations and the rich. To suggestions that health-care services can be delivered more inexpensively by private providers, unions furiously reply that quality and equity of care will be jeopardized. Associations and unions are adept at identifying some other jurisdiction in Canada (or in the United States) where providers are paid more. They warn that pay must be ratcheted up here and now or some personnel will flee elsewhere.

From 1998 to 2008, the cost of physicians' services jumped

6.8 percent a year. Just over half of that increase—3.6 percent—
came from higher fee schedules, the rest from a higher volume
of demand because Canadians used the system more. Canadian
nurses' incomes from 2000 to 2009 rose twice as fast (2.3 percent
after inflation) as the average wage of all workers (1.1 percent).

The jump in the cost of physicians' services from 1998 to 2008
is deceptive. The surge in yearly income began after governments followed the Romanow commission's suggestion and
poured more money into the system, starting in 2005. Predictably,
associations and unions mobilized to take what they could of
the new money. Payments to physicians, for example, rose
9.6 percent in 2008–2009, the highest gain in a decade. The
increase ranged from 3.9 percent in British Columbia,
Saskatchewan and New Brunswick to 13.4 percent in Quebec and
11.9 percent in Ontario.

In Ontario fee schedules for doctors rose 2 percent a year,
roughly in line with inflation, from 1993 to 2003. From 2009 to
2011, the fee schedule rose slightly above 4 percent a year, or
more than double inflation. The fee schedule provides only a
partial picture. Other financial incentives were offered to doctors
to practise differently, so many physicians' incomes rose far
beyond 4 percent a year. The Ontario Nurses Association reached
an agreement for a 9.25 increase from 2008 to 2010, with additional wage improvements for night shifts and weekend work.
Their benefits soared for dental work, vision care, hearing aids.
Five weeks of vacation were granted after twelve years of service
and six after twenty. These agreements unfolded as Ontario slid
into a deeper fiscal hole following the recession of 2008.

Some short-term relief for governments might be in store.
The Ontario Nurses Association settled for 3.75 percent over three
years, 2011–13, although again with substantial improvement
in benefits. Governments' post-recession fiscal frailties might

produce a recognition among providers that the previous decade's increases cannot continue. True, doctors train for many years—up to fifteen years for a surgical specialist. They don't make much money while interning and during residency. Their skills, and the time to acquire them, justify handsome payment, but not rates of increase of the kind the country recently experienced. What's needed is a long-term understanding that remuneration should rise at the rate of inflation. This kind of reasonable restraint would by no means solve medicare's sustainability challenge, but it would be an important element. The huge number of applicants for positions in medical schools, to say nothing of foreign doctors immigrating to Canada, suggests the country's supply of physicians would not be hurt by restraint.

Even if governments take a resolute line, pressures for spending on physicians and nurses will be intense. Canadians' use of the health-care system, already rising, will increase as the population ages. As it is, Canadians visit family doctors 151 million times a year, or about five times a year per capita. They use specialists' services 56 million times, consultations 36 million times, diagnostic and therapeutic services 18 million times and undergo about 600,000 surgeries.

Medical specialization grows, and specialists cost more money. The best-paid specialists are thoracic and cardiovascular surgeons, whose remuneration, depending on the province, ranges from $450,000 to $670,000, followed by ophthalmologists ($418,000 to $700,000), otolaryngologists ($393,000 to $539,000), obstetricians and gynecologists ($277,000 to $456,000) followed by urologists, neurosurgeons, internal medicine physicians, plastic surgeons and so on down to psychiatrists ($128,000 to $258,000). The average gross billing for all specialists in 2010 was $341,000, for family physicians $239,000. Today, Canada has as many specialists as family doctors, reflecting the increased allure of specialization—although Canada still has the highest ratio of family doctors to specialists apart from Australia and France.

Those who believe enormous cost-efficiency gains are as ripe as fruit on trees insist that cost pressure can be alleviated by substituting care from less-expensive providers. The example par excellence is nurse practitioners—nurses who have done extra training and are qualified to administer certain tests and procedures previously reserved for doctors. This substitution makes medical sense and policy logic. As with so many of these supposedly enormous efficiency gains, the advantage of nurse practitioners' enhanced role is overblown. Nurse practitioners doubled in number from 2004 to 2009, but they still represent only 0.7 percent of the total registered nursing population. It will be a very long time before their participation brings more than marginal cost relief to the system. Nurse practitioners would receive less money for delivering certain services than a family physician, but if their rate of salary increase tracked that of doctors, with no gains in productivity, the entire system would be only marginally better off from a cost perspective. On the theory, however, that every bit helps, and that in some cases nurse practitioners can deliver speedier service that is just as effective as that provided by family physicians, governments should encourage more of them—and even nurses-only clinics, as part of an overall thrust to keep people closer to home and farther from hospitals for simple ailments or the ongoing treatment of chronic medical conditions.

Nurses' unions naturally clamour for the training of more nurses, insisting that Canada needs additional thousands of them. That conclusion is not what international numbers show. According to the OECD, Canada has slightly more than the OECD average for number of nurses as a share of population, whereas the ratio of physicians to the population is the second lowest. The ratio of nurses to physicians is the second highest in the OECD, which rather gives the lie to the argument that Canada needs more lower-cost nurses to do the work of higher-cost physicians, because the ratio by international standards is already tilted toward nurses. But there will be demand for more nurses nonetheless as the population ages and if more care is delivered, as it should be, out of hospitals in nursing homes, long-term care facilities and in patients' homes.

Not just doctors and nurses have done well from the surge of money into medicare. Hospital administrations have been well served. Ontario publishes the salaries of all on the public payroll who earn more than $100,000, so it is possible to see the administrators' salaries. At the Ottawa Hospital, a major teaching institution highlighted earlier in the book, CEO Jack Kitts earned $642,000 plus another $60,000 in taxable benefits in 2010. He was assisted by fourteen vice-presidents with salaries from $219,000 to $449,000. Fifty-eight nurses took home more than $100,000. In total, the hospital had 308 persons on staff earning more than $100,000—and this figure does not include the doctors whose fees were paid by the Ontario government. All across the province, CEOs were doing well. At the small Collingwood General and Marine Hospital, the CEO earned $199,000; in Cornwall, $239,000; Dryden, $177,000; Guelph, $309,000; Kingston, $320,000. Being CEO of a hospital is a complicated job. Some CEOs are physicians (such as Dr. Kitts) and would have earned handsome amounts as medical practitioners. Nonetheless, these are very generous salaries for the public sector. The salaries reflect personnel cost inflation of recent years and make easy targets for those who work in the rest of the system—and for critics outside the system who believe that cost containment has been given short shrift in a sector where continuing cost increases outstrip governments' revenue growth. Some provinces are beginning to tie wage increases for senior personnel to delivery of improved patient outcomes and financial management, developments that should become the norm.

Figuring out how many providers the health-care system needs will always be an imperfect calculation. It was illustrated to be especially imperfect when Canadian provincial governments followed the advice some years ago of two veterans from the "rational planning" school of health-care economics. These economists instructed provinces, whose governments were only too eager to listen, that doctors cost the system money. Reduce their numbers, the experts recommended. Governments then lowered nationwide medical school enrolments—1835 in 1985, 1708 in 1990, 1578 in 2000—while the country's population rose. What unfolded was an utterly predictable shortage of doctors. The basic law of supply and demand thereafter favoured doctors' financial interest. Their numbers fell. Demand kept rising, so they were able to bid up the value of their services. Governments, having thought lower enrolments would save money, found that the laws of supply and demand worked the other way.

Belatedly, governments reversed course. Medical school enrolment nationally jumped 55 percent from 2000 to 2010. Once the first cohort of this new enrolment began practising, physician numbers grew twice as fast as the overall population. As more of these graduates enter the labour force, the supply-and-demand pressures that pushed up doctors' incomes will ease slightly. Demand for physicians' services, however, will continue to grow, since there is no price for accessing them (the moral hazard of overuse of a free good), the population is aging and medical services in the economic literature are considered to some extent a "luxury" good where the demand grows more than proportionately to income. Canada still remains far behind the OECD average of physicians per 100,000 of population—203 for Canada compared with the OECD average of 310. This low ratio partly explains why finding a family physician and getting to see a specialist are among the chronic conditions of medicare.

Increasing the number of doctors, however, doesn't translate precisely into easier access for patients. The feminization of the physician workforce has gathered speed, with consequences for hours worked per physician. Thirty-six percent of physicians are now women, compared with 29 percent in 2000 and 22 percent in 1990. Forty-one percent of family doctors are women. Younger physicians are more likely to be women. Among doctors under thirty years of age, women outnumber men seven to four, compared with those fifty to fifty-nine years of age where men outnumber women two to one. In medical schools today, well over half the students are women, reflecting the better grades that women consistently achieve in pre-medical university education. Ten years from now, the medical profession will be even more feminized than today, given the share of women in medical school.

Various studies have shown that female doctors work fewer hours per week than male doctors, because women in medicine, as elsewhere, try to juggle work and family. Younger male practitioners, too, seem less inclined to work the very long hours that their older counterparts did, many of whom were in single-earner families where the man worked and the woman looked after children at home. Today, young male practitioners, like female ones, seek a different work–family balance. Although more doctors are entering the profession, more of them are needed today to do the same work as a decade ago—at a time when overall patient demand is rising.

How about reducing demand by charging a fee for accessing the public health-care system? After all, CCF Premier Tommy Douglas designed public health care in Saskatchewan with premiums and user fees every time a citizen saw a doctor or entered a hospital. These payments were needed, Douglas said, to help finance the system and to remind people to use it responsibly. His government increased premiums and fees, although a later NDP government abolished them in the name of equity. Swedes think user fees necessary and normal. Swedish people on low incomes are exempted, and a ceiling is imposed on yearly payments. Swedes believe fees are needed to remind citizens to use the health care system responsibly, and direct them to the lowest-cost part of the system, since fees at family-practice clinics are lower than at hospitals. The Quebec government proposed a similar system in its 2010 budget, with each patient's visit included as part of year-end income-tax calculations. Since 40 percent of Quebeckers do not pay income tax, the poor would have been protected. Exemptions for those with chronic conditions could have been included. The Quebec proposal avoided the paperwork and messiness of payments in physicians' offices. A furor erupted over the proposal, however, and it was withdrawn, since it offended the critics' sense of equity.

Indicative, although not conclusive, evidence from studies in Canada and abroad suggests that even with exemptions, fees do tend to deter at least some people for whom a fee would be an economic hardship. Since the poorer the patient, the greater the likelihood that he or she will have poor health, the deterrence of payment, however limited, might keep people away from the system. If patients wait, because of being deterred by fees, their conditions risk worsening. When they eventually do present to the system, their health will have deteriorated, their treatment will be more expensive and positive outcomes less certain.

Once the poor (and possibly all seniors) and those with chronic conditions are exempted and a ceiling imposed on the total amount anyone pays in a single year, user fees would not raise much money. User fees would definitely not solve the financing challenge of health care. Even Swedes don't believe that argument. A small number of people who have acute or chronic conditions, and those near the end of life, place the largest financial burden on the health-care system. Fees would not restrain their use of the system, since they either have conditions that need constant and serious attention, or they would be exempted. If governments concluded that they need more money for health care—and they will—better methods of finding the money exist than user fees.

If pay displeases Swedish doctors, their options are limited. They can move to another country within the European Union, but the other Scandinavian countries don't pay doctors hugely better. Germany and the Netherlands do, but the German and Dutch languages are essential for practising. The Swedes are excellent linguists, but only a minority speaks German, and Dutch even less.

Canada sits beside the United States, where historically doctors have been better paid. Vast research budgets at some U.S. medical centres eclipse those available in Canada, so those centres attract talent from around the world, including Canada. Canadian physicians can get fed up and emigrate—surgeons who don't have enough operating time, researchers with inadequate budgets, family doctors with too many patients. Some recent orthopaedic surgical graduates emigrated because they could not find work in Canada where operating time in hospitals had been allocated to established surgeons.

In the 1990s, the U.S. economy boomed in a reprise of the Roaring '20s while Canadian health-care budgets grew in mid-decade at less than the rate of inflation for the first time since the introduction of medicare. An outflow of Canadian doctors ensued (mostly to the United States) — 777 in 1994, 674 in 1995 and 726 in 1996. Some Canadian doctors did return in those years, but the net yearly loss ranged from 418 to 508.

The net outflow continued at a lower rate until 2004, when Canada began to experience a net yearly gain. As Canadian phys-icians' incomes soared, and the federal government put more money into health care, including medical research, Canada didn't look so bad after all. Who knows how many Canadian expatriates could not abide political developments in the post-9/11 United States? A huge U.S. national debt, which exploded under President George W. Bush and was subsequently exacerbated by the 2008 recession and by congressional Republicans' refusal to co-operate with the Obama administration's deficit-reduction proposals, will now burden the country's future. President Obama has recom-mended sweeping changes to medical care. U.S. economic and health-care challenges seem likely to ward off a mass migration of Canadian doctors.

Saskatchewan's doctors drew a line in the sand at fee-for-service. That same payment system remained the unalterable demand of the physician representatives on the Hall Royal Commission that recommended national medicare. Without fee-for-service, the commission would not have reached a consensus report. Fee-for-service recognized that doctors were independent practitioners and business entrepreneurs, not salaried employees or glorified civil servants taking directions from people who knew little or nothing about medicine.

How can a hospital CEO control the costs to support the doctors' work — nursing and clerical staff, instruments, medicines, technologies—when the CEO cannot control how much doctors work, except by imposing top-down limits on their access to hospital service, which, in turn, leads to lengthy wait times and frustration for patients? Doctors as independent entrepreneurs, working inside a hospital that offers privileges but does not pay them, means a complicated governance structure: a medical staff with its own prerequisites, demands and outside paymaster, and an administrative staff with a board of directors responsible for everything else. Running such an institution requires ongoing negotiations, delicate labour management and a great deal of time.

Fee-for-service offered one great advantage: it encouraged more work. With doctors in short supply, every payment to a physician improves patient access, however slightly. Perhaps the negotiated fee schedule encouraged too much medicine—too many prescriptions filled out by family doctors who received a fee for each one; too many tests ordered by physicians paid to read and analyze them. Perhaps fee-for-service encouraged too little time spent with each patent. But fee-for-service did mean that the more patients a doctor saw, the greater his or her income. More patients, more income. Patients who got faster access were satisfied. They weren't paying, after all.

Fee-for-service remains alive but increasingly unwell. About 70 percent of all clinical billings are tied to fee-for-service, down from about 85 percent in 2000. Governments in some provinces are trying to lure doctors away from fee-for-service, because it has led to family doctors' working alone rather than in teams. New family doctors, especially females, want to move from fee-for-service to a system with regular and good income without the incentives to work extra hours. Every study of Canadian health care for a quarter of a century has urged family practitioners to work in teams with other doctors, nurse practitioners, pharmacists, nutritionists and other professionals to provide a kind of one-stop shopping for patients. This concept is much more easily implemented in urban settings where many professionals practise than in rural and isolated areas, so it will never be the model for the entire country. Since a majority of Canadians live in urban areas, however, it should be the model for most governments.

The hoped-for efficiency gains from clustering professionals has produced mixed results—another reason to beware of assertions that medicare's challenges can be solved by efficiency gains alone. The clustering of medical professionals, and new funding models for doctors, did not save governments money; in fact, short-term results suggest the opposite, as the Ontario example shows.

The Ontario government wanted professionals to group together, keep their premises open longer (thereby offering an alternative to emergency rooms), allow patients to be seen by the proper kind of professional (nurse practitioner or pharmacist instead of a higher-paid doctor) and give the government some cost relief from fee-for-service. Various kinds of family-health units were established—some offered more services than others. By the end of 2010, about 7500 of the province's 12,000 family physicians were enrolled in these schemes. Physicians' pay varied from scheme to scheme but, in essence, doctors received a salary with a smaller fee-for-service payment for each patient. The funding model attempted to marry the cost certainty of a salary, or a payment tied to a roster of patients signed up by the professionals, with an incentive to see more patients through fee-for-service. These alternative funding arrangements spread fast: the number of patients enrolled leaped 24 percent to almost 10 million. Far from restraining costs, government incentives for grouping, plus the attraction of the grouping model for patients, meant participating doctors wound up receiving 25 percent more money than those who practised only on a fee-for-service basis.

Another surprise: although the government's agreements with these family-health groups specified that they were to remain open beyond the traditional 9 A.M. to 5 P.M., a June 2010 survey found that 92 percent of all services were still being offered during traditional regular hours. This disappointment reflected a system still organized more around the conveniences of providers than patients. Another survey found that wait times were similar for patients wanting to see a physician working fee-for-service or under an alternative funding arrangement. The survey found that 40 percent of patients got to see a doctor within a day—a great advantage of the family-health grouping model—but the rest had to wait a week or more. The Ontario auditor general then uncovered a problem with people on the lists of rostered patients: doctors were being paid for a patient on his or her list, even when the patient went to another physician. The government was paying twice: once for the patients on Dr. A's list, a second time for those being seen or treated by Dr. B.

Alternative payment arrangements, originally conceived for family doctors, spread. Almost 50 percent of specialists now work under one of these blended payment systems, as do 90 percent of emergency physicians who used to work on salary. As a result of the change, payments to ER physicians rose 40 percent from 2006–2007 to 2009–10, although the number of emergency physicians increased only 10 percent and patient visits 7 percent, a classic case of cost inflation. Far from making an efficiency gain, the new system cost more without corresponding improvements in output.

Why not put every doctor on a salary, as in many parts of the British system, the great Mayo Clinic and some Health Maintenance Organizations in the United States? Salaries would bring cost certainty to governments or regional health authorities, but two challenges immediately present themselves. First, salaries offend the idea that physicians are independent practitioners. Any government that tried a quick switch to a salaried model would be in for an awesome fight, although the time might come when such a fight will be necessary if physicians' pay increases do not moderate. Second, a straight salary does not provide an incentive to see additional patients. The positive virtue of salaries is that a physician is not penalized for spending extra time with patients. With wait times already plaguing medicare, salaries would likely exacerbate those wait times as fewer patients were seen.

The clustering model for physicians and other professionals makes sense, but it has not yet produced relief from the health-care cost curve. Nor has it improved sufficiently the after-hours access that a "patient-centred" system needs, and that has to change. The public underwrites the costs of medical education, pays for the hospital facilities in which doctors practise and remunerates physicians at substantial rates. In exchange, the public has the right to require of family physicians something beyond nine-to-five, five-day-a-week delivery of medical services. Unless physicians and nurses show more flexibility in how they work, and unless they accept that their remuneration cannot continue to outstrip governments' revenue growth, it will be very hard to improve medicare's challenges of quality, access and cost.

SIXTEEN

Hospitals

Hospitals are the jewels of the health-care system. Within their walls, medical miracles and everyday competence are displayed; outside, hospitals are sources of civic pride. To them go fundraising dollars, not to home care or other forms of community care. The great and the good in communities serve on hospital boards, because these institutions are of such importance and prestige. In small communities, losing a hospital is a civic catastrophe; in large cities, they are confirmation of a city's status.

Hospitals became the focus of medicare to the eventual detriment of the entire system. Today, and even more so in the future, many more people must be treated outside hospitals, especially the frail elderly, those who show up at emergency departments with less than acute conditions and those with chronic conditions. Managing chronic conditions, and sometimes multiple chronic conditions, will be the single biggest challenge of the future. Hospitals are usually the wrong place to tackle that challenge. Given the unacceptably long wait times that plague the Canadian system, more straightforward procedures must be done outside hospitals. Medicare needs to be "dehospitalized" to the greatest extent possible, because we are asking hospitals to do too much, at too high a cost, based on a rigid funding formula.

Any health-care system has to be governed. Component parts cannot do their own thing, since patients flow in and out of the system at different points. Canadian provincial governments, for the most part, have found the correct governance structure for health care—on paper. Regional health authorities are institutions closer to populations than provincial governments and are best positioned to organize care. Regional authorities can coordinate care among various health-care institutions and systems—hospitals, home care, nursing homes, long-term care, family and specialist clinics. A hospital-centred system cannot achieve this coordination as effectively, because those who run hospitals will be principally concerned with their institutions and less concerned with the rest.

Provinces have added and subtracted health authorities. Alberta has changed four times, trying to find the optimal size. Nova Scotia has nine regional health authorities, whereas it only needs three or four. Leaving aside the number, the idea of having regional authorities is right—provided that they have the necessary powers and control over budgets.

Ontario created a dysfunctional halfway house: fourteen Local Health Integration Networks with their own administration and boards, but limited budgets and powers, although the government promised in 2012 to give the LHINs more power over family practitioners. Ontario's system looks integrated on paper but is not in fact.

What's needed—as in Sweden and Britain and some Canadian provinces—is a fully integrated structure that gives the regional authority control over budgets. The provinces' job is to set standards, organize overall financing to the regional authorities, regulate where necessary, then let the regional authorities administer the system. The result would be—or rather should be—a rise in the power of regional authorities but a concurrent reduction in the huge provincial health ministries, the end of hospital boards, fewer hospital administrators. There should be no net increase in bureaucracy, in other words. Of course, the real world likely would not work this way, because bureaucracies are inherently self-protecting. In Quebec, a regional system was put in place without a corresponding reduction in the other bureaucracies. Only a government of uncommon resolution would not allow an increase in bureaucracy.

Devolving power might make health care somewhat less politicized. Health care, being largely public, is always going to be political and partisan, but having unelected people administer the system locally—while of course being ultimately responsible to the legislature—can take some health-care issues out of the partisan arena. This kind of non-political arrangement is what physicians have wanted from their first fight over medicare in Saskatchewan.

Doctors cannot have it both ways: establishing a non-political body to administer the system while not answering to that body. Regional authorities should oversee paying physicians, to whom they would be responsible. The idea that physicians should be paid by a separate entity—a provincial health-care plan, which they bill for their remuneration—leads to moral hazard, lack of accountability for outcomes, bifurcated and confusing adminis- tration within hospitals and the absence of clear lines of authority. Physicians (and nurses) should be responsible for outcomes, contracts and work conditions to the health authorities who employ them.

Regional health authorities, in turn, should be held account- able for outcomes and costs to patients and governments. Their results should be published yearly, as in Sweden, so taxpayers can compare them to see which authority is doing best. Just publishing figures will not be enough to enjoin authorities to improve;

rewards should be offered to those whose results improve. Competition for dollars among authorities, although painful for the worst comparative performers, is one way of getting laggards to improve, which is what happens in Sweden where poor results get media attention, galvanize local soul-searching, and even a bit of anger, and cause health-care providers and their institutions to examine how they can and must improve. It is counter-intuitive in Canada to think this way, because the instinctive Canadian response is to fund the weakest-performing institution and hope for improvement. It was a pity that in the 2003–2004 health accord, the Martin cabinet dropped a demand that the prov-inces report wait times annually according to a common national definition—because Quebec objected and provinces opposed any comparative data that risked putting some of them in a poor light.

Canadians largely want a single-payer system in which their health care is "free" at the point of delivery by doctors and in hospitals, but they are increasingly indifferent about who provides the service, provided that the quality is high. Here, then, is the difficult political question for medicare: private delivery. The Canada Health Act specifically allows it. The documents prepared by civil servants at the time of the act's proclamation illustrate that those who drafted it contemplated private delivery if it was paid for publicly. A few such clinics exist, such as the Shouldice Hospital in Ontario, specializing in hernia repair, and a smat-tering of specialized surgical clinics in Saskatchewan, Alberta and British Columbia. Private diagnostic clinics exist in Quebec. Community health services use private companies to deliver nursing and home care. As part of making medicare more flexible and less costly, there should be an expansion of private providers of publicly paid for services, as is now the norm in Sweden and

Britain, assuming these providers can deliver comparable care with public institutions and at lower prices. This would be part of the badly needed "dehospitalization" of medicare.

The word *private* is hopelessly confused in Canadian health care. Too many defenders of the status quo have insisted that the word means patients must pay for their health care with the result that equity is diluted, standards fall and the much-vaunted "values" of medicare are eroded. These assertions represent the triumph of ideology over common sense, practicality, norms in comparable countries, patient satisfaction and service. *Private* can mean individuals paying for some services, as occurs to varying degrees in a majority of OECD countries, but it can also mean private delivery of health-care services paid for publicly.

A truly patient-centred system would have a regional health authority ask, without prejudging the answer, how and where can patients best be served at the lowest cost consistent with high-quality treatment and outcomes? The analysis should not be pre-empted by assuming the answer is always public institutions. Public regulation and accountability, absolutely. But if a private clinic for surgeries or a nursing home or home-care provider can better the outcomes or costs, or both, of public institutions, then a "patient-centred" system should be neutral about the deliverer of the service, private or public.

The single payer remains the state, which also monitors quality. The contract goes to the provider with the best service and cost. Other single-payer systems use this approach extensively. It's past time that provinces adopted it, where a plurality of providers competes for business with a single purchaser, the regional health authority. Obviously, the model won't work everywhere. Rural areas might not have enough providers to offer competition, so the public monopoly would remain. If a private provider failed to deliver either quality outcomes or lower costs, or both, the regional health authority could rescind or not renew the contract.

How can a large public system such as health care be made more innovative? Without being categorical, there are two schools of thought. The first school insists that innovation will arise and efficiency gains will occur through better rational planning by those running the public system. This well-intentioned position belies what we know about where innovation and efficiency usually arise, which is through some degree of competition. The second school believes efficiency gains will arise through some forms of competition. Private markets are obviously imperfect. They certainly are in private health-care systems, because patients often lack the medical information necessary to make wise choices.

When Canadians engage in public debates, they often discuss trade-offs and balance points between equity and efficiency. Reasonable people can disagree on those trade-offs and balance points, arguing for more equity or more efficiency, or a better blend of the two. Generally, citizens look to the market to create wealth through competition, innovation and efficiencies, but to the state to flatten some of the inequalities that the private market creates in the pursuit of wealth generation. The state and the private sector working together is a long-established model.

Imperfect as the trade-offs are, society uses both the private sector and public policies to seek a blend of efficiency and equity. Except in health care, where the "values" of equity have been bizarrely interpreted to exclude private enterprise in core areas of health care (hospitals and doctors) but to let it rip elsewhere. In the core areas, whatever efficiency gains and innovation we count on in other walks of life from the dynamics of private enterprise have been banned. Instead, we search for those gains from the least likely source, public monopolies. Public health systems in Australia, New Zealand and Western Europe have embraced mixed delivery, albeit in very different ways, whereas Canada remains wedded to a model that others have abandoned.

Day and night across Canada, people go to emergency rooms for assessment and treatment. Some of them should not be there. They should be seeing their family doctors, or visiting a family-health clinic or receiving information by Telehealth services. Sometimes, family doctors are not available, either because the patient lacks one, or the doctor's or clinic's office is closed. The triaging that goes on at the hospital is wrongly directed, at least in part. One of its purposes should be not to triage people within the hospital's emergency services but to direct some of those who present away from the hospital, ideally to a family clinic attached to the hospital (some of these already exist) or one nearby affiliated with it. Patients who present at emergency are triaged and told to wait. Often for hours and hours. Frequently, they are told little or nothing by staff; indeed, some emergency wards have signs telling patients, once triaged, not to ask staff about anything. In a properly run health-care system, family practitioners would be more widely available outside nine to five, and every family clinic would be open in the evening and provide weekend coverage (part of the explicit deal between practitioners and the state). Citizens would be on a rostered list at one clinic or another, where they could go or phone.

Across Canada, small hospitals serve shrinking rural communities. These are expensive to sustain as hospitals and, in some instances, could be converted into family clinics offering non-acute services. Or, within a regional health authority, they could become a clinic for repetitive surgeries. Just as people in outlying areas despised Canada Post for changing their daily mail delivery from home to post boxes, so too they will scream about closing or converting hospitals. Brave governments have done it in the past, including Premier Roy Romanow's in Saskatchewan. If medicare is to be sustainable, very hard decisions will have to be made. Because Canada's population has shifted toward urban areas, public services have to change with the shift. In the majority of cases, being directed away from the hospital to a less costly and more appropriate place will be better for patients.

In an entrepreneurial regional health authority, with a commitment to be patient-centred, a cluster of family doctors who choose to work outside normal hours could group themselves and emulate France's SOS Médicins model. In operation since 1966, SOS Médicins' approximately one thousand doctors answer 4 million calls and make about 2.5 million home visits a year. SOS Médicins call centres are open twenty-four hours a day, 365 days a year. Patients pay a fee for the service—in the range of $75 to $100—to get an SOS Médicins doctor to visit them at home. Patients can be reimbursed the cost if they are poor or according to their insurance.

"Dehospitalizing" a health-care system takes time and upfront money. Governments are spending to build new nursing homes and long-term-care facilities, and to train people to provide home care. Across OECD countries, an average of about 1.5 percent of the gross domestic product is being spent on long-term care, with Canada right on the OECD average. Although still a relatively small part of the total health-care bill, it's a fast-rising part, given the aging of the population.

The need for community care is greatest among those over eighty years of age, of whom there will be many more as the baby-boom population ages. Since women live longer than men, the majority of those needing long-term care will be women. Canada's challenge is that public money to build more long-term care facilities will be tight because provincial governments are burdened by deficits and face a decade of slower growth than in the ten years before the 2008 recession.

Under those circumstances, and given the urgency of creating more spaces quickly, regional health authorities should sign public–private deals for private enterprise to construct facilities under tendered contracts that might also include operating the facilities with a guaranteed number of patients at costs that would vary according to the severity of the patients' needs. Of course, these privately constructed and operated facilities would be regulated, monitored and paid for by the regional health authority, as custodian of the public interest. If we wait for everything to be done with public money, we will not move nearly fast enough to deal with the pressure to have more places for seniors who need long-term care to go. Again, practicality should trump ideology.

Critics will complain that a blitz to create institutionalized long-term or nursing facilities through private–public partnerships would mean bricks and mortar instead of more chances for elderly patients to remain at home. The critics are partly correct. In Canada, of the 1.5 percent of GDP spent on long-term care, 1.3 percent is for institutionalized care, but only 0.2 percent is for home care. In Denmark, by contrast, the ratio is $3 on home care to $2 on institutionalized care. In part this is explained by Denmark's decision a little over a decade ago not to build any more institutions but to focus all its efforts on home care. Other countries, including Nordic ones, France and Britain, give vouchers to the elderly so they can choose the care that best suits their needs. Vouchers, it is thought in those countries, encourage private and public providers to improve consumer choice through competition. We could learn from this example.

Obviously, it is desirable to care for as many people at home as possible, for their own sake and because it is less expensive. Some provinces have started offering tax advantages to the elderly, or disabled, who wish to fix their homes to make them more easily habitable. More such incentives might be required, as will more incentives for family members to take time off to care for people at home. The costs of such measures, although considerable, are still likely less than the cost of institutionalization. Still, home care has its limits, including the wear and tear on families, the nature of chronic and overlapping conditions, dementia and Alzheimer's mostly associated with old age, to say nothing of plain old physical frailty. The more people who can be cared for comfortably at home the better. Home-care advocates are right about that. But institutionalized care will still be needed, in larger quantities, and quickly. Relying exclusively on governments to finance and build facilities will take too long.

Clogged at entry and exit points, large hospitals cope as best they can. They have a confused management structure, with administrators and physicians operating according to different mandates and receiving their money from different parts of the provincial government. The majority of them operate within global budgets dictated by the government either directly or through regional health authorities. The hospital knows what its supply of money will be and tries to fit demand into that supply. Since the demand is always greater than the supply of space, machines and personnel, rationing and triaging are a way of life for administrators, doctors and patients. The hospital has no incentive, under the traditional financing model, to earn more money—that is, to soak up some of the unmet, or at least waiting, demand. It cannot charge patients for medical services. In many cases, it cannot increase the volume of patients beyond what the supply of money from the global budget will allow. It has no financial incentive to increase the volume of patients, except through efficiency gains. A patient is a cost to the hospital budget, not a revenue earner. A hospital operates on a Procrustean model—patients' needs fit into what's available. This financing model has been largely abandoned in other countries, but predictably it remains the dominant model in much of Canadian medicare. It's time for Canada to catch up.

Vilfredo Pareto was an Italian economist whose work gave rise to the theory of Pareto efficiency. Pareto efficiency means figuring out how to make one person (or more) better off while not adversely affecting the welfare of anyone else. Pareto efficiency makes no judgment about equality. If three people have ten apples each, and one person gets another apple, the common welfare is enhanced because one person is better off, provided that his or her additional apple did not come from one of the other two people. Everyone did not gain. Only one person did. But since no one lost, the overall situation is better. That's Pareto efficiency.

Applying Pareto efficiency is foreign to medicare. The idea of someone getting ahead causes Canadians to assume that someone will lose, as in dropping back in a queue. Nothing is more offensive to Canadians' view of health care than someone jumping the queue because of money or influence, or both. That is the main reason why governments outlaw or squeeze private medicine. But what if private payment does no harm to the system? What if a few gain but no one loses?

Consider hospital surgeries. Most large hospitals find themselves with many of their operating rooms unused most of the time. Earlier in this book, we saw that of the Ottawa Hospital's one hundred operating rooms, only four remained open 24/7. The remaining ninety-six were open for business (patients) from 8 A.M. to 4 P.M., five days a week. They were closed Saturdays and Sundays. Shortage of money and, to a lesser extent, staff and postoperative beds caused the closures. The result: long wait times for many surgeries. A first-year commerce student could remedy that disconnect with market tools, which of course Canadian health care forbids.

What if a hospital were allowed to use some of the operating time now going begging for private surgeries performed by staff at the hospital? The hospital would price the surgeries such that it made a profit, then plough the profit back into the hospital. Such surgeries would enhance equity, because they would free up more surgery time for others from 8 A.M. to 4 P.M. A critic would snort that the answer would be to give hospitals more money to fund additional surgeries, which is commendable in theory but doubtful in practice. The federal–provincial agreement of 2003–2004 allocated billions of dollars for five procedures, including hip and knee replacements. The money did nothing for the many other kinds of surgeries. It is extremely unlikely that governments will find the billions of additional dollars to ramp up the number of surgeries across Canada to reduce wait times across the range of surgical needs. If hospitals with spare capacity could earn some extra money by paid surgeries in the operating rooms *that would otherwise not be used,* Pareto's efficiency would result. The welfare of a few patients—those with the financial means to pay—would be enhanced, but other patients' welfare not adversely affected: the hospital would earn money for its public purposes; the state would not pay more.

Pareto's efficiency does not apply if someone's welfare is diminished by someone else's gain. So if a queue gets longer, or if a room is taken by a paying patient that would otherwise have gone to a non-paying one, then equity is offended. The biggest challenge with implementing such a system within a hospital would not be the shortage of operating-room time but where to put patients after surgery. Rooms are very often not available because of bed blockers. But if within a regional health authority there were institutions with spare capacity—from ORs to post-operative recovery beds—then the authority should be given the flexibility to graft on to the system, making money for the public good, provided that no one's welfare is diminished. After all, at least a few of these paying patients might go to the United States, so why not keep their money in Canada? Since surgeries are usually less expensive in Canada than in the U.S., why not let Canadian institutions operate on Americans (or others) and earn money, if there is excess capacity in these institutions? As for staffing, surgeons love surgeries. Many surgeons are frustrated by lack of access to operating-room time. Finding surgeons willing to do more surgeries at an appropriate price would not be hard. Nor would finding nurses and other staff who might wish to earn overtime money (assuming their union would allow it).

This surgical system would be a marginal change. It would not open the floodgates to private medicine. It would be an adjunct to the existing system, with money earned going back into the system. It would require an adjustment of philosophy already accommodated in public health-care systems elsewhere. In Sweden, about 1 to 2 percent of surgeries, mostly day surgeries, are private, in Britain about 10 percent, including people who come from abroad for operations.

Two other changes—both within the single-payer system—would be much more consequential. Both are already standard procedure in other single-payer systems. The first is part of dehospitalizing health care, because the more services that can be safely removed from hospitals, the more hospitals can focus on the work for which they are best equipped, acute and emergency care.

Various surgeries do not need to be performed in a high-cost hospital. These represent repetitive surgeries for such problems as cataracts, joint replacements, hernias; plus all sorts of out-patient treatments such as dialysis, radiation, diagnostic imaging, to mention a few. It should not matter who provides the service — public, private non-profit or profit — assuming that quality is maintained and the state pays. The job of the regional health authority should be to encourage the best service at the best price for patients. Some provinces have authorized clinics outside hospitals to perform repetitive surgeries, with encouraging reductions in wait times. Saskatchewan, in particular, is showing very good results from authorizing clinics for repetitive surgeries: shorter wait times and high-quality outcomes. A study in the *Canadian Journal of Surgery* reviewed the first two years of the Centre for Surgical Innovation (CSI) at the University of British Columbia Hospital, a thirty-eight-bed ward with two operating rooms. It was given a contract by the provincial government to perform sixteen hundred additional hip and knee replacements, and after two years the study found shorter wait lists, high patient and staff satisfaction and low post-operative complication rates.

In Quebec, the contract between Sacré-Coeur Hospital and the Rockland Clinic, which had been working well, with large volumes of surgery and high patient satisfaction, was abruptly cancelled by the provincial health minister in 2011. He succumbed to pressure from unions insisting that private delivery of publicly financed health care was an affront. It was an affront — to union rules, power and incomes, but not to patients.

The cost of contracts signed with clinics will have to be

adjusted for volume and price, since some surgeries such as cataracts have become so routine that costs have fallen dramatically, even if the medical fee schedules have not, although Ontario lowered a few fees in May 2012. Regional health authorities would have to be careful to ensure that the higher volumes anticipated from surgeries in clinics do not explode budgets because fees are set too high. These are details, albeit important ones. What counts most is the principle that public health care should be delivered by either private or public providers where quality and outcomes are better and costs are lower. This system, widely used elsewhere, will introduce competition among providers, help dehospitalize the system, reduce some wait times, lower costs and help hospitals focus on what they do best.

Hospitals also need to be financed differently. As has been noted, Canada has lagged behind practices elsewhere. Many hospitals across Canada—there are exceptions, as in British Columbia— are still largely financed from a global budget given them by governments directly or, in some provinces, through a regional health authority. This method of financing reflects the top-down, bureaucracy-controlled, politically influenced model too common in medicare. The global budget is based, more than anything else, on last year's budget. Sometimes hospitals are given incentives to do more in particular areas, such as additional joint-replacement surgeries, from special pots of money set aside for that purpose. Generally, however, they operate within global budgets that force hospitals to consider each patient as a cost. Hospitals cope with patient demand by limiting supply of services in order to fit within existing budgets. The results are long wait times when demand pressures hit inflexible supply.

Slowly, governments are introducing, or contemplating,

funding for hospitals based on how many patients they actually treat, or what is called activity-based funding (ABF). Almost every country in the OECD uses variations on the ABF model rather than global budgets, because ABF encourages hospitals to increase volume and to be innovative, not by squeezing supply but by trying to expand it. By increasing the volume of patients—by seeing them as revenue sources rather than costs—hospitals seek efficiencies. Almost every international study about ABF shows that patients move through hospitals faster, volumes increase and wait lists decline as hospitals respond to the incentives to do more. Some ABF formulas emphasize volume; others emphasize volume and improved outcomes; still others reward hospitals for quality improvements that presumably lead to greater efficiency and outcomes. Patient surveys report high levels of satisfaction in countries that use ABF models, largely because wait times drop but quality outcomes do not.

ABF models throw up new challenges, the most important being that if hospitals are rewarded for treating more patients, they earn more from the public purse. Total costs of health care will rise, because more patients will be seen. Under global budgets, governments can limit costs by curbing demand through limiting supply. Under ABF, supply increases but so does the cost of providing that supply: more fee-for-service procedures, more personnel to deliver services, more rooms being occupied. An ABF system is definitely more patient-centred; it can also be more costly. Therefore, ABF needs to be introduced gradually and blended within global budgets, as happens elsewhere. Even so, it likely will require a cap on volume; otherwise, budgets might explode. In addition, regional health authorities should price procedures properly, resetting payments downward when new technologies or methods make procedures cheaper.

Regional health authorities should use these blended ABF

models. It would help get more value for money from hospitals and move more patients through the system to reduce wait times. It would also be part of a redesign of care with a real emphasis on patients by stimulating competition among providers (hospitals, clinics, doctors) for public dollars, decentralizing delivery of care outside of hospitals, allowing hospitals to earn money from a few patients to help finance care for others; in short, ABF practices would be just one reform among many to get away from the traditional medicare model that has produced inadequate value for money. That Canada has been so reluctant to experiment with, let alone implement, reforms like these already undertaken elsewhere speaks to the chronic condition of Canadians' smug satisfaction with and reluctance to tamper with their iconic medicare.

SEVENTEEN

Drugs

Canadians pay too much for pharmaceuticals. Within the OECD, Canada pays the second-highest share of its GDP on prescription pharmaceuticals—$640 per capita compared with the OECD average of $487. Medicare cannot be made more sustainable without bringing drug costs—and the rate of increase in drug costs—down, because drugs now represent the second-largest cost to the health-care system after hospitals. Nor can medicare's founding principle of equity be achieved if drug coverage remains a patchwork across Canada. Drug coverage needs an overhaul based on a different conception of equity from one that defines obligations among people within today's generation (horizontal equity) to one that deals with obligations between today's and tomorrow's generations (vertical equity).

Canadians spent about $32 billion on drugs in 2011, about 85 percent of which was on prescribed drugs. This figure does not include the many billions of dollars for prescribed drugs in hospitals. From 1975, three years after the full implementation of medicare, to 2006, per capita expenditures on hospitals (adjusted for inflation) rose 51 percent, on physicians 98 percent and on pharmaceuticals outside hospitals 338 percent.

From 1999 to 2009, drug costs grew faster than any other part of the health-care system, although since 2005 pharmaceuticals' share of total health spending stabilized at around 16 percent, about double the share three decades ago. As the population ages, that share will rise appreciably, because it has been estimated that about 85 percent of people over sixty-five years of age use prescription drugs. Within the Ontario Drug Benefit Plan, for example, spending has been growing at 9.4 percent per annum over the past decade, with about two-thirds of the increase tied to seniors.

Drug coverage in Canada is a patchwork. Sixty-one percent of drug costs were paid privately, 39 percent publicly. For prescribed drugs only, private insurance plans paid 37 percent, citizens paid 18 percent out-of-pocket and public plans covered 45 percent, for an overall private–public split of 55–45. Two-thirds of private prescription drug spending was covered by insurance, usually through employer plans, but a third was out-of-pocket.

Canada ranked near the bottom of OECD countries for the share of drug costs covered by the state. As the OECD rather pointedly observed, this gap offers one explanation why, outside medicare coverage, Canadian health care resembles that of the United States—mostly private and very expensive.

Canadians are not only big drug users, but what they consume is comparatively expensive. Drug prices are 10 to 30 percent higher than in Australia, France, Germany, the Netherlands, Britain, Sweden and New Zealand. Generic drug prices have been the highest, or among the highest (depending on the study), in the OECD. So are drugs under patent, so-called brand-name drugs. Canada has the worst of all worlds: expensive drugs, extensively used, with almost no coordination among buyers and widely varying coverage among provinces and people.

Worldwide, the brand-name drug companies are in an innovation slump. Some drugs they discovered years ago, and from which they made huge profits—Lipitor, the cholesterol-lowering drug, for example—have lost or are losing patent protection. Those higher-priced patented drugs will be replaced by lower-priced generics. The savings for provincial drug plans, and for Canadians who use these drugs, will be considerable. Still, the long-term upward march of drug costs will continue. Other countries are struggling with the upward march, too, but none more than Canada. Other countries have far greater public coverage of drugs because they recognize that the continuum of health care ought to extend to drugs.

The challenge, therefore, is threefold: get the price of drugs down, expand coverage to end the patchwork and figure out how to pay the higher overall costs of expanded coverage with an aging population.

Provinces have always been responsible for pharmaceuticals. Each one has a formulary for pharmaceuticals used in hospitals and subsidy programs, mostly for seniors and the poor. Inside hospitals, drugs are covered as an essential service under medicare. Step outside those doors, and drug coverage varies widely from province to province according to age, income, marital status, medical need and listing on the formulary. Consider one study reported in the *Canadian Medical Association Journal* in 2008. A seventy-three-year-old patient with a heart condition and high cholesterol is married with a combined income of $44,806. He takes six medications. The cost of his drugs yearly is $1238. As a senior, however, his cost would vary from $60 in New Brunswick to $1332 in Manitoba and almost as much in Saskatchewan and Newfoundland and Labrador. Why so high in these three provinces? Because the man's income exceeded the provinces' low-income rate for a large subsidy. Or think about a twenty-three-year-old single woman with a child and an income of only $14,000. The two drugs she needs would cost $807, but her coverage would range from $252 in British Columbia to $849 in Nova Scotia. Every senior in Canada is covered by some sort of provincially funded drug plan, but the coverage differs considerably. Many provinces have special plans for low-income families, but these vary widely, too. Provinces have very different policies for expensive drugs needed by small numbers of patients. And, of course, each has a different formulary of drugs that it will finance inside public plans, so a patient might get access to a drug in one province but not in another.

Given this patchwork, it's past time to bring down pharmaceutical costs. The idea: make the federal government fully responsible for pharmaceuticals in Canada; at the very least, let Ottawa develop, negotiate and administer a national formulary. Those who have watched provinces guard their jurisdiction over health care will snort that provincial baronies would never contemplate such an idea. Except that for one brief inspiring moment, they did.

In 2004, the idea that Ottawa should take charge was raised not by the federal government but by the provincial premiers. British Columbia's premier, Gordon Campbell, spearheaded the attempt at the premiers' annual summer meeting to get colleagues to agree that the federal government was better positioned than provinces to finance a national pharmaceutical plan. Astonishingly, they all agreed with Campbell. His logic was impeccable. Since Ottawa has the constitutional authority for patents and drug safety under its criminal justice power, and since it decides which drugs should be available over-the-counter or only by prescription, and since it has excellent scientific expertise, it made sense for Ottawa to run the entire drug program. It could negotiate for better prices because it would be buying for the whole country. Canada would have a standard drug formulary, prices and availability instead of a patchwork. Best of all for the provinces, Ottawa would assume responsibility for the financing of drugs.

Alberta's Progressive Conservative premier, Ralph Klein, called the idea a "stroke of brilliance." Saskatchewan's NDP premier, Lorne Calvert, endorsed it enthusiastically, adding that "it's not every day the premier of Saskatchewan and the premier of Alberta are in agreement." Unanimously, the premiers called for Ottawa to take responsibility. Said Alberta's health minister Gary Mar, who had replaced Klein when the premier slipped away to the casino in Gatineau for long stretches, "There is no doubt the federal government is looking for improvement to the health-care system they can take credit for. This is their opportunity to put their money where their mouth is and do something that is an important part of our health system." Quebec premier Jean Charest, whose province has its own public drug plan, didn't want any part of a federal initiative—until he was persuaded that Quebec could run a parallel provincial one.

The idea of national pharmacare has been around for a long time. Medicare's founders dreamed that some day it would extend beyond hospitals and doctors. The Hall Royal Commission wanted it, with deductibles for citizens. In 1997, the federal Liberals' election platform promised a national pharmacare program. Various pro-medicare groups have called for it. The Canadian Federation of Nurses Unions lobbied the premiers before and during their 2004 meeting. The Romanow commission endorsed the idea as a long-term objective, recommending a form of public catastrophic drug coverage as a first step.

The premiers' timing in 2004 could not have been worse. The Liberals had changed leaders and were led by Paul Martin, who was preaching "transformative change." But Martin advanced so many changes—he was also beset by the sponsorship scandal that

Chrétien had bequeathed him—that he had no time to flesh out what would have been a radical, complicated change. In 2006, the Liberal era gave way to a minority Conservative government led by Stephen Harper, who expressed not the slightest interest in a national plan. The Conservatives' federalism doctrine was to keep Ottawa out of provincial jurisdiction. The party abhorred potentially expensive new social programs, preferring targeted tax cuts to achieve social and political objectives. Having flashed through the premiers' minds in 2004, the idea of national pharmacare never inspired them again.

The provinces, of course, could develop their own common formulary. On several occasions, premiers have promised to develop an interprovincial drug formulary. The best they could achieve, however, was an agreement to negotiate collectively for new drugs coming on the market. As with most things interprovincial, regional groups of provinces can sometimes act together; mostly, provinces go their own way. So it is with pharmaceuticals.

Each province negotiates separately with the drug companies, who are delighted with this arrangement. Instead of facing negotiators purchasing products for almost 35 million people, they face someone, say, from Nova Scotia on behalf of 950,000 people or Alberta with 3.8 million. The bigger the order, the greater the chance of a lower price, as every business person understands. By forgoing bulk purchasing for almost 35 million people, Canadian health care is missing a chance to secure lower prices for drugs.

A national formulary negotiated by one buyer, Ottawa, makes logical sense. Since 2002, the Common Drug Review (CDR), agreed to by the federal and provincial governments, has provided recommendations on the listing of new drugs to the provincial drug plans. An independent committee of eleven professionals (plus two members of the public since 2006) considers the safety and clinical and cost effectiveness, in and of itself and in comparison with existing therapies. The CDR recommends; it remains for the provinces whether to follow the advice, which they do more than 90 percent of the time. It would be much more efficient if Ottawa continued to run the CDR, did the scientific analysis (instead of different provinces having their own clinical analysis) and then implemented the recommendations in a national formulary, a variation of what is done everywhere else in the world for public drug plans.

New Zealand has its Pharmaceutical Management Agency, Britain its National Formulary. The United States uses formularies for the Department of Veterans Affairs and Medicaid. Perhaps the most relevant comparison for Canada is Australia, another federation. There, the Pharmaceutical Benefits Pricing Authority issues a schedule of drug benefits after receiving advice from scientific experts, then negotiates the purchase of the drugs on behalf of the entire country. It is impossible to say by how much a single negotiator could get lower prices from manufacturers, but basic economics suggest some savings would accrue from bulk purchasing. Drug companies could not play one province off against another, or cut special "secret" rebate deals, as they do now. Many factors influence the price of drugs, but having such an ineffective method of negotiating price and volume is certainly one.

If provinces could not agree to allow the federal government to act, they could do so collaboratively, as happens with the Canadian Blood Services. The CBS is a national organization, based in Ottawa, that controls the country's blood supplies—on behalf of the provinces with a budget provided by them. By all accounts, it has been a great success: timely supplies and safe supplies of blood for all parts of Canada, a hugely better system than ten blood services could provide. (Quebec, predictably, runs its own service, although it piggybacks purchases of pharmaceuticals for blood diseases onto those made by the CBS.)

Canadian drug prices are out of line with international prices. A 2011 study of generic (off-patent) drug prices for the Patented Medicine Prices Review Board, a federal government agency, found that French prices were 73 percent lower than Canadian, Germany's 62 percent lower, Sweden's 42 percent lower, Britain's 54 percent lower and the United States' 57 percent lower. Only Switzerland's generic drug prices were higher than Canada's. For most provincial drug programs, the study concluded, "potential cost savings of 40–50 per cent seem quite feasible." As for patented drugs, another 2011 study for the Review Board found that Canadians' prices ranked third-highest of seven countries studied.

Consider little New Zealand, population 4.4 million, which is the heroic country for those hungering for a national formulary because it has one. New Zealand uses one national agency, established by the country's District Health Councils, to bargain with companies for the best price in exchange for their drugs being listed on the formulary. One Canadian study looked at four widely used drugs, compared their prices in New Zealand and British Columbia, and found that New Zealand's prices were 21 to 79 percent lower. From this rather small sample, the authors concluded that Canada, with a national formulary and a single negotiator, could achieve a 50 percent saving in drug costs. Such a saving could pay for a national pharmaceuticals plan in Canada. Other studies focusing on such a plan have reached similar conclusions.

The New Zealand comparison doesn't fit Canada. New Zealand has no brand-name drug companies. Its market is too small and its geographic location too distant for drug companies to consider setting up shop there. New Zealand accepts this reality and can design a drug policy around cost, quality, of course, and not much else. Canada and many other Western countries want companies to invest in research, development and manufacturing. For Canada to adopt a New Zealand strategy would essentially be to exclude the brand-name drug industry, largely concentrated in Quebec and Ontario.

Canadian policies to stimulate research and development by brand-name companies have produced mildly disappointing results. The industry promised, in exchange for improved patent protection for their products in 1987, to spend 10 percent of sales revenues on research and development by 1996. The industry initially kept that promise: by 1996, companies were spending 12.5 percent. Starting in 2003, however, the share dropped below 10 percent and has remained below ever since, hitting 8.2 percent in 2010. Over an eight-year period, 2003 to 2010, the companies fell $1.2 billion short of their 10 percent commitment, although the companies insist that their commitment was only to reach the 10 percent target in 1996, not to maintain it. Moreover, they would argue that the Canadian regulatory system is costly and decentralized, which is true. Big breakthrough drugs have been discovered elsewhere, although Singlar, an asthma drug, was largely pioneered in Canada. So was Vioxx, a drug that was subsequently withdrawn from the market because of adverse side effects. Statistics Canada has estimated that 28,000 people are employed in the pharmaceutical industry, with other jobs tied to but not directly part of the industry. Sales and marketing personnel, however, vastly outnumber researchers and other highly trained medical personnel. Companies spend more money selling product than researching, and a lot of their research budgets are in routine clinical trials.

One way of measuring research efforts is to compare spending on research and development with domestic sales. In Canada's case, for the brand-name companies the ratio in 2008 was 8.1 percent, compared with 19.5 percent for France, 18.2 percent for Germany, 25.6 percent for Sweden, 42.3 percent for Britain, 19.4 percent for the United States and 120 percent for Switzerland, home to some of the world's largest brand-name companies. Only Italy had a lower ratio than Canada's, and Canada's ratio was lower in 2008 than in 2000. Research and development spending appears to be associated with where pharmaceutical head offices are located. That none is in Canada explains in part the disappointing research and development performance. Canada is a branch plant, and it shows.

So, although Canada's brand-name prices are, on balance, higher than in many countries, Canada has not received the full industrial benefits promised by extended patent protection for brand-name drugs. Giving them more patent protection, or throwing even more tax credits their way, isn't likely to improve performance. The brand-name industry will hate a national drug policy of any kind. The industry will threaten layoffs, declining investment, less research and development. It will certainly lobby Quebec and Ontario to oppose anything national, since that is where the bulk of the industry's jobs are located. It will argue that Canada is a small market internationally, and, therefore, it should not overestimate its bargaining leverage, because companies can pack up and go elsewhere. There will be threats, but in the balance between trying for more sustainable drug costs and the possibility that some threats might be realized, the gains lie in facing the threats, since the money potentially saved for taxpayers will in the long run outstrip the potential job losses. For example, if prescription drug costs fell by 20 percent, the $5 billion saving at $100,000 a job would produce twice as many jobs as brand-name companies do now.

The irony of high brand-name drug costs is that prices have actually not risen. By law, the price of a patented drug cannot rise by more than the consumer price index (CPI) over any three-year period. This policy is monitored by the Patented Medicine Prices Review Board. In almost every year since 1988, price increases of patented drugs stayed below the CPI. What happens, however, is that companies apply for patents for new drugs that are very similar to older ones facing the loss of patent protection, sometimes called "me-too" drugs. These are intended, in part, to forestall the entry into the market of cheaper generic drugs. If companies are successful in securing a patent, the price for the slightly newer drug remains high. As new blockbuster drugs have been in short supply, these look-alike drugs are increasingly important to maintain profits.

Brand-name companies and generic manufacturers fight like the feuding Montague and Capulet families in *Romeo and Juliet*. They sue each other endlessly over loss of patents and patent infringement. (In one celebrated struggle between AstraZeneca and Canada's largest generic firm, Apotex, litigation continued for seventeen years, the Federal Court issued fifty-five decisions, the Federal Court of Appeal fifteen decisions and the Supreme Court one. Since 1997, Apotex has been a party to 432 different cases in the Federal Court and the Federal Court of Appeal, plus seven in the Supreme Court.) They issue studies and counter-studies arguing the perfidy of the other. They incessantly lobby Ottawa over drug approvals and provincial governments over formulary and other policies. The companies within each industry are always trying to influence physician and pharmacist decisions over which drug to prescribe. Governments have put in place regulations and laws to try to stop some of the most egregious practices to influence medical decisions, but if there is a way around such practices, it will be found. The profits to be made are too great to completely stifle the ways of profit seeking. No doubt, lobbying efforts would continue if there was a national formulary. It would just be more focused—on the national government, or on whatever body the provinces might collectively assemble to work on their behalf.

The Montagues and Capulets of the drug industry can occasionally co-operate. Brand-name companies will contract with generics to manufacture a product. (They can also produce their own generic to compete with new entries into the field once patent protection is removed.) Protecting patents or challenging them is a costly legal business, but the profits in the pharmaceutical industry can be large. Similarly, getting drugs on provincial formularies is critical, because provincial drug plans soak up large volumes and signal prices to private insurance plans. Getting drugs onto formularies involves pricing deals, often secret, whereby companies will ostensibly sell a drug for a given price (the list price) to a province but then offer secret rebates. Private insurers use the list price but do not benefit from rebates, the extent of which remain secret, so people privately insured pay higher prices than those on provincial drug plans. Companies do not want rebates to become known, because the list price is the one they use internationally and with other provinces.

Other deals involve paying rebates and allowances to pharmacies to get them to stock product, except that these rebates don't affect the price paid by consumers, including provincial drug plans, as the Competition Bureau of Canada noted in studies in 2007 and 2008. Provinces, notably Ontario, followed by British Columbia, have been stripping away some of these rebates and lowering the price they will pay for generic drugs.

Then there is the distortion caused by Quebec's drug plan. It stipulates that no supplier may sell to another province at a lower price than in Quebec, or risk its place on the Quebec formulary. This threat means that smaller provinces—and that means all but Ontario—cannot negotiate a price lower than Quebec's because pharmaceutical companies would fear losing business in the country's second-largest province. British Columbia, for one, gets around the Quebec threat by publishing only the list price it ostensibly pays, while negotiating secret rebates, blocking any transparency in the process. If a national plan were put in place, but Quebec opted not to participate, Quebec's stipulation would collapse because companies would no longer be blackmailed by losing market share in Quebec when they could gain more in the larger rest-of-Canada market.

A national formulary is about better prices. What about use—the volume of drug use that has been driving up drug costs? Pharmaceutical sales rose 6.4 percent a year from 2005 to 2010, and sales track overall drug consumption. A little of that growth, perhaps a tenth, comes from the current increase in number of adults, which includes the boomers. Some comes from the fact that certain ailments can now be treated by drugs rather than in hospital. When this happens, drugs actually save the health-care system money. In other instances, drugs help keep people with chronic conditions alive longer, and that increases the cost to the health-care system, although it is excellent news for the patient. There are new drug treatments for which none existed previously. A handful of these are immensely expensive—new cancer drugs, for example—and every province wrestles with deciding whether to finance them. Even when a province looks at all the available evidence and concludes that it should not finance the drug because the cost is so high, the prolongation of life so short and the number of patients affected so limited, once the negative decision is announced, the patient(s) take(s) their story to the media. Headlined and heartbreaking stories of human tragedy are flung in the government's face. The opposition parties join in the generalized outrage and, invariably, the government retreats, thereby adding another very costly drug to the formulary. If this happens in Ontario, as it has, the manufacturers of the drug are delighted, since listings by Ontario formulary are the ones against which other provinces judge theirs. Companies can immediately lobby the other provinces, whipsawing them against the Ontario decision.

The biggest looming drug-cost challenge, however, comes from an aging population. Seniors, per capita, use many more drugs than the rest of the population. They cost provincial drug plans more than does any other segment of the population, and their numbers are rising. These plans account for about half of all prescription-drug expenditures in Canada, and seniors are the biggest driver of those expenditures. In some provinces, seniors pay small deductibles or co-payments; in others, they pay nothing. In 2009, a study of public drug plans in six provinces showed 63 percent of seniors were claiming five or more drugs, and 23 percent had claims for ten or more. Five of the top ten drug classes were for high blood pressure or heart failure. Various studies have shown that inappropriate prescriptions account for some of this large volume, but most of it comes with age and the availability of drugs that did not exist a while ago. Overall, provinces spent an average of $1311 on drugs outside hospitals for seniors in 2009. And, of course, seniors are much more likely to be hospitalized—they make up 14 percent of the population but 40 percent of acute hospital stays—and drugs in hospitals are all publicly funded. Three of four seniors reported having at least one chronic condition; one in four reported having three or more.

The baby-boom generation, born between 1946 and 1965, started turning sixty-five in 2011. By 2031, the boomers will have all turned sixty-five. The shift toward an aging population has already started. We ought to have planned for this shift years ago, but we did not.

When these seniors exit the labour force, they will leave behind a smaller share of the population working. Seniors' growing health-care costs will therefore have to be supported by a relatively smaller number of people in the workforce. That burden can be financed in only two ways: higher taxes on the next generation, or contributions by everyone now, including those who will be among the seniors in the next twenty years.

Canada has always financed health care within generations. That is, taxes are levied on everyone today to pay for today's health-care costs. Already, this financing is straining provincial budgets. Tomorrow, when fewer taxpayers will be in the work-force relative to retirees, the budgetary strain from health care will grow. If we continue to finance all of health care in the usual way, taxes in the future will certainly have to rise or other programs will certainly have to be cut—even if we achieve the much-vaunted but hard-to-realize efficiency gains. There are plenty of taxes we could raise for health care. All political leaders need to do is come clean with their electors and say we need more money for health care, and we are raising the following taxes by this much for that purpose.

There are at least four problems with this approach. First, higher taxes can have negative economic consequences. At the very least, these consequences on savings and investment have to be considered. You can argue for higher taxes on grounds of equity or deficit reduction, or both, but you cannot wish away possible adverse, aggregate economic consequences. Second, just raising money for health care does not necessarily buy cost-efficient changes because, as Canadians have learned, providers eat up most of the cash. They become better off, not necessarily the patients. Third, Canada is already among the top-spending countries for health care. There is no correct amount to spend on health care; and the richer the country, the more its people want to spend on their health. But when a country is already spending a lot, more spending tends only to bring marginal gains in outcomes and quality, unless the new money brings major productivity gains. Fourth, the political appetite for more taxation is almost non-existent, not just in Canada but throughout the OECD countries. Taxes have been raised in some European countries that faced a sovereign debt crisis, or feared facing one. But it took that kind of crisis to include tax increases in financial rescue packages for countries such as Greece, Italy, Ireland, Spain, France and Britain. Short of such a crisis, electorates are decidedly against paying higher taxes.

It is very easy to say that taxes should be increased; it is almost impossible to be elected promising to do so. Even if taxes are raised after a campaign, the furor is intense—witness the attempt to introduce the HST in British Columbia or health-care premiums in Ontario. Tax revenues as a share of total economic activity have declined since the late 1990s, so it can be argued that there is room to raise them again. Politically, however, the majority of people have become accustomed to the lower taxes. They are very loath to see them rise, especially as Canada enters a period of slower real growth.

It is more likely—although this is unproven in practice—that citizens might be inclined to support additional money for public health care if it were tied directly to a particular benefit that they would definitely receive, if not right away, then in the future. This is how the Canada Pension Plan operates. People pay a contribution into the CPP throughout their working lives, knowing that at a certain age a pension will await them. It's a kind of social contract, or social insurance, based on the principle of paying now for a guaranteed benefit later. It is a mandatory, transparent prepayment for a defined benefit everyone will use, except those unfortunate enough to die before the benefit kicks in. The politics around pensions is about contribution rates, not about the principle underpinning pensions. That debate was settled decades ago.

We know in Canada that as the population ages, demand and costs of drugs for seniors (and other services for seniors) will grow. We know that if we keep funding seniors' drug plans in the traditional way that the relatively smaller group of people in the labour force will be required to pay more from their pockets for these higher additional costs for seniors. Their tax rates will have to go up, or they will have to decide to have fewer other services from government. Something will have to give for the next generation to pay the additional costs for the seniors' health care, including drugs.

Here is where the idea of intergenerational equity enters the equation. If we don't tax ourselves enough today to pay for the services we demand, we punt costs until tomorrow through deficits and debt. We once assumed that economic growth would be robust, government revenues would swell and tomorrow's generation would finance the debt bequeathed by today's generation. None of these assumptions remains valid. A better, fairer way of preparing for these additional costs—and one that would expand public health-care coverage, thereby enhancing equity goals— would be to start a social-insurance fund, as with pensions, to build money for the additional costs of seniors' drugs. Depending on political will, and the taxpayers' willingness to pay, the fund could also store up money for community-based health services that seniors will need. Of course, there would be instantaneous political opposition to any additional social-insurance payment, because people are not accustomed to think about intergenerational equity. If the plan involved contributions by employers (in addition to taxpayers and governments), they would claim that contributions would be a drag on their competitive position. It would take a lot of persuading of Canadians, to be sure, but the alternative is to pay higher taxes, cut other government programs, or both. Start paying now through social insurance or pay later with a smaller tax base is the straight-up choice.

Canada needs a national plan, not today's patchwork. So logic and practicality dictate that the social-insurance plan should be run federally, just as the Canada Pension Plan is (except for Quebec), with the same benefits and contributions all across the country. In fact, the simplest of all seniors' drug plans would be to add the extra insurance payments to the existing CPP, turning it into the Canada Pension and Drug Plan (CPDP). The CPP has proven its worth; it is administered well and is understood and trusted by Canadians. It could be expanded to include contributions for drugs that seniors would receive at a fixed age. The contributions should be tied to income because that is the most progressive system, but also because as a general rule people who are more affluent live longer and will likely be consuming more drugs.

A federal drug plan for seniors, based on income-related contributions, would fit nicely with a national drug formulary that would likely secure lower prices for drugs than today's provincial formularies. The gaps in the existing provincial drug plans would vanish. Seniors would be covered, in exchange for having contributed throughout their working lives. Health risks would be pooled, as they are within medicare, and therefore be consistent with the values of all public health-care systems, not just the Canadian one. Private insurance companies would not complain, since seniors whom they are now obligated to cover are among their most expensive customers. Provinces, if they thought about it (as the premiers briefly did in 2004), would be relieved of a major expense, and one that is going to grow. In exchange for no longer having to finance a seniors' drug plan, Ottawa would obviously transfer less money to them, because it would need that money to contribute to the social-insurance scheme, again as with the Canada Pension Plan. Quebec would object to all this on jurisdictional grounds. To which, the rest of Canada would reply, fine, go ahead, keep running your own plan. It should be noted, however, that the idea of a social-insurance model was recommended by the Clair Commission on health care in Quebec in 2001.

The federal government, in addition to bargaining hard through a national formulary for lower prices, would have to keep drug costs down by all means consistent with trying to secure investment in research and development for pharmaceuticals in Canada. It should invite tendering for bulk purchases, end many of the occult practices between pharmacies and drug companies and use other strategies to keep costs low. It should put the administration of the plan in an arm's-length agency. As in every country, seniors should pay a portion of the drugs in the form of modest deductibles to prevent overuse.

Would Canadians accept prepaying for health-care benefits? At the moment, no, because politicians have continued to hoodwink them into believing future costs can somehow be paid for without affecting other government services or tax increases. But if presented with fiscal facts instead of illusions, Canadians would likely prefer prefunding to higher taxes. At least that is what a Canadian Medical Association poll suggested in 2010. Asked about more funding for health care, about two-thirds of respondents preferred a contribution-based plan such as the Canada Pension Plan, and about one-third favoured higher taxes.

Obviously, many details would have to be worked out, including the transition costs to a new program. If a seniors' drug plan worked satisfactorily, and the public understood the rationale for paying into such a social-insurance fund, contributions could be extended to finance community care. The political reason to start with seniors' drugs is that the certainty of seniors' needing drugs outstrips the likelihood of some form of community care. Politically, a seniors' drug plan has the biggest constituency. If the federal government removed from provincial shoulders the burden of seniors' drugs, the provinces might find the financial room to develop catastrophic drug coverage, which is needed by a small share of their populations.

At the heart of this argument about drugs is whether Canadians agree to be prepared for the future. If not, if they blind themselves to future costs and assume things can continue as they are, with money coming from somewhere but not their pockets, we will continue to stumble along, squeezing other government programs. If they think about the future, they will realize that the way health care is delivered within medicare today needs to be shaken up and that the growing health-care needs of tomorrow will require more money, even after efficiency improvements, and that is better to get ready for these needs through a social-insurance scheme, starting now.

EIGHTEEN

Conclusion

A tourist in an Irish joke asks a farmer for directions to a faraway village, to which the farmer replies, "I wouldn't start from here." The punchline applies to Canadian health care. Canada could have opted for a social-insurance model as in Germany and the Netherlands, a model that produces good health-care results with short wait times, although not necessarily lower costs. Or Canada could have chosen the French system, a national public plan augmented by private insurance. Canadian medicare's creators looked instead to Britain's National Health System, a single-payer model financed by tax revenues with core services delivered by the state. The model is now too deeply entrenched to be uprooted. And anyway, no single public health-care model stands so far above the others for quality, access and cost that other countries have been scrapping theirs for this clearly superior one.

Noble in aspiration and principle, anchored in history, framed within a certain conception of Canadian values, made rigid by powerful provider groups, administered by enormous bureau-cracies, buttressed by ideology, embraced as an icon, medicare has changed less than systems elsewhere. The love and fear with which Canadians envelop medicare make change difficult in practice and dangerous in politics. Election promises make sane people cringe: "Cut emergency wait times in half!" "Double the number of family doctors!" "A fix for a generation!" "A patient wait-time guarantee!" "Save medicare!" Promises are formulaic, simplistic, ideological and sometimes stupid.

The first and most important lesson about health care is that simple solutions to complicated problems are invariably wrong or deeply suspect. Health care, an extremely complex system that is encumbered with so much national emotion and self-definition, cannot be changed quickly or easily. Nor, as Canadians have seen over the past decade, do large amounts of additional money necessarily buy change. Most of the money reinforced the status quo, which is what one would expect in a provider-driven, bureaucratically administered system. Canada poured tens of billions of dollars into health care, following the Romanow commission recommendation, but got a poor return on that investment. Those tens of billions of dollars represented the costliest lost public-policy bet of this generation.

Partisan debate about health care invariably revolves around which party promises to spend more money on a system that is already among the most expensive in the world but produces only middling results by international standards.

The resistance is rooted in fear that change will inexorably lead to U.S.-style medicine. It is hardened by constant declarations that medicare is the best system in the world. It is ossified by constant invocations that medicare incarnates "Canadian values," as if only one health-care model—the Canadian one—exists to incarnate those "values." There is nothing unique about these much-heralded Canadian values. Every industrial democracy that finances health care largely with public money shares these values of equity and fairness based on risk sharing and public financing. All that is unique is the Canadian system, not the values.

More money into the existing system would reflect the folly

of having learned nothing. That risk remains, since the Harper government has committed to raising transfers to provinces, while indexing these increases at 6 percent for another five years, after which indexation will fall to perhaps 4 percent a year. Here is a possible repeat of the post-Romanow period: additional sums that buy little change. For fifty-five years, since the Diefenbaker government in 1957 agreed to contribute half the costs of hospital construction (a plan previously negotiated by the Liberals), federal governments have wanted to have at least some role in health care. Harper ended that tradition. That he ended it temporarily does not mean it will not be revived. Politicians do come and go, after all. It should be an abiding ambition of federal opposition parties and intelligent provincial governments to rethink health care in the context of the Conservatives' abandonment of the traditional federal interest in medicare. Some of the ideas in this book, including a national pharmaceutical strategy for seniors and national clinical institutions, might be part of filling the void left by the Harper Conservatives.

The decade ahead will feature slower economic growth in Canada and the rest of the Western world. Slower economic growth will coincide with an aging Canadian population. The first of the baby boomers began retiring in the first years of this decade. The growing number of them leaving the workforce will likely mean a lower level of productivity confronted by greater demands for social spending, especially health. Governments therefore will face more straitened fiscal circumstances in the decade ahead than in the sunny one before the 2008 recession. Health care, the biggest social program, cannot remain immune from these new circumstances—unless governments make more severe cuts to programs other than health care and/or raise more revenues and/or shake up the way medicare is organized. Choices will be inescapable and hard.

The three urgent health-care objectives are improving quality outcomes for patients, hastening access and lowering the long-term increase in health-care outlays. These goals are easy to state but difficult to accomplish. Maybe, just maybe, a period of reduced fiscal circumstances might lead, or force, Canadians into a serious discussion of health care. This hope assumes—likely against hope—that political actors will level with citizens about the difficult options ahead. If political leaders do not explain the facts of life to citizens—engage them, in other words, by informing them—then Canada will not appreciably improve its health-care system or lower cost increases, but sail along toward indifferent results and higher costs. Mark this, though. Even if the rhythm of cost increases is reduced, overall health-care costs will still rise as a share of the national economy in the long run. The important question is, by how much, followed by the most polit-ically charged question, how should society pay for the higher costs? Every advanced industrial country is wrestling with these questions. Canada will be no exception. The proposals in this book are intended to help Canadians think about quality, access and cost. And if political actors will not deal straight up with these health-care issues, then third-party actors such as medical asso-ciations, think tanks, media outlets and informed individuals need to lead debates, as Jeffrey Turnbull tried to do as president of the Canadian Medical Association—as long as these debates do not lead us into the quicksand of arguing that all we need is to "buy change" with additional dollops of money.

The changes that might give Canada a chance to achieve those three objectives will challenge every part of the system and the interest groups within it. The changes will affect doctors and their associations, health-care unions, the respective roles of the federal and provincial governments, hospitals, pharmaceutical companies, regional health authorities. The changes will require different thinking about ways of organizing care, inspired by other advanced industrial countries that allow private delivery of health care, either paid for privately or publicly. The changes will challenge citizens to recalibrate their deeply entrenched definition of equity. This important value has been defined as sharing risks between the citizens of today regardless of their economic circumstances. Call it horizontal equity. But there is also what we might call vertical equity, or intergenerational equity—the idea that we owe solidarity not just to our fellow citizens today but to the adults of tomorrow by not burdening them with our debts. As our society ages, with the health-care costs associated with aging, equity would be mocked if the older generation offloaded its inescapably greater health-care costs onto those who follow. We will need, therefore, to think ahead to contemplate the mixture of the rights of health care with the responsibilities of paying for it fairly, not just within this generation but between generations.

History shaped Canada's medicare: comprehensive public coverage for hospitals and doctors, a patchwork beyond those services. The future lies in making what is comprehensive work better and at lower cost increases by shaking up the way services are delivered, and by extending public coverage to replace the patchwork outside medicare for growing demands for drugs and community care. Elsewhere, these changes would be considered the norm; in Canada, they would be considered radical. There will be some areas where public monopolies should be challenged but others where a greater role for the state as buyer and provider should be encouraged. What Canada needs is to modernize the vision of medicare's founders by using more flexible means to deliver services through hospitals and doctors while expanding public health care to include the burgeoning demands of tomorrow. We need to expand public health-care coverage where it is weak but deliver it by new means where it is present. Ideology, inspired by vacuous slogans about "Canadian values," should be replaced by a more functional framework of what works best at a lower cost for patients. Personnel, hospitals and drugs are the three largest drivers of health-care costs and the biggest determinants of better health-care outcomes. Changing them is the key to the future of health care.

It will take political leadership of the highest order to alert Canadians to what is happening to their health-care system and what should be done to improve it—and it will take contributions from many non-political actors. Leadership of this sort will require being willing to admit that we need to talk about health care, not with slogans and ideology and wishful thinking but with straight talk. The talk will mean tackling the two most difficult tasks in public life. First, place unpalatable truths in front of the people. Second, alert people to looming problems that will require hard decisions today and outline options for those decisions.

Canadians are so wedded to the medicare status quo, so fearful of change lest medicare somehow slip away and so ignorant of what other countries are doing that the political risks of candid talk, let alone serious reform, are intimidating. We are clinging to a system that exists nowhere else in the world: narrow and statist for hospitals and doctors, U.S.-style private and public health care for everything else. Countries with largely public systems have been shaking up the statist approach for hospitals and doctors, while ensuring that public coverage extends beyond these services to other patient needs, especially elderly ones. That is the trade-off that other countries have made; that is the trade-off Canada needs.

Canadian health care is not in crisis, if by that we mean that it cannot continue without collapse. There is much that is good about it, and many excellent people who work within it. Medicare, rather, manifests chronic conditions—perpetual financing squeezes, long wait times, dysfunctional decision making, federal–provincial bickering and wrong incentives— and a system that is not what everyone believes it should be: patient-centred. Public institutions, like individuals, can exist with chronic conditions for a long time. There are means of lessening some of medicare's chronic conditions if we have the courage to talk about them, banish foolish fears of sliding into a U.S. model and understand that the only two options that will ensure the deepening of chronic conditions is to do nothing or to spend more doing the same.

EPILOGUE

It is never easy to change a complicated public system that is encrusted with existing patterns of behaviour, made rigid by the established interests of provider groups and unions, frozen by ideology and supported by a population fearful of anything that might take from them elements of what they have come to know. And yet, over time and under the hammer blow of cascading realities, a public system can change, albeit slowly, which is what is happening to that most iconic of Canadian institutions: health care.

Those who govern and operate Canada's health-care system are finally facing facts. Myths are being banished. Reality is replacing rhetoric. Old prescriptions have been found wanting. Reforms, long discussed, are beginning to occur. Many more changes are still needed, but changes are happening. For this development, we can only be glad.

The publication of *Chronic Condition* in the fall of 2012 coincided with the beginnings of change and modestly contributed perhaps to some fresh thinking about the health-care system. It tried to awaken Canadians to some evident but unspoken truths— and truth, as any politician knows, can be a dangerous intellectual gamble when it confronts long-established mythologies.

Health ministers, who used to quake at telling the truth,

or perhaps did not know the truth themselves, now speak the previously unspeakable: that Canada's health-care system by international standards is expensive but under-performing. An informed audience today will hoot off the stage anyone insisting that Canada has the best health-care system in the world—a comfortable staple of political speech-making not long ago.

This line of defence for Canadian health care has crumbled in the face of recent international evidence. The international studies referred to in *Chronic Condition* are now widely known in health-care-policy circles. They shatter the myth, put about for so long by defenders of medicare, that the system favourably compares with other largely public health-care systems in the world—a myth propagated by the influential Romanow commission of 2002. The myth was wrong then, and it remains wrong.

The Commonwealth Fund study of 2010 ranked Canada's health care sixth out of seven countries, with the U.S. last. Another Commonwealth Fund study of the use of technology by family doctors placed Canada ninth or tenth out of ten countries in every category. OECD studies, the gold standard for number-crunching, showed the Canadian system in the top five for per-capita spending but with middling outcomes.

Governments, following the Romanow commission and the federal–provincial accords of 2004, poured money into health care: $41 billion in additional funds, indexed at 6 percent annually. A huge injection of money was needed, in Romanow's words, to "buy change" or, in then–Prime Minister Paul Martin's language, to produce "transformative change" and to "fix medicare for a generation." It did nothing of the kind, as could easily have been predicted.

The money bought time but not change, or at least not nearly enough change to justify the cost. Big chunks of the money went to organized and mobilized providers—doctors, nurses and health-care staff. Their wages went up, but because they worked as they had always done, productivity, always hard to improve in health care, actually went down. Spending more money largely reinforced the status quo. The new money bought peace, but not change.

Recently, therefore, two of the pillars underpinning the mythology of medicare cracked. The international comparative evidence eroded claims about the putative excellence of Canadian health care, and the infusion of large additional amounts of public money did not significantly improve the system. These two assertions had blended into the Romanow prescription—that lots more money would stabilize and improve the existing system, which was, after all, the best in the world. The evidence is now in: the Romanow diagnosis was wrong, so the prescription predictably failed.

Even if governments wanted to try another Romanow–Martin fix and pour large additional sums into health care, the money isn't there as it was a decade ago. The terrible financial recession of 2008–2009 weakened public finances. Whereas in the early 2000s governments enjoyed surpluses, the recession and its aftermath plunged all of them, except Saskatchewan, into deficits from which they had not recovered half a decade later. The impact on health-care budgets was severe.

From 2004 to 2010, health-care spending had increased at about 7 percent a year. That yearly increase was much faster than economic growth plus inflation and population growth. Seven percent, in the words of the Ontario finance minister, Greg Sorbara, in 2004, was "unsustainable," although his government then drove up health care by 7 percent every year from 2004 to 2011, while the province's deficit mounted.

In province after province, health-care spending had been squeezing almost every other part of the budget by stealth, because citizens did not realize the yearly leaking of money from other programs to buy more health care. Perhaps because so much money was being spent for such modest results, citizens became more skeptical that more money was the answer to what ailed health care.

A Focus Canada survey in December 2012 by the Environics Institute about what was needed to improve health care revealed that by a 2.5-to-1 margin respondents chose efficiency over money. A decade ago, the same survey had shown efficiency and money with roughly the same level of response. The general public, this survey suggested, had gotten wiser: endless amounts of more money would not fix what ailed medicare.

From 7 percent, health-care spending increases dropped in 2011 and 2012 to an average of 3 percent across Canada. Increases might go lower still, what with New Brunswick and Newfoundland and Labrador announcing spending freezes in 2013, Ontario dropping its health-care budget increase in 2012 and 2013 to 2 percent, and Alberta wrenching its yearly increase from 9.5 percent yearly over the last decade to 3 percent.

The unanswered but critical question is whether these lower, reasonable rates of spending increases can be maintained or whether after a period of restraint, cost pressures will bubble up, provider groups and unions will mobilize again, and politicians will revert to their old ways of promising more money for health care, willy-nilly. A period of restraint followed by a surge happened before in the mid-1990s; it must not happen again.

Lower rates of health-care spending, decried in some quarters, actually mean more innovation and system change. When more money is no longer readily available, people have to use their brains instead of their bargaining power. And so, with varying degrees of speed, changes long discussed are happening.

Pharmacists and nurse practitioners are being given new

responsibilities to deliver certain medical services such as flu shots and prescription refills at a lower cost than if provided by physicians. More family physicians are grouping together and working with other professionals. Physician and nursing wages are settling down to something like the inflation rate. Money is being redirected to home care and long-term institutionalized care, the greatest need for an aging population. For example, in Ontario the budget for hospitals is being frozen while that for home care is rising by 4 percent.

New systems are being introduced to curtail wait times, which in Canada are among the longest in the Western world. The evidence from OECD countries is clear: throwing more money at waiting times, as Canadian governments did, will fail every time. At best, it might buy shorter lists temporarily; at worst, the money is wasted.

Provinces are negotiating collectively to buy a few generic drugs, thereby slicing costs. In several provinces, the funding formula for hospitals is changing to offer incentives to do more surgeries in order to modify the global budget straightjacket described in *Chronic Condition*'s opening chapter about the available but unused operating rooms at the Ottawa Hospital and large hospitals across Canada. Saskatchewan is leading the way with day surgeries being done in private clinics under contract with the state, a step towards reducing wait lists for certain surgical procedures. Saskatchewan, like parts of the health-care system elsewhere, is introducing LEAN management techniques to improving efficiencies. Nova Scotia, whose emergency departments are described in *Chronic Condition*, has improved their look and the speed with which people are being treated.

An imposing list of big changes still lies ahead. It remains to be seen if the political will exists to pursue it. The de-hospitalization of the system is inching ahead, but of course hospitals remain the crown jewel of the system in the eyes of many communities. We have done very little about the rising pressures from an aging population on seniors' drug plans, including introducing a social insurance method of paying for them throughout a person's life. Too many governments are still locked into ideological rigidities (that do not exist in other countries) about the private delivery of public-insured services where private delivery can maintain quality, lower and cost and hasten access.

Slowly, but still too slowly, people in the health-care world are turning their eyes to what we can learn from other countries that spend less per capita on health care and deliver better outcomes. They know more now about Sweden delivering services privately but with public payment. Or about the split between purchasers and providers within Britain's National Health Service. Or the French mix of a basic public system topped by extensive private insurance. Or the Australian model of buying drugs nation- ally for a health-care system essentially run by the states. That other countries with largely public health-care systems do better than Canada is finally dawning on more and more people in the Canadian health-care systems. Modesty about the virtues of the Canadian system is itself a welcome virtue. It also contributes to a better starting point for an "adult conversation" about medicare that the repetition of the mythology that Canada had found the best health-care system in the world.

Certainly the pressure on provincial budgets will not diminish. Every economic forecaster predicts that growth in the decade following the 2008–2009 recession will be slower than in the decade before the recession. Prime Minister Stephen Harper's government has already announced that the index on federal transfers to the provinces will fall from 6 percent to something around 4 percent in 2016 when the Paul Martin accords expire. That reduction will cost the provinces billions of dollars. Existing deficits, higher debts, slower economic growth, smaller transfers from Ottawa and aging populations will be straining provincial budgets for every public service, including health care.

Even though spending increases on health care did diminish after the recession, the smaller increases still pinched provincial budgets. In province after province, departmental budgets were reduced and civil service wages were frozen. The share of total provincial spending devoted to health care continued therefore to rise. Put another way, if health care was only rising at 3 percent instead of 7, but provincial spending overall was frozen or being reduced, the health care share continued to grow.

What about higher taxes? Defenders of medicare, when confronted with the evidence of pinched budgets in many areas of public policy to make room for health care, reply that the problem lies with governments' decisions to lower taxes. The dwindling number of those who hold this view—those whom we might call the "Romanow School"—sometimes insist higher taxes are needed but, sensing the public antipathy to those higher taxes, say, no; making society less unequal is the long-term answer, which would inevitably mean higher taxes on somebody to provide the additional revenue for social programs. So the argument is really about the reduction of income inequality rather than more money for health care. Income inequality is an important debate to have but a more complicated and fraught one than merely spending more money for health care. The sad fact for the hewers to this line of argument is that the public appetite in tough economic times for higher taxes is so limited that even NDP parties are reluctant to advance it, except for hitting higher-income earners. And with health-care spending in Canada already among the highest per capita in the world, why would even more spending on health care, financed by higher taxes, make the system better?

An important piece of unattended business lies in the federal dimension of health care. Apart from health care for aboriginals and the military, provinces are responsible for organizing, delivering and largely financing health care. Nonetheless, federal governments stretching back to the government of Prime Minister Louis St. Laurent believed Ottawa should play some role. Often the federal desire was rebuffed by provinces or produced unseemly rows, but the desire remained. It also reflected what polls suggested Canadians desired: medicare was a national program that, to a fault, reflected what it meant to be Canadian.

Prime Minister Stephen Harper adopted a different view. For him, federalism was a classical system of divided powers. Provinces did their constitutional thing; Ottawa did its. Politically, he saw no gain for his Conservative Party in injecting itself into health care because it would lead to squabbles with the provinces. Just write cheques and let provinces run the system, hopefully with much experimentation.

The Harper position is constitutionally quite defensible. It is neat, clean, in keeping with traditional federalism principles and practice, but it is also politically vulnerable. It breaks with history in the sense that previous governments for more than half a century had sought some role in health care; and it breaks with how Canadians see medicare. It creates, if you like, a double vacuum, and politics hates one vacuum let alone two.

Opposition parties and civic society are therefore facing an opportunity to craft a sensible role for Ottawa in health care beyond the more limited one the Harper Conservatives have created. The worst response for any party would be to revert to the old rhetoric and promise to spend heaps of additional money, to out-bid the Conservatives. This is what public sector unions want, but public opinion suggests Canadians don't believe in that answer any more. Moreover, only fools make the same mistake twice, let alone repeatedly.

Instead, the federal role should be to create one national council to assess health-care quality, instead of the proliferation of provincial ones. It should be to have one national buyer, the federal government, for one national drug formulary for public drug plans. It should be to graft a seniors drug plan, paid for by social insurance contributions, onto the Canada Pension Plan. Among other possibilities. Public health care is just that—public— and it is entirely appropriate to debate its shape, cost and future in public forums, including during and between election campaigns.

The ice that encrusted discussion of Canadian medicare is melting. Everywhere in the system and in informed circles beyond, the status quo has been found wanting. The remedies of the post–Romanow period have been tried and have largely failed. Fresh thinking is around. And it is about time.

APPRECIATION/
ACKNOWLEDGMENTS

Canada's health-care system has been poked, diagnosed, analyzed, monitored and otherwise subjected to more scrutiny than a patient with multiple ailments. These reviews have taken many forms: government-sponsored commissions, books and articles from health-care academics and former practitioners, submissions from lobby groups ranging from the Friends of Medicare to professional medical associations and health-care unions. Think tanks, too, have weighed in. Legislative committees toured provinces and reported their findings. Pollsters have taken the pulse of public attitudes. There is also a huge and rich literature about health care internationally.

Anyone trying to analyze the Canadian health-care system starts with three building blocks: Statistics Canada, the Canadian Institute for Health Information and the Organisation for Economic Co-operation and Development. Data from these sources pepper the book. To these must be added provincial budgets, a weird fascination of mine that has caused many would-be guests to decline dinner invitations lest I expostulate on spending and revenue trends. Provinces have also commissioned studies: Fyke in Saskatchewan, Mazankowski in Alberta, Clair and Castonguay in Quebec, Drummond in Ontario. There were the national studies: Roy Romanow's *Building on Values*, which has done much to frame today's debates, and the Senate's five-volume study under Michael Kirby. The Canadian Health Services Research Foundation publishes good research with original ideas. Useful studies have been published by the C.D. Howe Institute, the Institute for Research on Public Policy, the Mowat Centre, among others.

Many university research institutes—I am grateful to so many that I cannot list them all—have enriched understanding of health-care policy. I have borrowed liberally from scholars at these institutes. I greatly benefited from the insights of other scholars and commentators, only some of whom I can list here: Mark Stabile, Jacqueline Greenblatt, Harvey Lazar, Paul Grootendorst, Aidan Hollis, Livio Di Matteo, Steve Morgan, Herb Emery, Don Drummond, David Dodge and Richard Dion, Ann Snowdon and Jason Cohen, Will Falk, Philippe Couillard and the country's leading health-care journalist, André Picard of *The Globe and Mail*.

For the history of medicare, the two foundational books are David Naylor's *Private Practice, Public Payment: Canadian Medicine and the Politics of Health Insurance, 1911–1966* and Malcolm Taylor's *Health Insurance and Canadian Public Policy: The Seven Decisions That Created the Health Insurance System and Their Outcomes*. Many monographs supplement these eminent works. I relied for my account of the arrival of medicare in Saskatchewan on the books written about that momentous time and about Tommy Douglas from authors such as Dennis Gruending, Frederick Vaughan, A.W. Johnson, Robin Badgley and Samuel Wolf. Monique Bégin is a wonderful woman for whom I have had a long and deep respect. She was customarily lively and generous in recounting events that led to the Canada Health Act. Her book about the act provides a lively summary of those debates. I spent many hours over the years talking about health care with premiers and other politicians and with senior civil servants, none of whom wanted to be quoted owing to the extreme political sensitivity of the subject.

I do want to thank the physicians and administrators who are named in the book for the time they shared with me and for their insights. I am also deeply appreciative to those who read some or all of the manuscript as it progressed: Owen Adams, Bill Tholl, Richard French, Charlotte Gray, David Dodge, Dr. David Naylor, Dr. Chris Carruthers, Dr. John Ross. Peter Nicholson treated the manuscript to a brilliant, detailed critique—and suggested the title! Don Drummond, the country's leading policy polymath, somehow found time to offer detailed and customarily constructive suggestions. Cathy Beehan, the redoubtable leader of Action Canada, a program that deepens the understanding of Canada for some of our brightest young minds, arranged a day-long seminar on health care at Mount Sinai Hospital in Toronto. I want to thank the hospital's CEO, Joseph Mapa, and especially an Action Canada fellow, Dr. Samir Sinha, for explaining to me his innovative methods of treating older patients. I also appreciated the insights of Action Canada fellows in the health-care field who came to Toronto that day: Jan Stefan Eperjesi, Rebecca Comley, Ali Okhowat, Nadine Caron, Ben Fine, David Kelton and Scott Robertson. Good luck to them all in their respective medical fields. Australian, Swedish and British experts helped me to appreciate their countries' systems. I also thank Ryan Lebons and Michael Coda, my two research assistants from the Graduate School of Policy and International Affairs at the University of Ottawa, where I am privileged to be a senior fellow.

I owe a very special debt to Dr. Jeffrey Turnbull, who allowed me to spend a week with him in and around the Ottawa Hospital. He is an exceptionally dedicated physician, a past president of the Canadian Medical Association, a person with an anchored commitment to social justice and someone who cares passionately about the issues discussed in the book. I do not know if he would agree with the analysis and conclusions, but our conversations were stimulating, at least for me. I am also thankful to the Ottawa Hospital senior staff (especially CEO Jack Kitts) and physicians at the hospital for allowing me to spend time there. I am also indebted to people at the Champlain LHIN for helping me to better understand regional administration: Dr. Wilbert Keon, Dr. Robert Cushman and Alex Munter.

Penguin Group (Canada) decided that perhaps Canadians would indeed read a book on the most important public-policy issue in the country, health care. I am grateful to Penguin, and especially its publishing director, Diane Turbide, for the company's confidence. Any errors of fact, interpretation and analysis are entirely mine.

As always, my wife, Wendy, offered only quizzical looks and a resigned sigh when I disappeared to read or write. This is the latest in a long string of books for me, and she has always been supportive in this, as in the rest of our lives' journeys. She remains for me, *sine qua non*. And I think always of our children, now fine adults whom we love: Tait, Danielle and Brook.

Ottawa and Point Comfort,
Quebec, 2009–12

INDEX

A

accessibility. *See also* wait times
  principle of medicare, 124, 150
  of private care, 295
Ackerby, Stefan, 287
Act Respecting Health Insurance, 65
activity-based funding, 343–44
acute-care hospitals, 37, 48, 50
addicts, medical care for, 44–48
aging population
  in British Columbia, 188
  and drug use, 358–59, 361
  effects of, 3, 14
  emergency department use, 32
  and equity in health care, 242–43
  and health care, 3, 25, 188–89
  health-care costs of, 188–89, 243
  and long-term care, 336
  and pressure for private health care,
    244
  and timeliness of care, 243
  and wait times, 243–44
Aglukkaq, Leona, 168
AIDS and the homeless, 47
Alberta
  balanced billing in, 136
  cataract surgery in, 201
  funding health care, 175–79
  and health-care premiums, 190
  health-care study in, 64–66
  and Health Council of Canada, 166
  hip and knee replacements, 199, 200
  joins medicare, 127
  patient charter, 168
  physicians' remuneration demands,
    137
  private clinics in, 201–6
  private health care recommendations,
    249–50
  public consultations on health care,
    276–79
  regional health authorities in, 217–18,
    329
  wait times in, 200, 277
Alberta Bone and Joint Health Institute,
  195
Alberta Health Act, 276
Alberta Health Services, 201, 202, 203
Alberta Premier's Advisory Council on
  Health, 249
alcohol addiction, 25
  medical care for sufferers, 44–48
  psychology of, 45
alternative level of care designation,
  27–28
angioplasty, 234, 235
Annell, Anders, 294
Apotex, 355
AstraZeneca, 355
Australia
  drug plan in, 304–5
  equity in system, 302–3
  financing of hospitals, 305
  funding of health care, 303–4
  health-care ranking, 158
  health-care spending, 236
  health outcomes, 302
  medicare initiated, 303
  pharmaceutical costs, 302
  pharmaceutical plan in, 351
  private health care in, 239, 302–4
  and private health insurance, 251, 302
  private hospitals in, 303
  similarities to Canada, 300–1
  as single-payer system, 239, 286
  spending on health care, 301
  taxation in, 303
  wait times in, 301

automobile use, and health status, 264–65

B

Bachand, Raymond, 5, 182
balanced billing, 136
Baltzan, David, 101
Baltzan, Marc, 141–42
Baumol's cost disease, 214
B.C. Medical Association
    on Hall report (1980), 141
    and health insurance debate, 62
bed blockers, 28
    effect on emergency departments,
        33–34
Bégin, Monique, 99
    background, 132
    and Canada Health Act, 132, 145–47
    concerns over medicare, 137–38
    conflict with provinces, 143–44, 146
    criticisms of Crombie, 140
    enters political arena, 133–34
    on expectations for Canada Health
        Act, 151
    and extra billing, 142
    and Hall report (1980), 141, 142
    health-care meeting with Trudeau,
        146
    and health promotion, 258
    interest in public service, 132–33
    and move to save medicare, 139
    and provincial spending of health
        funds, 140
    social policy interests, 134
    and user fees, 142
    white paper on medicare, 145–46
Bennett, R.B., 63
Bethune, Norman, 67–68
Beveridge, Sir William, 69, 81–82, 114
Beveridge Report (1942), 69, 81–82, 113
Binnie, Justice Ian, 247–48, 250
Bismarck, Otto von, 58
Blair, Tony, 306–7, 308
Blakeney, Allan, 225
Blohm, Lisa, 299
Blue Cross, 72
body mass index, 263
Bracken, John, 68, 97
Branson, Sir Richard, 307
Breau, Herb, 144
Britain. See also National Health Service
    (U.K.)
    annual statement of health-care use,
        285
    costs of health system, 305–6
    doctors in, 309
    drug prices, 352

health-care ranking, 158
health insurance introduction, 59
health spending, 310
home care in, 336–37
model of health care, 286–87
pharmaceutical plan, 351
private health care in, 239, 307, 332,
    340
reforms to health system, 306, 307,
    308
as single-payer system, 160, 239, 286
wait times in, 307–8, 309–10
British Columbia
    cutting of taxes, 190
    doctors' remuneration demands, 137
    drug purchases, 357
    funding health care, 187
    funding of hospitals, 52
    health insurance debate in, 61–62
    joins medicare, 127
    private clinics in, 224, 239
    regional health boards in, 217
British Medical Association, 59
Broadbent, Ed, 143
Brommels, Mats, 287–88, 296
budgets
    and aging population, 189
    in Alberta and health care, 176–77,
        179, 204–5
    in British Columbia, 187–88
    deficits in, 131, 139
    and doctors' remuneration, 162
    of Douglas government, 75, 79
    and drug costs, 162
    global, 28, 40, 51, 209, 222, 293, 305,
        308, 309, 337, 338, 342–43
    health care, 3–4, 5, 14–15, 110, 131,
        152, 166, 172–74, 186, 187–88,
        191–92, 193, 224, 235, 258, 323,
        359
    of hospitals, 22, 51, 164, 342–43
    of Ministry of Health Promotion and
        Sport, 258
    in Nova Scotia, 209
    in Ontario, 182–83, 185, 274
    of Ontario Health and Long-Term
        Care Ministry, 258
    in Quebec, 180, 181, 321
    of regional authorities, 329, 342
Bush, George W., 323

C

Calvert, Lorne, 349
Cambie Surgery Centre, 224
Cameron, David, 306
Campbell, Gordon, 348

Canada
    challenges facing, 193–94
    compared to Sweden, 288, 294
    compared to U.S., 8–11, 81, 156
    drug costs in, 345–48
    economic growth, 367
    fear of private delivery, 295–96
    health-care ranking, 156–62, 167
    health-care spending compared to
        other countries, 236
    health outcomes and income, 255
    health outcomes ranking, 255
    home care in, 336
    insurance choices in, 250–53
    obesity rates in, 255
    and OECD report, 252–53
    pharmaceutical sales in, 354
    population shift in, 335
    primary care doctors in, 293
    similarities to Australia, 300–1
    smoking rates in, 255
    spending on health care, 156, 157,
        193–94, 301
    sport participation by citizens, 255
Canada Assistance Plan, 130
Canada Health Act (1984)
    accessibility principle, 150
    challenges to, 151
    and extra billing, 132, 204, 227
    and facility fees, 150–51
    and health promotion, 258
    interpretation manual, 148–49
    negotiations over, 145–47
    passing of, 147
    PC's opinion of, 151
    penalties under, 150
    portability principle, 149–50
    principles of, 124, 276
    and principles of medicare, 148–49
    and private health care, 224, 227, 331
    public administration concept,
        148–49
    size, 147
    success of, 151, 152
    and user fees, 297
Canada Pension Plan, 130
Canada's Food Guide, 265–66
Canadian Blood Services, 351–52
Canadian Council on Social Development,
    68
Canadian Federation of Nurses Unions,
    349
Canadian Health Coalition, 139
Canadian Health Measures Survey, 263, 264
Canadian Institute for Health Information,
    13, 165, 191, 198, 203

Canadian Institute for Health Research,
    200
Canadian Journal of Surgery, 341
Canadian Medical Association, 136,
    270–71, 272
    challenge to Canada Health Act
        (1984), 151
    creation of, 58
    health-care system campaign, 23
    and health insurance, 59, 70
    hearings on public attitudes, 284–85
    opposition to public health care,
        116–17
    and patient-centred care, 168
    request for Royal Commission, 96–97
    submission to Hall commission, 102–3
    support for public health care, 163
Canadian Medical Association Journal,
    347
Canadian Nurses Association, 163
Canadian Policy Research Networks
    (CPRN), 280–83
Canadian public
    belief in efficacy of efficiencies, 283,
        284
    desire for more from health system,
        283–84
    desire for quality, 331
    dichotomy between taxes and
        services, 276, 278–79
    distrust of health system management,
        282
    identity and medicare, 2
    and individual responsibility, 285
    support for public health care system,
        96, 270–71
    survey of health (1953), 115–16
Canadian Radiation Oncology Services
    (CROS), 226
Canadian Radio and Television
    Commission, 133, 134
Canadian Sickness Survey (May 1953),
    115–16, 117
Canadian Taxpayers Federation, 184
Canadian Triage and Acuity Scale, 33
Cancer Care Ontario, 226
Cancer Commission (Saskatchewan),
    76, 79
capitation model of payment, 233, 293,
    294, 299
cardiac bypass surgery, 165
case managers, 195
Castonguay, Claude, 155, 180, 221–24
Castonguay report, 229–34, 249
cataract surgery, 52, 165, 184, 201, 203,
    205, 341, 342

Catholic Church, 64, 68
Centre for Surgical Innovation (B.C.), 341
Champlain Health Authority, 53
Chaoulli, Jacques, 245, 246
Chaoulli case, 239, 245–49, 250, 251
Charest, Jean, 181, 349
Charter of Rights and Freedoms, 245
children, fitness rates in Canada, 263
Children's Hospital of Eastern Ontario, 37
Chrétien, Jean, 6, 10, 11
Citizens' Reference Panel (Ontario),
    283–84
Clair, Michel, 155
Clair Commission on health care, 363
Clark, Joe, 108–9, 144
collective wealth concept, 231
Common Drug Review, 350–51
Commonwealth Fund surveys, 157–59,
    163, 200
Community Health Councils (B.C.), 217
competition
    in health-care systems, 286, 291–92,
        293, 295
    and innovation, 333
Competition Bureau of Canada, 356
comprehensiveness principle, 103, 105,
    108, 122, 123, 124, 140, 148, 369
computers
    e-health system, 44
    use of and health status, 264
    use in hospitals, 42–43
continuum of care, 235–36
Co-operative Commonwealth Federation,
    62
    birth of, 66
    budgets of, 75
    conflict with doctors, 83–84, 86
    lack of influence in Parliament, 116
    popularity of, 70
    public health-care plan, 70–71
    and Regina Manifesto (1933), 76
    and role of government, 86
    support for public hospitalization,
        120
    wins power, 66
costs
    control of, 259, 323–24
    of health care, 1, 2–3, 4, 26, 28–29,
        49–50, 85, 114, 131–32, 162, 172,
        212
    of health care and economic growth,
        259
    of health care in Nova Scotia, 212
    of health care in Sweden, 298–300
    of health care under private
        insurance, 252

increase in health care spending,
    14–15, 193
of National Health Service (U.K.),
    305–6
of pharmaceuticals, 345–48
public's understanding of, 274, 275
reducing through efficiencies, 195–96
"Creating a Healthier Canada: Making
    Prevention a Priority," 254
Crombie, David, 139, 140, 141

D

Dagnone, Tony, 170
data, about health care system, 198–200
Davey, Keith, 121
Dawn of an Ampler Life, The (Whitton),
    69
Day, Dr. Brian, 239
deficit budgets, 131–32
dehospitalization, 48, 328, 335, 341, 342
delisting services, 4, 185, 235, 273
demand and supply of health care, 215
dementia, 25
demographics. See aging population
Denmark
    health-care spending, 236
    home care in, 336
Deschamps, Justice Marie, 247
Di Matteo, Livio, 177, 178
Di Matteo, Rosanna, 177, 178
diabetes, 47, 161, 184
diagnostic testing, 26, 161
    demands for by patients, 26
    overuse of, 198
    private delivery of, 331
    wait times for, 33, 165
Diefenbaker, John, 89, 96, 97, 367
    friendship with Hall, 99
    and Hall Royal Commission, 129
    introduction of public hospitalization,
        121
    wins second election, 121
diet, and health status, 265–66
doctors. See also family doctors;
    remuneration
    annual visits to by Canadians, 316
    attitude to health insurance, 59, 64
    attitude to nurses, 58
    British, and Saskatchewan strike, 92
    capitation model of payment, 233, 293,
        294, 299
    conflict with federal government,
        131–32
    conflict with Saskatchewan
        government, 86, 87–94
    demand for services of, 319–20

disagreement with CCF government,
83–84
in early Canada, 57–58
emigration of, 136–37, 322–23
employment conditions in
Saskatchewan, 83
as entrepreneurs, 225–26, 323, 324, 327
and extra billing, 136, 137
falling incomes, 135
and fee-for-service, 149, 323
and Great Depression, 63, 64, 66
hours worked by, 320
immigrants from U.K., 83
insurance plans run by, 84–85
lack of access to, 33
limits on, 58
livelihood during Great Depression,
63
in NHS (U.K.), 309
opinion of public health care, 70,
82–83
opt out of OHIP, 136
pay freeze in Ontario, 51–52
payment for specialists, 36
primary care in Canada, 293
ratio to population in Canada, 317–18,
320
salaried, 326–27
shortage of, 319
specialization of, 316
strikes by, 63–64, 74, 91–94
support for medicare, 142
in Sweden, 293, 294–95
and user fees, 135–36
women as, 320
working in teams, 281, 324–25
Dodge, David, 3
Douglas, Tommy
career as minister, 78
childhood illness, 77
defeat in federal election, 89–90
early years, 77–78
enters politics, 78
experience with health-care system,
77
goal for health-care system, 168
as Greatest Canadian, 79
Hall opinion of, 99
implements early health-care policies,
78–79
influences on, 77–78
introduces medicare, 86–88
and premiums, 321
support for medicare, 74–75
and user fees, 321
drug-information system, 167

drugs. *See* pharmaceuticals
Drummond, Don, 183, 186
Duncan, Dwight, 5, 182
Duval, Dr. Nicholas, 224, 237, 238, 240,
241
Duval Orthopedic Clinic, 238–39

E

economic growth, and health-care
spending, 231–32
Economist Intelligence Unit survey,
159–60
education
and obesity link, 266
spending on compared to heath care,
193
efficiencies
and activity-based funding, 343
advantages of finding, 199–200
belief in efficacy of, 274, 277–78, 283,
284
challenges to implementing, 213–19
changing nurses' scope of practice,
196–97
and closing of hospitals, 196
and competition, 333
and cost reductions, 50, 195–96
as cure for health-care system
problems, 280
e-health services, 197
and governance, 218
and group clinics, 325, 326
in hospitals and surgeries, 339–40
improving, 232
increasing hospitals', 222
and Local Health Integration
Networks, 50–51
and nurse practitioners, 317
Pareto principle, 338, 339, 340
and patient satisfaction, 195
proposals for implementing, 210–11
role in funding health care, 12
and savings, 199
suggestions for, 218–19
and sustainability, 196
in Swedish health system, 288
tardiness in implementing, 209–10
e-health system
Canada's rank, 167
and efficiencies, 197
in Ontario, 44, 186
public support for, 281
electronic health records. *See* e-health
system
emergency departments
bed blockers in, 33–34

misuse of, 34, 206–7, 208–9, 334
in Nova Scotia, 211
triage in, 31, 33–34, 35
use by seniors, 31, 32
volume of patients in, 32
wait times, 31, 35, 206
Emergency Wait Times Strategy
(Ontario), 167
employment conditions. *See* social
determinants of health
Epp, Jake, 151
equalization payments, to Quebec, 180
equity
in Australian system, 302–3
under mixed private-public system,
222–23
and premiums, 321
and private health care, 224, 225,
333–34, 339–40
threat to, 242–43
and user fees, 321
Established Programs Financing Act
(EPF), 139, 142, 146
Euro-Canada Health Consumer Index,
160–61
Evans, Iris, 250
exercise, and health status, 264–65
extra billing
Bégin and, 143–44
and Canada Health Act, 132, 224, 227
cost of, 145
debate over, 136, 140, 147
and facility fees, 204
and Hall commission, 108, 140–41, 221
and medicare principles, 137–38, 140
Ontario doctors strike over, 152
penalties for, 150
refund to patient, 146
support for abolition, 142
eye surgery, 201, 205

F

facility fees, 150–51, 204
family doctors
alternative structures, 334, 335
in Australia, 304
availability of, 185, 334
lack of access to, 33, 205
method of payment, 324, 326
number of female, 320
in Ontario, 50, 185, 218, 329
in Quebec, 232–33
rate of visits to, 316
ratio to specialists, 316–17
remuneration, 293, 299, 314
role in medicare, 334

in Sweden, 293, 299
use of electronic health records, 186
working in teams, 324–25
federal-provincial relations, 63, 69
accord of 2003–2004, 215
conflicts over medicare funding,
138–39
confusion about medicare plan, 126
and health care, 117, 118, 119, 142,
143–44
health-care conflicts, 63
Rowell-Sirois commission, 71
fee-for-service
advantage of to doctors, 203, 324
decrease in, 324–25
and emergency room doctors, 207
and Hall commission, 101, 108, 140
moving away from, 216
in private clinics, 202
and Saskatchewan doctors, 149, 323
support for in Saskatchewan, 84
Firestone, Dr. O.J., 98, 101, 104
First Ministers' Accord on Health Care
Renewal, 200
First World War, 60, 70
fitness, of Canadians, 263
France
drug prices, 352
health-care spending, 236
home care in, 336–37
private delivery of care, 335
private health insurance in, 251
SOS Médecins, 335
Frank, Dr. Cy, 195, 197–200, 201, 212
freedom of choice
in Canada, 292–93
in Sweden, 292
Friends of Medicare, 204
Frontier Centre for Public Policy, 160
Frost, Leslie, 119, 120
funding
activity based, 343–44
of Australian health care, 303–4
Canadians' opinions on methods,
273–74
of drug plans, 361–62
guarantees of, 191–92
of health care, 12, 13–15, 69, 82, 108–9,
122–23, 163, 185, 188, 281–82, 285
of health care in Quebec, 229, 230
of hospitals, 337–38, 342–44
of medicare, 359–60
proposed by Douglas, 321
public *versus* private services, 278
Fyke, Kenneth, 155–56, 196, 197
Fyke report, 155–56, 197

G

gambling as source of health-care funding, 108, 109, 185, 188
generic drugs. *See* pharmaceuticals
Germany
  drug prices, 352
  health-care ranking, 158
  health-care spending, 231, 236
Getty, Don, 204
Gordon, Walter, 121, 124, 126
governance
  challenges of and health care, 216–17
  changes to, 218
  desire for, 233
  and efficiencies, 218
government actions/policies, effect of, 257–58, 267–68
Great Depression, 63, 64, 66, 70, 72, 73, 75–76, 82, 100, 113, 130
Greater Winnipeg Relief Plan, 64
Grossman, Larry, 146
group clinics, 325–26

H

Hall, Emmett, 149, 221, 257
  attitude to health-care system, 101–2
  background, 98
  education, 98–99
  and health-care charter, 104–5
  hearings of 1980, 139–41
  legacy of, 111
  opinion of Douglas, 99
  political aspirations/beliefs, 99
  report of 1980, 141–42
  and Royal Commission, 99–104
Hall Royal Commission, 99–104, 112, 123, 141, 257, 323, 349
  concern about abuse of system, 106
  dental services recommendation, 106
  and doctors' remuneration, 108–9, 140–41
  drug payment recommendation, 106
  on extra billing, 108
  eyeglasses recommendation, 106
  fee-for-service recommendation, 101, 108, 140
  financial miscalculations of, 109–10, 130
  financing recommendations, 108–9
  and health-care charter, 104–5
  home care recommendation, 107
  and individual's responsibility for health, 105–6
  makeup of commission, 98
  medical group submissions to, 102–3, 104

Hansen, Colin, 5
Harmonized Sales Tax, 188
Harper, Stephen, 14, 350, 367
Heagerty, J.J., 114
Heagerty report, 114
Health and Social Service Regional Councils (Quebec), 217
Health Care in Canada (survey), 272
health-care reforms, 219–20
health-care tax (Quebec), 224
"Health Care Transformation in Canada" (CMA), 23
Health Consumer Powerhouse (Sweden), 160
Health Council of Canada, 159, 166, 167
health insurance
  Alberta study on, 64–66
  in Britain, 59
  changing attitudes to, 60–61
  CMA attitude to, 59
  coverage before medicare, 102–3, 115–16
  during Depression, 72
  doctor-run, 72, 84–85
  doctors' attitude to, 59, 61, 62, 64, 72
  early proposal for in B.C., 61
  in Germany, 58–59
  Heagerty report and, 114
  and health-care costs, 252
  introduction of state, 86
  King on, 60–61
  opposition to, 62
  premiums in early medicare, 79–80
  private, in Quebec, 245–49
  public attitude to, 61, 62, 64, 72
  in Saskatchewan, 84
  types of, 64, 65
  and wait times, 252
  workers' voluntary, 59–60
health-quality councils, 216
health status
  automobile use and, 264–65
  of Canadians, 263
  computer use and, 264
  diet and, 265–66
  exercise and, 264–65
  factors affecting, 264–66
  and income, 255
  inequality and, 48–49, 162, 260, 263
  poverty and, 48–49, 194, 255, 298–99
Hebert, Dr. Guy, 30–35
Herle, David, 270, 274, 275
Heurgen, Mona, 298
hip and knee replacements, 165, 184, 199, 200, 339, 341
Holm, Lars-Erik, 290–91, 298

home care
    in Britain, 336–37
    in Canada, 336
    in Denmark, 336
    desire for as part of health coverage,
        119
    in France, 336–37
    lack of funding for, 120
    private delivery of, 331
    in Sweden, 300
homeless people, 44–48
Hospital Insurance and Diagnostic
    Services Act, 120
Hospital Services Plan (Saskatchewan),
    80, 85
hospitals
    acute-care, 37
    administrators' salaries, 318
    bed blockers in, 28
    budget stresses, 28, 53
    challenges facing, 337–38
    closing in Alberta, 204–5
    closing for efficiency, 196
    computer use by, 42–43
    cost controls, 323–24
    effect of hospital bill on, 120
    family-health clinics at, 34
    financing in Australia, 305
    financing of, 51–52, 342–44
    increasing efficiency of, 222
    misuse of, 29
    origin in Canada, 57
    overcrowding and patient release,
        42
    private, in Australia, 303
    and private care in, 222
    role in medicare, 328
    in rural areas, 211, 334–35
    and Saskatchewan medicare, 79
    surgeries and efficiencies, 339–40
    in Sweden, 293, 300
    teaching hospitals, 22
    user fees in, 152
    volume of patients in, 35
    working with private clinics, 202
House, Wallace, 146
housing. See social determinants of
    health
Howard, John, 303

income, and health status, 255
Independent Labour Party (Ontario), 60
indexing, of health-care transfers, 13–14
individual responsibility, for health care,
    105–6, 257, 268, 277, 285

inequality. See also social determinants
    of health
    and health status, 48–49, 162, 260
infant-mortality rate, 161
inflation, effect on health care costs, 14
influences on health care system,
    168–69
Inner City Health, 44, 45, 48
innovation in health care, 333
"Integrated Pan-Canadian Health Living
    Strategy," 256
internal medicine, and aging population,
    25

J

Japan, 236

K

Karolinska Institute, 287, 296
Keep Our Doctors (KOD), 90, 91, 92, 93
Kennedy, John F., 121
Kent, Tom, 121
    interest in health care, 122
    plan for medical care financing,
        122–23
Keon, Dr. Wilbert, 256
Kherani, Dr. Amin, 201, 202, 203
King, Mackenzie, 60–61, 62, 68, 73
    creates Royal Commission (Rowell-
        Sirois), 71
    early support for public heath care,
        112, 113
    health plan, 71
    inaction on health care, 114–15
    and Paul Martin Sr., 117
Kirby, Michael, 155, 228, 256
Kirby Senate committee, 155, 228, 256
Kitts, Jack, 32, 318
Kjoller, Hanne, 291
Klein, Ralph, 204, 250, 349

L

labour relations. See unions
Lalonde, Marc, 132, 133, 134, 139
    and wellness agenda, 259
LaMarsh, Judy, 121, 124
    on M. Sharp, 125
Lavoie, Jean-Noel, 134
law and health care, 245–49
Lazar, Harvey, 219
League for Social Reconstruction, 66
Lemne, Carola, 294–95
Lennartson, Fredrik, 289–90
Lévesque, René, 142
Liberal Party
    dissension over medicare, 125–27

King's support for public health care, 112
Kingston conference (1960), 122
National Liberal Rally, 122
Pearson minority governments, 124–25
Pearson's support for public health care, 112–13
"Plan for Health," 122–23
in Saskatchewan, 75
support for medicare, 122, 123, 129
Liepert, Ron, 176
life expectancy, of Canadians, 162
Lloyd, Woodrow, 88–89, 92, 93, 95
Local Health Integration Networks (LHINs), 50–51, 53, 218, 329
long-term care
Canada's ranking, 162
increasing facilities for, 335–37
lotteries, 108–9, 185

M

MacEachen, Allan, 125–26, 127, 145
Mackenzie, Ian, 113–14
Manitoba
cutting of taxes, 190
funding health care, 187
governance of health care, 217
joins medicare, 127
regional health authorities in, 217
Manning, Ernest, 124
Mar, Gary, 349
Marchand, Jean, 125
Marleau, Diane, 150–51
Marmot, Sir Michael, 260–61
Martin, David, 152
Martin, Paul, 13, 163, 349–50
Martin, Paul, Sr., 127
dedication, 118
as proponent of public hospitalization, 117–20
Matthews, Deb, 168
Mazankowski, Don, 155, 249
McCutcheon, Wallace, 98, 100–1
McGuinty, Dalton, 184–85
McIntosh, Major J.W., 61
McLachlin, Chief Justice Beverley, 247, 248
means test, 103, 104
Medical Care Insurance Act, 113. See also medicare
Medical Reform Group of Ontario, 142
medical school
enrolments in, 216, 319
in Quebec, 180
women in, 320

medicare
and Canadian identity, 2
components of system, 212–14
controlling costs, 173
debate over in Saskatchewan, 90–92
and deficit budgets, 131–32
endorsed by Liberal Party, 122
exclusion of pharmaceuticals from, 86
and extra billing, 140
fee-for-service model, 101
financing of, 79–80, 119, 131–32, 138–39, 175, 359
hospital role in, 328
increases in costs, 173
initiated in Australia, 303
introduced by Douglas, 86–88
Kent financing plan, 122–23
as national symbol, 270–71
payment methods, 94–95
and pharmacare, 349
principles of, 86–87, 124, 148, 152
private health care within, 149, 225
(See also private clinics)
and profit, 227
provinces join, 127
and provincial plans, 119
public administration of, 148
public support for, 92, 271–72, 275
purpose of, 258
Quebec opposition to federal, 125
and the Regina Manifesto (1933), 76
rising costs of, 135
Robarts's view on, 129
and stagflation, 131
supported by doctors, 142
sustainability of, 174–75
two-tier health care and, 140–41
use of by Canadians, 316
and user fees, 140
white paper on, 145–46
Medicare Australia, 304
Ministry of Health Promotion and Sport, 258
Mitchell, Dr. Robert, 201, 202, 203
Mode Three Billing, 137
Montreal Group for the Security of the People's Health, 67
Moore, Michael, 8
moral hazard, 15, 26, 285, 319, 330
mortality rates, 159–60
Muckle, Wendy, 44–48
Mulroney, Brian
and Canada Health Act, 147
support for Canada Health Act (1984), 151
Murray, Father Athol, 91, 93

N

National Energy Program, 142
National Health Service (U.K.), 94
    budget changes, 308
    changes to, 52
    costs of, 305–6
    doctors leaving, 83
    financing of, 306–7
    as model for Canada, 286–87
    reforms to, 306, 307, 308
    remuneration to doctors, 225
    wait times in, 52
National Institute for Health and Clinical
    Excellence (U.K.), 308
National Liberal Rally, 122
National Pharmaceuticals Strategy, 167
Netherlands, the
    health-care ranking, 158
    health-care spending, 231, 236
New Brunswick
    joins medicare, 127
    regional health corporations in, 217
New Democratic Party
    Douglas leads, 88
    support for medicare, 129
New Zealand
    drug prices, 352
    health-care spending, 236
    national formulary in, 352
    pharmaceutical policy, 351, 352–53
    private health care in, 239
    as single-payer system, 239
Newfoundland
    joins medicare, 127
    regional health boards in, 217
Nielsen, Jim, 146
Nixon, Richard, 121
Northwest Territories, 127
Norton, Keith, 151
Norway, health-care spending, 236
Nova Scotia
    district health authorities in, 217
    funding health care, 187
    health care costs, 212
    joins medicare, 127
    problems in health-care system,
        207–11
    regional health authorities in, 329
    wait times, 212
nurse practitioners, 43, 317
nurses
    doctors' attitude to, 58
    in private clinics, 202–3
    ratio to doctors, 317–18
    ratio to population in Canada, 317–18
    remuneration, 315

and scope of practice changes, 196–97
    unions, 202–3, 317–18
    working in teams, 281
nurses' unions
    and nurse training, 317–18
    and private clinics, 202–3

O

Obama, Barack, 9, 323
obesity rates
    in Canada, 255, 263
    link to education, 266
OECD
    ABF model use, 343
    average pharmaceutical costs, 345–46
    on Canadian system, 10, 50, 161–62,
        167, 195–96
    on doctors' remuneration, 314
    health promotion study, 266–67
    long-term care statistics, 335
    on members' health systems, 195–96
    nurses and doctors to population ratio,
        317–18
    on private health insurance, 250–53
    report on future, 3, 4
    research, importance of, 161
    taxation, 268, 360
    wait times, 53, 251, 310
Ontario
    budgets, 182–83
    cataract surgery in, 342
    Citizens' Reference Panel, 283–84
    compared to other countries, 186
    cutting of taxes, 191
    delisting of services, 235
    doctors opt out of OHIP, 136
    doctors' remuneration, 51–52, 137, 315
    doctors' strike over extra billing, 152
    e-health system, 186
    family doctors in, 185
    funding health care, 176, 182–87
    funding of hospitals, 52
    group clinics in, 325–26
    joins medicare, 127
    Local Health Integration Networks,
        50–51, 218, 329
    premiums introduced, 173
    private clinics in, 226, 239
    public's ignorance of costs, 275
    regional health authorities in, 329
    wait times in, 53, 167, 184, 185–86
Ontario Drug Benefit Plan, 346
Ontario Health and Long-Term Care
    Ministry, 258
Ontario Health Insurance Plan (OHIP),
    136

Ontario Health Quality Council, 185–86
Ontario Medical Association, 136
    challenge to Canada Health Act
        (1984), 151
    fight over extra billing, 152
    on Hall report (1980), 141
Ontario Nurses Association, 315
operating rooms. *See also* surgeries
    capacity of, 39–40
    demand and supply problems, 39–40,
        41
    hours of use, 40–41
    in Ottawa Hospital, 40
Organisation for Economic Co-operation
    and Development. *See* OECD
Ottawa Hospital, 37
    administrators' salaries, 318
    budget, 51
    and Dr. J. Turnbull, 21–25
    emergency room wait times, 31–32
    operating rooms, 40
    and patient flow monitor, 27–28
    surgery statistics, 39
out-of-country medical treatment, 9
out-of-province treatment, 149–50
out-patient treatments, 341
overuse of health-care system, 15, 198

P
Page, Kevin, 174–75
Pareto, Vilfredo, 338
Pareto principle, 338, 339, 340
Parti Québécois, 142, 145–46
Patented Medicine Prices Review Board,
    352, 355
path dependency, 213, 214
Patient First Review (Saskatchewan), 170
patient flow monitor, 27–28
Patient Wait Times Guarantee, 166
patients
    and activity-based funding, 343
    alternative level of care designation,
        27–28
    attitude to health-care system, 275
    as centre of health-care system, 168,
        170
    continuum of care, 235–36
    demands by for tests, 26
    desire for charter, 277
    desire for private clinics, 239–40
    equity under mixed private-public
        system, 222–23
    fees paid by in Sweden, 297–98
    flow of, 27–28, 202
    health-care coverage, 235–36
    in health-care system, 168–69

    need for case managers, 195
    opinion on health-care system, 170
    payment for private services, 241
    and private delivery of care, 332
    in reformed NHS (Britain), 308
    volume in emergency departments, 32
Pearson, Lester, 132
    announces financing of health plan,
        123–24
    leads Liberals, 121
    medicare ultimatum to caucus, 126
    and minority government, 124–25
    support for public health care, 112–13
pharmacare, 349–50. *See also*
    pharmaceuticals
pharmaceuticals
    in Australia, 351
    in Britain, 351
    bulk purchasing of, 350, 351
    Common Drug Review, 350–51
    companies' influence, 355–56
    companies' opposition to national
        drug plan, 354–55
    cost of, 26, 345–48
    coverage for, 26
    coverage in Australia, 302, 304–5
    drug costs in Canada, 162
    drug-information system, 167
    drug plan in Quebec, 357
    effect on health care costs, 14
    exclusion from medicare, 86
    as federal responsibility, 348–50
    funding use of, 361–62
    generic, 347, 356
    insurance coverage, 346
    national formulary, 348, 350–51, 352,
        356, 357, 363
    need for national plan, 362–64
    in New Zealand, 351
    patent protection, 347, 353, 354, 355,
        356
    practices of companies, 356–57
    prescribing of, 26
    prices in Canada compared to other
        countries, 352
    prices of, 352–58
    profits in, 356
    as provincial responsibility, 347–48,
        350–51
    replacing hospital procedures, 235
    research and development in, 353–54
    sales in Canada, 354
    slump in, 346–47
    in U.S., 351
    use by seniors, 358–59, 361
    use of, 357–58

Pharmaceuticals Benefits Scheme (PBS) (Australia), 304
pharmacies, in Sweden, 292
pharmacists
　enlarging role of, 197
　working in teams, 281
physical activity, and health status, 264–65
physician assistants, 43
physicians. *See* doctors
"Plan for Health," 122–23
Podger, Andrew, 303
politics
　and health care, 96, 310, 330, 365–66
　need for leadership, 370
portability principle, 140, 148, 149–50
poverty
　and health status, 48–49, 194, 255, 298–99
　reducing, 194
　in Sweden, 298–99
Praktikertjänst, 294, 295
Premier's Council for Economic Strategy (Alberta), 179
premiums
　in Alberta, 177
　in early medicare, 79–80
　for health care, 85
　in Ontario, 173, 185
　opposition to, 80
　supported by Douglas, 87
PricewaterhouseCoopers, 283
Prince Edward Island, 127
private clinics/health care
　in Alberta, 201–6, 331
　arguments for, 242
　in Australia, 302–4
　in Britain, 332, 340
　in British Columbia, 224, 331
　and Canada Health Act, 224, 227, 331
　Canadians' attitude to, 224–25, 228, 272–73
　Castonguay support for, 222
　and Chaoulli, 246–49
　controversy over in Sweden, 295
　"creaming" of patients, 241–42
　criticism of, 241–42
　and equity, 333–34, 339–40
　eye procedures in, 201, 202, 203
　and facility fees, 150–51
　fear of in Canada, 295–96
　in France, 335
　and Kirby Senate committee, 228–29
　within medicare, 225
　nurses in, 202–3
　office staff salaries in, 203
　in Ontario, 226, 239

opposition to, 151
　pressure for, 244
　public opinion on, 281
　in the public system, 222
　in Quebec, 223, 224, 226, 238–42, 331
　recommended by Mazankowski, 249
　and Romanow commission, 6, 228
　in Saskatchewan, 331
　spending on, 236–37
　status in medicare, 149
　support for, 155
　and surgeries, 339
　in Sweden, 239, 292–96, 331, 340
　and two-tier health care, 149
　and unions, 223, 228
　working with hospitals, 202
private health insurance
　accessibility of, 252
　advantages and disadvantages, 250–52
　in Australia, 251, 302–4
　in Canada, 249
　in France, 251
　OECD research on, 250–53
　in Quebec, 245–49
　in Sweden, 296
　and wait times, 248–49
private-provider/public payer model, 300
　flexibility of, 331–32
　for long-term care, 336–37
　in OECD countries, 332
　in Quebec, 341
　for repetitive surgeries, 341
　in Sweden, 292–96, 297
　and unions, 341
private sector, compared to public sector, 214
privatization, of select services, 185
profit, and health care, 227
Progressive Conservative Party, 68, 69
　and health-care policy, 97
　loss of interest in public health care, 116
　support for medicare, 129
　support for public hospitalization, 120
Progressive party, 60
provinces. *See also individual provinces*
　accusations by Bégin against, 140
　conflicts with Ottawa, 139
　cutting of taxes, 190
　health-quality councils in, 216
　medicare financing agreement with Ottawa, 138
　and pharmaceuticals, 347–48, 350–51
　raising of taxes, 190
　role in funding medicare, 138–39
　transfers to, 138, 139, 144, 150–51, 163, 173, 176, 180, 193, 204, 367

public administration, 50, 148
public consultations, 276–79
public health insurance. *See* health insurance
public hospitalization, 117–21
public sector, compared to private sector, 214

Q

Quality of Death Index, 159
Quebec
    and blood services, 352
    Castonguay report, 229–34
    comptes de la santé, 180
    doctors' remuneration demands, 137
    drug plan, 357
    family doctors in, 232–33
    funding health care, 176, 179–82, 229
    growth rate of spending on health, 180
    health-care tax, 173, 190, 224
    and Health Council of Canada, 166
    joins medicare, 127
    local health authorities in, 217
    opposition to federal medicare, 125
    and portability principle, 149–50
    private clinics in, 223, 224, 226, 238–42
    and private delivery of health care, 341
    and private health insurance, 245–49
    regional health authorities in, 330
    relations with Ottawa, 142
    remuneration to doctors, 141
    sovereignty-association, 138
    and user fees, 15, 182, 321
Quebec Charter of Human Rights and Freedoms, 245
Quebec Federation of Women, 132
Quebec Pension Plan, 130

R

radiation therapy, 53, 165, 226
rationing of health care, 9
reform of health care system, challenges to, 170–71
Regina Manifesto (1933), 76, 86
regional health authorities
    accountability, 330–31
    and activity-based funding, 343–44
    advantages of, 218
    in Alberta, 217–18, 329
    in British Columbia, 217
    budgets, 329, 342
    changes needed to, 329–30
    and doctor remuneration, 330
    and long-term care, 336

    in Manitoba, 217
    in New Brunswick, 217
    in Newfoundland, 217
    in Nova Scotia, 217, 329
    in Ontario, 218, 329
    and private delivery of care, 332–33, 336
    in Quebec, 217, 330
    role in health system, 329
    in Saskatchewan, 217
    in Sweden, 330, 331
remuneration
    balance billing, 136
    during Depression, 63, 64, 66
    for doctors, 293, 299, 313–16
    doctors', effect on budgets, 14–15, 162
    doctors' dislike of salaries, 83
    fee-for-service, 140, 149, 203, 207, 225–26
    fee schedules, 58
    in group clinics, 326
    Hall's hearings on, 108–9, 140–42
    hospital budgets and doctors', 51
    increases for doctors, 137, 215
    and inflation, 135
    method and wait times, 327
    for nurses, 315
    public payment of, 227
    by regional authorities, 330
    salaries, 14, 299, 318, 326–27
    Saskatoon Agreement, 94–95
    for Swedish doctors, 288, 293, 299–300, 322
    for U.K. doctors, 308
revenue reductions, and sustainability, 192
Robarts, John, 129
Rock, Allan, 151
Romanow, Roy, 6, 13, 105, 256, 307, 335
Romanow commission, 156, 164, 271–72, 279–80, 281, 283, 315, 366, 367
    "buy change" assumption, 214–15
    on health-care spending *vs.* other services, 189
    and pharmacare, 349
    and private health care, 228
    on sustainability, 174, 230
    on taxation, 192–93
Ross, Dr. John, 207–12
Rowell-Sirois Royal Commission, 71
Royal Society of Medicine, 159–60
Russell, David, 151

S

salaries. *See* remuneration
Salvation Army, 47

Saskatchewan. *See also* Douglas, Tommy;
    medicare
    Cancer Commission, 76, 79
    clinics and repetitive surgeries, 341
    direct billing of patients by doctors,
        136
    doctors and Great Depression, 66
    doctors' remuneration demands, 137
    doctors' strike in, 74
    and extra billing, 137
    funding health care, 187
    government-physician conflict, 86,
        87–94
    hardship in, 75
    health care before CCF, 76
    joins medicare, 127
    and medicare, 73
    and Mode Three Billing, 137
    Patient First Review, 170
    pre-CCF health care, 76
    regional health districts in, 217
    support for medicare, 275
    wait times in, 341
Saskatchewan College of Physicians and
    Surgeons, 74, 86
Saskatoon Agreement, 74, 94
Second World War, 70
    effect on policy makers, 113
Sharp, Mitchell, 124, 125, 126
Shouldice Hospital, 331
Sicko (film), 8
Singlar, 353
single-payer system. *See* Australia;
    Britain; New Zealand; Sweden
smoking rates in Canada, 255
Social Credit, attitude to public health
    care, 66
social determinants of health, 260–64
social insurance, 58–59
socio-economic status, and health, 260–
    62, 267, 268–69
sodium intake, 263–64
Soldier Party, 61
SOS Médecins (France), 335
SOS Medicare Conference, 139
South Alberta Eye Centre, 201, 202, 204,
    205
sovereignty-association, 138
Special Planning for Canada (League for
    Social Reconstruction), 66–67
spending, on health care, 115–16, 152,
    156, 157, 162, 191. *See also* costs
Sport Canada, 255
sports, participation rates in Canada, 255
St. Laurent, Louis, 116, 117–18
stagflation, 131

standard of living, 260–64
Statistics Canada, 198
Stelmach, Ed, 177
Stiernstedt, Goran, 289, 290
Strategy for Patient-Oriented Research,
    168
strikes
    over extra billing in Ontario, 152
    by physicians, 63–64, 74, 91–94
Stromberg, Lovisa, 298
structure
    of health-care system, 168–69
surgeries. *See also* operating rooms
    effect of lack of beds on, 39
    repetitive, 341
    wait times for, 39
sustainability
    of Alberta's system, 177–79
    of Canadian system, 314
    and efficiency, 196
    of health-care system, 231–32, 282–83
    of public health care, 174–75
    and quality, 196
    of Quebec's system, 179–82, 230–31
    and revenue reduction, 192
Sweden
    accountability of regional authorities,
        330, 331
    compared to Canada, 288, 294
    competition in health system, 291–92,
        293, 295
    controversy over private clinics, 295
    cost of heath-care system, 288
    coverage offered by health system, 288
    doctors and clinics, organizing of, 293
    drug prices, 352
    efficiences in health system, 288
    health-care spending, 236
    health-care system, 287–300
    health outcomes in, 194
    and health system changes, 293–94
    health system organization, 289
    home care in, 300
    hospitals in, 293, 300
    increase in cost of health care, 287–88
    pharmacies in, 292
    poverty in, 194, 298–99
    private health care in, 239, 294–95,
        331, 340
    private insurance in, 253
    private-provider/public payer model,
        292–96
    remuneration of doctors, 293, 322
    as single-payer system, 160, 239, 286
    spending on health care, 298–300
    taxation in, 288

user fees in, 297–98, 300, 321
wait times in, 289–91
Switzerland
drug prices, 352
health-care spending, 236

T

taxation
in Alberta, 176–77, 190
amount dedicated to health care, 236
in Australia, 303
in British Columbia, 188, 190, 191
cutting of, 173, 175–76, 189–90, 191, 192
effect on behaviour, 257, 268
as funding source for health system, 1, 2, 12, 69, 70, 80, 86, 108, 122–23, 192–93, 227, 281–82, 359–60
and Harmonized Sales Tax, 188
increasing, 85, 92, 109, 173, 176, 178, 179, 185, 190, 192–93, 232, 243, 282, 284, 285, 314
level of, 191
in Manitoba, 190
as method to improve health outcomes, 257
for national drug plan, 122, 363–64
in Ontario, 184–85, 190, 191
provincial and medicare, 4–5, 6, 103, 173
in Quebec, 173, 179, 180, 181, 182, 190, 224, 321
resistance to increasing, 4, 7, 15, 110, 135, 163, 175, 177, 196, 272, 274, 276, 278–79, 360
Romanow on, 192–93
and spending squeeze, 189–90
in Sweden, 194, 288, 300
on unhealthy foods, 257, 268
Taylor, Lord, 94
Taylor, Malcolm, 104
TD Financial Group, 186–87
teaching hospitals, 22
team clinics, 325–26
technology. *See also* e-health system
and wait times, 205
Telehealth, 277, 334
television, as health factor, 264
testing. *See* diagnostic testing
Thatcher, Margaret, 306, 308, 309
Thatcher, Ross, 93, 135
Thor, Johan, 287
timeliness of care, 243–44
Trans-Canada Medical Plans, 72
triage
difficulties with, 334

in emergency departments, 31, 33–34, 35
and wait times, 164
Trudeau, Pierre, 133, 138
belief in federal government, 144
and Canada Health Act, 145
and health care, 146
support for Bégin, 144
Turnbull, Dr. Jeffrey, 21–25, 27, 28–30, 41–48, 49–50, 52–53, 163, 368
views on medicare, 23
two-tier health care
Canadians' attitude to, 7, 273
and extra billing, 140–41
and private clinics, 149
and private insurance, 245–46

U

unions
and health care, 233–34
membership, 70
nurses', 317–18
and private health care, 223, 228, 341
and sustainability challenge, 314
and wage agreements, 51
United Farmers of Alberta, 60, 65
United Farmers of Saskatchewan, 78
United States
drug plans in, 351
drug prices, 352
health care in 1940s, 81
health-care system compared to Canada, 8–11, 81, 156
spending on health care, 9, 156
universality principle, 62, 86, 102, 103, 105, 106, 116, 119, 123, 124, 129, 140, 141, 148, 158, 230, 276, 277, 287, 301
user fees
advantages of, 136
and Bégin, 142
in Canada, 297
and deficits, 135–36
in early medicare, 79–80
and federal transfers, 150
in hospitals, 152
as method of reducing demand, 321–22
public's resistance to, 15, 145, 281
in Quebec, 182, 321
reimbursement for, 146
in Saskatchewan, 135
in Sweden, 297–98, 300, 321
as threat to medicare, 140

V

value for money of system, 7–8
Vioxx, 353

W

wait times
    and aging population, 243–44
    in Alberta, 200, 277
    in Australia, 301
    in Britain, 307–8, 309–10
    in Canada, 53, 200, 309–10
    Canada's ranking, 159, 161, 163–64
    challenge of, 164
    for diagnostic tests, 33
    for doctor's appointment, 209
    effect of clinics on, 341
    effect of increased funding on, 13
    effect of public health insurance on,
        252
    in emergency departments, 31, 35
    and funding, 163–64, 165, 166–67
    in group clinics, 326
    increases in, 166, 205, 242
    in Nova Scotia, 212
    in Ontario, 53, 184, 185–86
    Ontario strategy, 167
    in Ottawa, 52–53
    in Ottawa Hospital emergency
        department, 31–32
    and private insurance, 248–49
    reducing, 165–66, 241
    and remuneration method, 327

    resistance to publishing data, 331
    in Saskatchewan, 341
    for surgeries, 39, 339
    in Sweden, 289–91
    triage and, 164
Wait Times Reduction Fund, 165
wellness agenda, 254, 256–57, 258–60,
    264, 268
Werier, Dr. Joel, 36–39, 41
Weyburn Labour Association, 78
Whitton, Charlotte, 68–69, 97
Williams, Danny, 10
Williams, Dr. Geoff, 201, 202, 203
Wilson, Dr. Lawrence, 136
Winnipeg General Strike (1919), 60,
    78
Winnipeg Medical Society, 70
Woodsworth, J.S., 67, 78
Workers' Compensation Board, 239
working conditions. See social
    determinants of health

Y

Yom Kippur War, 130–31
Yukon, 127, 129

Z

Zeliotis, George, 245